T0329802

Emerging Issues in Bi

An Annual

Emerging Issues in Biomedical Policy

An Annual Review
Volume I

Edited by

Robert H. Blank
Andrea L. Bonnicksen

Columbia University Press   New York

Columbia University Press
New York   Oxford
Copyright © 1992 Columbia University Press
All rights reserved

Library of Congress Cataloging-in-Publication Data

Emerging issues in biomedical policy
edited by Robert H. Blank, Andrea L. Bonnicksen.
p. cm.
Includes bibliographical references.
ISBN 0-231-07410-7 (alk. paper)
1. Medical technology—United States—Moral and ethical aspects.
2. Medical ethics—Government policy—United States.
3. Medical policy—United States.
I. Blank, Robert H.   II. Bonnicksen, Andrea L.
[DNLM: 1. Delivery of Health Care—United States.
2. Genetic Engineering—trends—United States.
3. Health Policy—United States.
4. Technology, Medical.
W 84 AA1 E45]   R855.5.U6E44 1992   362.1'0973—dc20
DNLM/DLC   for Library of Congress
91-40654   CIP

Casebound editions of Columbia University Press books
are Smyth-sewn and printed on permanent and durable
acid-free paper.

Printed in the United States of America

c 10 9 8 7 6 5 4 3 2 1

Contents

General Introduction to Emerging Issues in Biomedical Policy: An Annual Review

A couple conceives a baby in order to donate the child's bone marrow to an older sibling with leukemia. A man sues his surgeon for using cells from his spleen to develop a patented and valuable cell line without his permission. The Supreme Court holds that the nasogastric tube cannot be removed from a permanently comatose young woman if she had not clearly made known her wishes about what to do if ever on life-support systems. An elderly man sues a hospital for wrongfully reviving him with electric shock when he had a heart attack. Surgery is performed on a twenty-four-week fetus, while still in the uterus, to correct a usually fatal condition of a herniated diaphragm. Such medical innovations, dilemmas, choices, and decisions as these are steady companions of the late twentieth century, and the issues arising from rapid advances in science and technology are frequent, varied, and provocative.

Today's biomedical technologies open doors to the presence of medicine in all facets of life. Ivan Illich has written of the "medicalization" of the western world, in which each life stage—from pregnancy to adulthood to death—calls for medical "tutelage" (1976:78). Individuals are born into a medical culture in which eye charts, vaccinations, dental hygiene, medical claim forms, blood pressure checks, medical referrals, and other tasks are a normal part of life. Advanced biomedical technologies extend the stages of life subject to medical care, and they increase the number of maladies for which intervention and treatment are expected.

Medical technologies offer powerful sources of hope in today's society. The expectation of answers and cures is deeply rooted in our technological (and optimistic) culture. The same techniques that tantalize bring with them, however, questions and uncertainties as they venture into fields without direct precedent. The freezing and micromanipulation of embryos raise questions about what an embryo is, how it should be treated, and what manipulations of it are morally appropriate. We cannot look directly to precedent, however, because only recently have embryos survived outside the body to become a topic of discussion. The costs of advanced technologies have introduced the issue of medical "rationing," but little precedent guides the first tentative steps into limits on and redistributions of medical benefits.

Medical technologies also bring unsettling ironies that resist easy understanding. For example, we see new technologies as promoting choice, but this may be an illusion if the techniques create a sense of obligation to use them. Similarly, we have worked hard to mainstream children with handicaps into our society and to understand that they are not, at root, different from children without handicaps, but prenatal screening places a value on preventing the birth of children with medical disorders in the first place. A legacy of Supreme Court decisions points to the struggle to uproot discrimination based on physical traits such as skin color and gender, yet the array of diagnostic tests in genetics opens possibilities for new discriminations based on an individual's genetic status.

Until recently, decisions about medicine lay almost entirely in the private realm between physician and patient. Yet the speed of new technologies, their scope, and the dilemmas they raise have all contributed to the idea that public officials ought to be involved in making decisions about who should have access to technologies and whether the techniques should be developed in the first place. The unveiling of the sphere of medical privacy can be traced, in part, to institutional review boards set up in the 1960s, which gave "outsider" oversight to medical protocols involving human subjects. Then, in the "right to die" case of Karen Ann Quinlan, a contested decision about whether to withdraw life-support systems gave no clear answer, and the parents and hospital turned to the courts for guidance. This decision underlay the growth of biomedical ethics as a distinct field. Today bioethicists, who are routinely consulted in hospital decision making, seek a philosophical framework for balancing biomedicine's promise with the broader social welfare.

Biomedical policy, as is bioethics, is rooted in rapidly accelerating biomedical innovations. It builds on the principles of biomedical ethics and moves into still further uncharted domains. The task of biomedical policy is to create principles for framing public decisions when the form of these decisions, or even the need for making them, is elusive. Biomedicine has brought with it a range of public decisions, some hasty, some ill-thought, some creative, and some quietly effective. All are experimental. The study of public policy gains new vitality when its topics are phrased in terms of "What if?" in addition to "What is?" What if states passed medical redistribution laws modeled after that proposed in Oregon? What impact would this have on public notions of "rights"? Or, what if judges concluded that a person's cell line were his or her property? How would that affect a person's decisions about surgery or the scientist's ability to obtain material for research?

Public decisions by judges, legislators, civil servants, and other officials have special significance for our daily lives and influence the way we see things and define issues. What distinguishes public policy is that public decisions imply the use of public funds, and they thereby broaden the interested constituency. Even when only small amounts of public money are at stake, public decisions are significant because they subsume the backing of the state. Policy decisions are commitments. They are statements that respond to emerging concerns and enthusiasms among citizens. When the government allocates hundreds of millions of dollars to map and sequence all the genes in a human cell, it gives genetic inquiry a new legitimacy. When a public hospital develops criteria for deciding who should receive scarce organs, it legitimates the priorities underlying those criteria.

Biomedical policy has a special importance in contemporary politics because it challenges keenly held societal values relating to privacy, discovery, justice, health, and rights. Biomedical techniques involve the human body and, with it, a deep-seated expectation of privacy. The idea of government action in decisions involving the body provokes vigilance. Some of the more forceful Supreme Court passages are set in the context of bodily privacy, where, for example, the Court has held that excessive intrusions by state officials violate ordered liberty (*Rochin v. California*, 342 U.S. 165 [1952]). The expected zone of privacy also extends to family decisions. The United States Supreme Court's decision in *Cruzan v. Director, Missouri Department of Health* involved the ordering of a nasogastric tube against the presumed wishes of Nancy Cruzan and against the expressed wishes of her parents (111 L.Ed.2d U.S. 224 [1990]). The conflict in that case—between the family's zone of privacy and the state's interest in protecting Nancy Cruzan as a person who could not speak for herself—attracted intense public attention.

Biomedical policy also challenges the value placed on technology as a vehicle for progress. René Dubos writes of Westerners' proclivity to experiment, improve, and inquire: "It is the desire for change which has set man apart from the rest of the living world, . . . and it is this desire that will continue to generate the most creative forces of his future" (1959:229–230). Amitai Etzioni is less compassionate, referring to reliance on technology to solve problems generated by technology as a technological fix (1973). Policy proposals often set limits on the development and use of medical techniques. This raises the protective instincts of those who see technology as a source of answers, not problems. That the first gene therapy protocol was reviewed fifteen times before approval while subsequent gene therapy protocols were approved with surprising speed illustrates the dual skepticism and trust with which we view technology. Our views about technology are ambivalent and in flux.

Public decisions about biomedicine also revolve around various interpretations of distributive justice. Equity is a prized value, but controversy surrounds the notion of equality in the disbursement of medical resources. Policy raises questions about the government's affirmative role in biomedicine as a funding source for research and development and as an agent of reimbursement for patients. Should sophisticated treatments that offer hope to small numbers of people speedily be made available? Or should priority be given to providing basic medical care for people without resources to pay for their own? Are the two goals necessarily at odds? The distribution of medical resources provokes conflict over who ought to benefit from medical innovations, whether rights to health care are inherent in our concept of liberty, and to what extent the government should take an active role in redistributing medical benefits.

Policy touches on health as a valued social good. The elevation of health as a perceived requisite to a happy and productive life is largely a twentieth-century phenomenon fueled by the promises of rapid scientific discovery. Whereas health was once primarily associated with the treatment of disease, the meaning of health now carries expectations of diagnosis, treatment, and cure, and of vigorous primary research to advance all three. Biomedical policy can either affirm or question the value placed on health.

Individual rights are another valued part of the Western heritage. Medical technology has greatly expanded the range of claimed rights and, in the process, has brought with it a veritable quagmire of questions about who has the right to do what. Among the seemingly antithetical rights now envisioned are the right to be born, the right not to be born, the right to conceive, the right not to conceive, the right of access to life-prolonging apparatuses, and the right to be freed from life-prolonging apparatuses. Compounding this are newly claimed obligations such as the obligation to learn whatever there is to learn about genetics for the benefit of future generations versus the obligation not to explore avenues of inquiry that might change the genetic makeup of future generations. Biomedical technologies engage our notions about rights amid a complex brew of obligations and responsibilities.

Because basic values are at stake, biopolicy proposals elicit emotional responses as well as intellectual curiosity. This makes the juncture at which private acts cross the line of public choice especially sensitive. Two general categories of error in policy judgment are possible. In the first, public decisions are not made when action is warranted. Although some techniques merely raise ironies, as discussed above, others raise dilemmas in which injuries might occur and the correct course of action is uncertain; crises in which serious injuries do occur in isolated cases; and chronic conditions in which dilemmas and crises repeatedly arise and the situation appears intractable. Generally, the need for policy escalates as the issues raised by new technologies move from dilemma to chronic condition. For example, a crisis arises if one vital organ is available and several people are vying for it. This decision has life-and-death implications and it warns that norms must be developed in the event a similar crisis appears. The crisis escalates to a chronic condition if there are perpetually too few organs available for too many people and organs are allocated in a way that promotes neither health nor justice. Here policy inaction has serious societal consequences.

In the second type of error, public action is taken but it is not in fact warranted. This is most likely to occur in the aftermath of a highly publicized but idiosyncratic crisis. Hasty and premature policies produce rules and laws that are easily outdated, inappropriate, and therefore ineffective, and also create barriers to the efforts of groups of individuals to resolve such problems by private action. This type of error is also destabilizing, especially if the policy itself, rather than the original problem, becomes the central issue.

Biomedical controversies are generally debated for their ethical and moral implications for some time before they become part of the policy agenda. When a commitment to act seems inevitable, varied types of policy are possible. Some public choices stop certain inquiries altogether, as in the federal government's refusal to review for funding projects involving the manipulation of human germ-line cells. Others, which are far more common, regulate the conditions under which activities are practiced, as in the National Organ Transplant Act, which sets forth conditions under which organs may be made available to prospective recipients. Still others are affirmative policies that aid biomedical research, provide disbursements, or set up commissions to study the implications of research.

A challenge for biomedical policy is to identify models for public action. Ideally, policy is continually responsive to emerging issues and conflicts. Public decisions are not only answers to problems but the starting point for new and more challenging levels of discussion. According to one observer, "indeterminancy [is] . . . an achievement, not a mishap" (Jabbari 1990:37). Public decisions are incomplete, experimental, and rooted in different levels and branches of government. Biomedical policy enters unexplored territory in that the substance of the issues—organ donations, embryo biopsies, genetic manipulations—is new. In other ways, however, the landmarks have been laid in existing rules, procedures, cases, and laws. Biomedical policy is partly a matter of applying new interpretations to the existing order, and the "living" Constitution of the United States testifies to our ability to weave contemporary meanings into guidelines framed in distant times. All this adds to the range of models to examine in developing new public choices.

At least four basic questions, then, must be asked in deciding when private acts ought to involve public choice. Among the more central are these: (1) What *values* are challenged by the prospect of public choice? (2) At what point is there a *need* for public choice? If public choice is desirable, two additional questions need to be addressed: (3) What *type* of public choice is appropriate: prohibitive, regulatory, affirmative? (4) To what should one look to find policy *models?*

Figure 1 presents a stylistic overview of biomedical policy. In general, the momentum for public choice grows when one or more central values are threatened by the absence of policy decisions and when the issue moves from a dilemma to a chronic condition. Many other factors, such as the rate of technological change, the success of past policies, and the willingness of lawmakers to become involved, influence the policy-making process. The figure illustrates the complexity of the policy context but it also suggests the need, at some point, to move beyond analysis and turn to policy enactment as a way of clarifying the issues.

The Emerging Issues Series

H. Tristram Engelhardt, Jr., has written that "what might appear an isolated biomedical choice will in the end be found to be embedded in a matrix of public policies, rooted in concepts of the good life, the nature of rights and duties, and the standing of moral objects and subjects" (1986:17). This series is initiated to provide a forum for the unfolding matrix of biomedical policies. We, as editors of the series, are guided by several assumptions. First, we assume that biomedical policy is a field

SOCIAL VALUES	NATURE OF ISSUES	NATURE OF TECHNOLOGY
privacy discovery justice health rights	dilemmas crises chronic condition	rapid change cumulative change purpose: prevent, treat, cure

PERCEIVED NEED FOR POLICY

↓

BIOMEDICAL POLICY
(public choice)

TYPE	PLACE	DEGREE OF INNOVATION
prohibitory regulatory affirmative	private/public mixed local state federal courts legislatures regulatory agencies	new interpretation of existing policy newly framed policy

Figure 1. Framework of Biomedical Policy

warranting its own voice. The literature devoted to biomedical ethics is relatively centralized, with specific journals and indexes. The literature in biomedical policy is growing but more decentralized, with pertinent articles dispersed in ethics, law, science, and policy journals rather than in a central place. This series is designed to provide a central gathering place for biomedical policy articles.

Second, we believe that biomedical policy draws its creativity from the merged perspectives of people from varied disciplines. Our first volume attests to our success in bringing together lawyers, scientists, physicians, legislators, and civil servants to write from points of view that, we may assume, are distinct as a result of the perspectives they gain from their disciplines. All authors readily agreed to address policy questions at some point in their essays, some saying they were interested in policy but did not normally have a chance to write about it. This confirmed our belief that a multidisciplinary approach to biomedical policy is both possible and welcome.

Third, we believe that although biomedicine encompasses a range of techniques, these techniques give rise to recurring themes. A longevity of the issues, in other words, holds even when technological and value changes occur. This series seeks to highlight the themes that reappear so that we may gain a richer historical understanding of what makes biomedical policy a comprehensive area. In this way we counteract the technique-by-technique exposé in the media at large.

Fourth, we are persuaded that biomedical policy is cumulative. This means that the policy successes of today can provide models for policies of tomorrow. Similarly, failures can be rooted out lest they become a cumulative burden that generates a mentality of hopelessness about resolving complex issues. Progress comes from paring, adding, experimenting, and exchanging. Biomedical policy sorts through public actions to cull burdensome policy and to integrate promising alternatives that become the essence of workable public choice. This series is geared to seeing, over time, how the policy models are developing—what themes recur, what models arise, and what acts succeed. Our interest, then, lies not only in emerging issues but also in emerging policy.

Volume 1 in the Emerging Issues Series

Our premiere volume covers two substantive areas that demonstrate the challenges facing our society as we move into the last decade of the twentieth century. In part I, respected scholars offer perspectives on how society sets priorities in the allocation of scarce medical resources in an era of escalating demands on those resources. Only reluctantly some observers are concluding that the present allocation plans have become a chronic condition which drains the strength of the medical system. Allocation is an especially fascinating area because its public choice model rises from the basically different paradigm of presumed scarcity rather than expected abundance. Because this paradigm is new (to this society at least), models of choice are elusive but, as the readings show, in formative stages.

Part II, on reproductive and genetic technologies, is in some ways the antithesis of the first. Whereas various commentators on allocation have concluded that limits to growth are necessary, participants in reproductive and genetic technologies have concluded that exciting and innovative techniques deserve new priorities and public commitments. This section combines the essays of well-known scientists, physicians, and lawyers writing about both the promise of new techniques and the dilemmas that the prospect of public choice raises.

Advanced reproductive technologies relate to the beginnings of life. Once highly controversial, they are becoming a stable part of medical life. With this stability comes a renewed need to keep alive the debate as potentially controversial refinements are quietly perfected and applied without the widespread media attention of earlier years. The "new genetics" stand where reproductive technologies were a decade ago, with spiraling applications prompting debate about whether and how fast we want to commit to the techniques. Genetics promises a new range of diagnoses and cures that will change the shape of medicine. The selections in part II show the mixture of anticipation and uncertainty with which we combine genetic discovery with clinical application. Among other things, the authors describe policy models developed in the private sector. Historically, around twenty years span the time when a technique is born and the first public act is taken. If this is still the case, biomedical policy is only now entering its bloom.

References

Dubos, René. 1959. *Mirage of Health: Utopians, Progress, and Biological Change.* New York: Harper.

Engelhardt, H. Tristram, Jr. 1986. *The Foundations of Bioethics.* New York: Oxford University Press.

Etzioni, Amitai. 1973. *Genetic Fix.* New York: Macmillan.

Illich, Ivan. 1976. *Medical Nemesis: The Expropriation of Health.* New York: Pantheon.

Jabbari, David. 1990. "The Role of Law in Reproductive Medicine: A New Approach." *Journal of Medical Ethics* 16(1):35–40.

I

Setting Policy Priorities for Allocating Scarce Medical Resources

Introduction: Setting Policy Priorities for Allocating Scarce Medical Resources

Robert H. Blank

It is becoming increasingly clear that major alterations in the health care system of the United States are necessary if we are to avert a crisis of immense proportions. Many seemingly unrelated demographic, social, and technological trends are converging to accentuate traditional dilemmas in medical policy making. The aging population, the proliferation of high-cost biomedical technologies designed primarily to extend life, conventional schemes of retroactive reimbursement by third-party payers, and the realization that health care costs are outstripping society's perceived ability to pay, all lead to pressures for expanded public action to resolve the problem. At the same time, public institutions appear both unable and unwilling to make difficult decisions in an area traditionally viewed as outside the political arena.

The constraints on medical resources already apparent in the United States are bound to be compounded by the confluence of the trends noted above. Even with all that is being done to contain costs, health care expenditures are expected to reach $650 billion in 1990 and $1.9 trillion by 2000, representing almost 15 percent of the gross national product (Blendon 1986). Moreover, annual per capita health care costs in the United States are over $2,500; the comparable figure for Britain is $800. Increased competition for scarce resources within the health care sector will necessitate resource allocation as well as rationing decisions (Blank 1988). In turn, these actions are certain to exacerbate the social, ethical, and legal issues and intensify activity by affected individuals and groups.

Further policy complications arise from the fact that distribution of medical resources is skewed toward a very small proportion of the population. More and more medical resources have been concentrated on a relatively small number of patients in acute care settings. Substantial questions about the just distribution of scarce resources in a society are accentuated in the establishment of biomedical priorities. For instance, in 1980, 1 percent of the population accounted for 29 percent of all health care expenditures; 5 percent accounted for 55 percent; and 10 percent accounted for 70 percent.

Elderly people are the leading users of hospital care and have the highest expenditures for health care per capita. Ironically, because of medical improvements and technologies that prolong life, chronic disease requiring frequent medical care has become a greater problem. Moreover, the demand for such care will continue to increase in an aging population. At present, 11.4 percent of the U.S. population, or approximately 25.6 million people, are sixty-five years of age or older. By the year 2035 the elderly population will double in size. Moreover, it is estimated that by the year 2000 the number of elderly age eighty and over will increase by about 50 percent, and that by 2035 approximately one out of every ten Americans will be over eighty-five years of age. This aging population already has put a tremendous strain on the health care system to provide acute- and especially chronic-care facilities for a population that is heavily dependent on these services, leading Callahan (1987) to suggest setting limits on the use of life-prolonging technologies for the elderly.

The Value Context of Setting Social Priorities

Observers of American society since Alexis de Tocqueville have commented on the uniqueness and internal diversity of values among its citizens. As a society, we emphasize individual autonomy, self-determination, personal privacy, and a shared belief in justice for all humans. Individuals in a liberal society are free to determine for themselves what is their preferred lifestyle and then, as long as they do not harm others, to live it. With this general consensus of support for abstract values, however, the belief has developed that each person's views should be heard and that all interests should be represented. The result has been a proliferation of competing interests on issues of public concern. Despite this diversity of viewpoints, several cultural themes that enjoy near-consensual support work against setting constraints on health care.

First, the prevailing value system places heavy emphasis on the notion of rights. Although the United States Constitution makes no mention of a right to health care, the courts have interpreted the right to life to include an inherent claim of all citizens to health care and to autonomy in making decisions concerning health. Although there has always been friction between individual rights and the common good or societal welfare, when they conflict the individual's claims to health care generally have taken precedence. Conflict over the limits of rights is intensified by the introduction of technologies that contrast rights and responsibilities across a variety of divisions in society. Basic questions focus on the scope of individual rights, the extent to which society ought to intervene in these freedoms, and how such constraints, if any, might be justified. Also, how far ought the concept of community be expanded to take into account the rights of, and responsibility toward, the unborn, toward future generations, toward other species?

The emphasis on the individual's right to medical care is also reflected in the patient-physician relationship, which has been seen largely as a private one, beyond the public realm. Although in the aggregate we are willing to cut costs, when it comes to the individual patient we have been ready to expend all resources without consideration of costs. There is a not-so-implicit assumption that every person has a right to unlimited expenditure on his/her behalf, despite the understanding that in the aggregate this is unfeasible. The problem of unlimited individual claims in the context of finite societal resources produces the dilemma of health care today. As stated by Schramm, "If society's task is to improve the health of the many, disproportionate spending on acute care for a small number of persons must come into question" (1984:730).

The suggestion that we somehow limit medical expenditures on an individual in order to benefit the greatest number, however, contradicts the traditional patient-oriented mores of medicine. There are strong pressures for intensive intervention on an individual basis, even in the last days of life; this pressure persists, despite the enormous cost for very little return in terms of prolonging the patient's life. In addition, supporting this maximalist approach to medical care, we have created an intricate mechanism for minimizing the amount any single individual will pay for these benefits. Private health insurance allows individuals to protect themselves by spreading the risk of requiring expensive medical treatment across many persons. The real cost of the services is thus obscured, because individuals seldom must bear the costs directly or fully. This insulation of the individual patient from cost encourages the maximalist approach and reinforces the presumption that cost should not be a concern in the treatment of the patient. No matter how much is spent on the patient, the payment will usually be made by the amorphous third-party payer.

The belief that individuals have the right to unlimited medical care should they so choose it; the traditional acceptance of the maximalist approach by the medical community; and the insulation of the individual from feeling the cost of treatment together place severe limits on the extent to which proscription of expensive and often ineffective intervention is possible. Arguments in favor of containing the costs to society of health care, while acceptable at the societal level, tend to fail when applied at the individual level. Although a large proportion of the population supports some type of cost containment in theory, traditional beliefs in the maximalist approach remain strong when their own health or that of their family is at stake.

One barrier to the creation of effective societal health care priorities centers on expectations of unlimited availability of medical technology both among consumers and providers. These expectations fuel unrealistic public demands which, in turn, are encouraged by many providers of health services. The LORAN Commission report by the Harvard Community Health Plan reprinted here emphasizes the need to moderate public expectations if "insurers, providers, and government are to fulfill their respective missions."

A second value of the American public which shapes demands for expansion of health expenditures is its obsession with prolonging life. Franz Ingelfinger concludes that too much money is spent to "convert Western octogenarians to nonagenarians" (1980:143). The determinants of death are many, and to pour untold millions into defeating only one merely shifts the opportunity to others. Saving an elderly person from one illness might very well expose that person to an even more debilitating disease. Although the quality of life of many persons at advanced ages is low and extensive technological intervention might prolong life only briefly, American society has an excessive concern with keeping alive at all costs. Although there is considerable evidence that this perspective is quickly changing, by far the most expensive year of life for most people is the terminal year. Still, we are hesitant to withhold treatment, no matter how costly, if it extends life.

In addition to the significant emphasis in the liberal tradition on individual autonomy and a broad range of rights, American culture is also predisposed toward progress through technological means. This value extends to medical technology through a deep commitment to the belief that medicine will progress and give us even greater powers over disease. This heavy dependence on technology to "fix" our health problems, to the exclusion of nontechnological solutions or prevention, is also tied to a tendency of Americans to look always for the easiest solutions. As David Mechanic states the case,

> As a culture, we do far better in the application of a "technological fix" than in building complex social arrangements that must be sustained over time in coping with expressive, frustrating, and often intractable problems. (1986:207)

The quest for increasingly higher levels of technology in order to avoid difficult changes in lifestyle continues, even when it becomes obvious that technology cannot provide the sought-after panaceas.

Setting Priorities: Allocation and Rationing

Long-term solutions to the health care crisis require a reevaluation of traditional orientations toward medicine in the United States. Considerable reevaluation of our social priorities is crucial at three levels. First, we must come to some consensus as to how much of society's limited resources we are willing to allocate to health care. As a society we continue to expend vast sums of money on goods and services that we can largely agree are less worthwhile than health care and some that actually are costly to our health. What priority do we place on health care as compared to education, national defense, housing, automobiles, and leisure activities? How much are we willing to take from these competing areas and transfer to medical care? These first-level "macroallocation" decisions entail politics at its rawest as the funding pie is apportioned on the basis of societal priorities.

Second, once a consensus is reached as to how high a priority ought to be put on health care vis-à-vis other spending areas, the finite resources (money, skilled personnel, blood, organs, technologies) available for health care must be distributed among various areas within health care. Assuming that society refuses to make major alterations at the macroallocation level, hard decisions will be necessary to ensure use of these limited medical resources in a just and equitable way. This is the allocation level where the tradeoffs must be appraised and choices made that will drastically revise prevailing assumptions of both the health care community and the public. Here again conventional givens are challenged—givens that appeared to be reasonable when resources were plentiful, but which now, in the era of fiscal constraints, are obsolete.

Some of the clearest tradeoffs currently debated in the health policy literature are:

Disease prevention/Health promotion	v.	Curative or rescue high technology
Improved quality of life	v.	Prolongation of life
Marginally ill	v.	Severely ill
Young	v.	Old
Morbidity	v.	Mortality
Cost containment	v.	Individual choice

Whether contrasting a preventive with a curative or rescue approach, care for the young or for the old, or an emphasis on quality of life against extension of life, the debate, unfortunately, often is framed in either-or terms. It would be more comfortable to place high priority on all categories or, alternatively, to balance them out in an equitable way. Unhappily, the options are narrowing, and resources dedicated to one category do reduce health resources committed to the others. The stakes in how these resources are allocated among the possible categories, therefore, have become quite high, particularly for those elements of society that lack the personal resources essential to protect their own interests. This situation makes the need for establishing meaningful social priorities in health care allocation even more critical and forces us to make rationing decisions of some type.

Recently, there has been considerable activity at the national level on the need to shift social priorities toward disease prevention and health promotion. In his article in this volume, Dr. J. Michael McGinnis, Director of the Office of Disease Prevention and Health Promotion of the U.S. Department of Health and Human Services, discusses the major federal initiative *Healthy People 2000*, developed under his direction. This extensive report identified three national goals: to increase the span of healthy life, reduce health disparities, and achieve universal access to preventive services. In his essay, Michael A. Stoto, Senior Staff Officer, Division of Health Promotion and Disease Prevention, at the Institute of Medicine, critically analyzes *Healthy People 2000*. He argues that while it is the "most clearly articulated statement" of what might be regarded as national health priorities for the 1990s, it fails as a national health priority statement.

As difficult as it is to set priorities among these tradeoffs, the third level of health care policy is even more painful because it deals with identifiable patients. Although there are a disparate multitude of definitions for the term *rationing*, each entails a choice between the claims of specific individuals who are competing for resources defined as limited because society has allocated fewer resources than are necessary to treat all affected individuals. Some criteria, therefore, must be established to determine when to use the resources and when to withhold or withdraw them. Rationing then, takes place within the context of prior allocation decisions which create scarcity.

Rationing has always been a part of medical decision making. Table I.1 presents a spectrum of ways in which health care can be rationed. Whether imposed by a market system in which price determines who has access; a system in which care is distributed on the basis of need as defined by the medical community, litigation, and corporate benefits managers; or a queue system in which time and the waiting process becomes the major rationing device, medical resources always have been distributed according to criteria that contain varying degrees of subjectivity. Although the United States to date has rejected any explicit rationing system, these less obvious forms are commonplace. In the words of David Mechanic,

> Although rationing is sometimes evoked by critics of change as a new impending threat and aberration, rationing of health care has always existed but it has remained sufficiently embedded in common modes of thinking to attract little attention. . . . Given the complexity and generosity of the American system of care, we have successfully maintained the illusion that rationing is foreign to it. (1986:63)

In almost all instances, rationing criteria are founded in a particular value context that results in an inequitable distribution of resources based on social, as well as strictly medical, considerations.

Instead of focusing on whether some form of rationing is necessary, the debate more properly should be directed toward the extent to which the government and its agents should take a direct role in establishing rationing procedures and structures. Should the haphazard, inequitable, and often contradictory rationing continue, or should the government accept responsibility for the allocation and use of medical resources and take active steps to design and implement a comprehensive rationing system?

No matter what allocation scheme is used, some elements of society will benefit and others will be deprived. Philosophical debate has long been devoted to what criteria ought to be used to determine whether or not a particular policy is just or fair. Do we select those policies that maximize the good of the greatest number, help those who are least well

Table I.1   Forms of Rationing

Form	Criteria Used
1. Physician discretion	Medical benefit to patient Medical risk to patient Social class or mental capacity
2. Competitive marketplace	Ability to pay
3. Insurance marketplace	Ability to pay for insurance Group membership Employment
4. Socialized insurance (i.e., Medicaid)	Entitlement Means test
5. Legal	Litigation to gain access and treatment
6. Personal fundraising	Support of social groups Skill in pubic relations Willingness to appeal to public
7. Implicit rationing	The queue Limited manpower and facilities Medical benefits to patient with consideration of social costs
8. Explicit rationing	Triage Medical benefit to patient with emphasis on social costs and benefits
9. Controlled rationing	Government control of medicine Equity in access to primary care Social benefit over specific patient benefits

off, or concentrate goods in a small elite on the assumption that somehow benefits might trickle down to those on the bottom? Ever since Plato first argued that health resources should not be wasted on the sickly and unproductive, the distribution of these limited resources has been part of a public policy debate.

The ethical issues involved in setting health care priorities, therefore, continue to be of central importance. How can society limit lifesaving resources among its citizens? What system of allocation is most justifiable, and by what ethical criteria? Moreover, because explicit government rationing usually applies only to persons dependent on public support, ethical questions of equity and fairness are inherent in any societal attempts to ration medical resources. In their essays chosen for this volume, Paul T. Menzel, a philosopher at Pacific Lutheran University and author of *Strong Medicine,* and John Moskop, a professor in the Department of Medical Humanities at East Carolina University School of Medicine, explore the ethical dimensions of rationing.

Making Hard Policy Choices

Despite their disagreement on how it ought to be done, the authors here agree that there is an urgent need for objective priority setting that takes into account the fact that we cannot afford to proceed full speed ahead on the development and use of all biomedical technologies. As a society, we must realize that the rapid advances in biomedicine, and the many real benefits that accompany them, carry with them problems and costs just as real. We cannot afford any longer to blindly embrace technology for its own sake and must carefully assess the long-term implications of each application prior to its use. Daniel Callahan, Director of the Hastings Center and author of *Setting Limits* and *What Kind of Life?*, offers his views in an essay on how we as a society ought to proceed to better set priorities for a healthy existence.

The rapid diffusion of biomedical technologies, in conjunction with social and demographic trends, is leading to the need for increasingly arduous decisions about how to best use them. As we come to realize that we cannot afford to do everything for everybody, we are thrust into policy dilemmas that deal directly with human life and death. Ironically, these dilemmas are all the more difficult because we are now at the brink of developing remarkable capacities to intervene directly in the human condition, from preconception to life extension. Just when we have the technical capacity to do things we only recently dreamt about, rising expectations and scarce resources combine to limit their availability. The resulting need to allocate biomedical technologies, in turn, raises critical concerns over whose needs take precedence, what individual rights and responsibilities entail, and when societal good justifies restricting individual good. These policy issues, although by no means new, take on a new importance within the context of the emerging conflicts accentuated by our technological successes in biomedicine.

There has been a clear strategy in the United States to avoid making the difficult decisions regarding the distribution of scarce medical resources. Most often the "solutions" merely shift costs from the government to the individual or from one level of government to another. Henry Aaron, a senior fellow at the Brookings Institution, and William B. Schwartz, Vannevar Bush University Professor at Tufts University, argue in their joint paper that elimination of inefficiencies in the health system can only provide temporary fiscal relief and that current cost-containment measures ultimately must give way to rationing. They provide a very useful contrast of the American experience with that of Great Britain, where explicit rationing is practiced.

Although there is a tendency to place emphasis on federal policy to deal with the health care crisis, innovation often comes at the state and local levels. Most states and localities are currently facing major budgetary problems centered around rapidly escalating health care costs. In the late 1980s Oregon's legislature initiated a controversial and sweeping attempt to set health care priorities. In his article, Dr. John Kitzhaber, President of the Oregon Senate, describes his state's pioneering effort and the difficulties of implementing an explicit rationing scheme within the current social context. Likewise, local governments are not immune from the devastating effects of the health care crisis and, in reality, often bear the heaviest burden of paying for the costs of a growing indigent population. In another paper, David J. Kears and Rodger G. Lum, Director and Assistant Director, respectively, of the Alameda County Health Care Services Agency, discuss the Alameda County, California experience in trying to provide a more comprehensive, fair, and rational system of allocating health resources.

All the essays that follow examine critical elements of the difficult policy issues that surround the setting of priorities in health care. The authors, from academia, government service, and the private sphere, espouse a broad range of positions. Their backgrounds span the fields of medicine, ethics, and the social sciences. All are astute observers and well-respected experts in their fields. Although the perspectives they offer on setting societal priorities in health care vary, particularly regarding rationing, it is significant that all reach the similar conclusion that the U.S. health care system is very ill and that vigorous and urgent attention is essential if we are to avert a major breakdown of the system in the future.

References

Blank, Robert H. 1988. *Rationing Medicine.* New York: Columbia University Press.
Blendon, Robert J. 1986. "Health Policy Choices for the 1990s." *Issues in Science and Technology* 2(4):65-73.
Callahan, Daniel. 1987. *Setting Limits: Medical Goals in an Aging Society.* New York: Simon & Schuster.
Ingelfinger, Franz J. 1980. "Medicine: Meritorious or Meretricious." In Philip H. Abelson, ed., *Health Care: Regulation, Economics, Ethics, Practice,* pp. 141-145. Washington, D.C.: American Association for the Advancement of Science.
Mechanic, David. 1986. *From Advocacy to Allocation: The Evolving Health Care System.* New York: Free Press.
Schramm, Carl J. 1984. "Can We Solve the Hospital-Cost Problem in Our Democracy?" *New England Journal of Medicine* 311(11):729-732.

1

Investing in Health: The Role of Disease Prevention*

J. Michael McGinnis

Health care during 1990 is estimated to have cost Americans more than $630 billion, which, if distributed equally among all individuals, would cost every four-person family in the nation over $10,000. Nearly 60 percent of these expenditures were handled privately, either by patients or through private health insurers, and 40 percent came from public sources—federal, state, or local governments, largely through the Medicare and Medicaid programs (HCFA 1990). Since 1965, health care spending has grown almost twice as fast as the gross national product—a broad-based measure of society's ability to pay for that care.

This ever-increasing national health bill does not necessarily translate into better health for Americans. It is true that Americans are living longer. Life expectancy in the twentieth century has increased by almost twenty-seven years to its current level of about seventy-five years. Since 1980, life expectancy has increased 2.4 years for males and 1.6 years for females. In the last quarter of a century, mortality rates for stroke declined approximately 58 percent and for coronary heart disease, 48 percent (NHLBI 1989:36).

Despite these changes, more than half of Americans currently die before their time—that is, before age seventy-five. In addition, relative

*This essay is a revised and updated version of an article published in *Issues in Science and Technology*. The capable assistance of Amber Barnato, Mary Jo Deering, Marilyn Schulenberg, and Christina Wypijewski is gratefully acknowledged.

to some other nations, Americans' "time" might itself be considered premature. In overall life expectancy, the United States ranks fifteenth among thirty-nine selected nations for women and nineteenth for men— more than three years below the rate for the leader. For infant mortality, we rank twenty-second of thirty-nine, with a rate nearly twice that of Japan, the nation with the lowest rate (NCHS 1990:116, table 20).

In the United States, these early deaths carry a heavy toll in economic as well as human terms. More than twelve million potential years of productive life were lost to the nation in 1988 as a result of deaths that occur before age sixty-five (CDC 1990). The costs of medical care and lost productivity for some of the country's leading health problems run as high as an estimated $135 billion for heart disease (NHLBI 1989:6) and $158 billion for injuries (Rice et al. 1989:3). The aggregate cost of illness for Americans is staggering, yet many of these illnesses are preventable.

Indeed, for each of the leading causes of death and disability in this

Table 1.1   The Five Leading Causes of Death in the United States and Associated Risk Factors

Cause of death	Risk factors
Cardiovascular disease	Tobacco use Elevated serum cholesterol High blood pressure Obesity Diabetes Sedentary lifestyle
Cancer	Tobacco use Improper diet Alcohol Occupational/environmental exposures
Cerebrovascular disease	High blood pressure Tobacco use Elevated serum cholesterol
Accidental injuries	Safety belt noncompliance Alcohol/substance abuse Reckless driving Occupational hazards Stress/fatigue
Chronic lung disease	Tobacco use Occupational/environmental exposures

SOURCE: National Center for Health Statistics/U.S. Department of Health and Human Services. *Health United States: 1987* (DHHS publication No. (PHS) 88-1232).

Table 1.2   Costs of Treatment for Selected Preventable Conditions

Condition	Overall magnitude	Avoidable intervention*	Cost per patient[+]
Heart disease	7 million with coronary artery disease 500,000 deaths/yr 284,000 bypass procedures/yr	Coronary bypass surgery	$ 30,000
Cancer	1 million new cases/yr 510,000 deaths/yr	Lung cancer treatment Cervical cancer treatment	$ 27,000 $ 26,000
Stroke	600,000 strokes/yr 150,000 deaths/yr	Hemiplegia treatment and rehabilitation	$ 22,000
Injuries	2.3 million hospitaliza- tions/yr 142,500 deaths/yr 177,000 persons with spinal cord injuries in the U.S.	Quadriplegia treatment and rehabilitation Hip fracture treatment and rehabilitation Severe head injury treatment and rehabilitation	$570,000 (lifetime) $ 40,000 $310,000 (lifetime)
HIV infection	1–1.5 million infected 118,000 AIDS cases (as of January 1990)	AIDS treatment	$ 75,000 (lifetime)
Alcoholism	18.5 million abuse alcohol 105,000 alcohol-related deaths/yr	Liver transplant	$250,000
Drug abuse	Regular users: 1–3 million, cocaine 900,000, IV drugs 500,000, heroin 375,000 drug-exposed babies	Treatment of drug- affected baby	$ 63,000 (5 years includes social services)
Low birth weight babies	260,000 LBWB born/yr 23,000 deaths/yr	Neonatal intensive care for LBWB	$ 10,000
Inadequate immunization	Lacking basic immunization series: 20–30%, ages 2 and younger 3%, ages 6 and older	Congenital rubella syndrome treatment	$385,000 (lifetime)

*Examples (other interventions may apply).
[+] Representative first-year costs, except as noted. Not indicated are nonmedical costs, such as lost productivity to society.
SOURCE: Office of Disease Prevention and Health Promotion; Department of Health and Human Services.

country, epidemiologic and biomedical research have identified risks that can be reduced to improve health prospects (table 1.1). Measures such as early detection, intervention, and changes in individual behavior could eliminate an estimated 45 percent of cardiovascular disease deaths, 23 percent of cancer deaths, and more than 50 percent of the disabling complications of diabetes (Amler and Dull 1987:50, 79, 40). Attention to even a few risk factors such as poor diet, infrequent exercise, the use of tobacco and drugs, and the abuse of alcohol, could prevent between 40 and 70 percent of all premature deaths, and one-third of all cases of acute disability (Kottke 1986:3). In contrast, technologically oriented medical treatment currently promises to reduce premature morbidity and mortality by no more than perhaps 10 to 15 percent (Institute of Medicine 1982:3).

Each individual's chance of dying ultimately is 100 percent, but proven preventive practices can decrease suffering, decrease disability, and improve quality of life by thwarting problems before they occur or become irreversible. More than 95 percent of the approximately $630 billion spent in 1990 for medical care in the United States went to treat rather than prevent disease. Many of the interventions purchased with this sizable investment were for conditions that could have been avoided (table 1.2). A better balance is clearly in order.

Successful Precedents

Prevention strategies have already proven their merit (U.S. Preventive Services Task Force 1989). One of the best known and best accepted of these is the immunization of infants against childhood diseases. Diphtheria, whooping cough, and polio have largely disappeared in the United States, along with their once considerable burden of death and permanent disability. Although measles has almost been completely eliminated, recent outbreaks among some inner-city preschool children and children of migrant farm workers around the country demonstrate that vaccines are not reaching everyone. In this area we cannot afford complacency.

Campaigns designed to raise public awareness of health risk factors, including behavioral risks to health, have also shown their worth. One of the most successful has been the National High Blood Pressure Education Program, an extensive effort to teach the public and health professionals about the relationship of high blood pressure to stroke, and about the habits that influence high blood pressure's onset and severity. Initiated in 1972 by the National Heart, Lung, and Blood Institute (NHLBI), in collaboration with public and private organizations at the national, state, and local levels, the program promotes, among other things, drug therapy, dietary change, weight loss, smoking cessation, and exercise. Due in part to this program, stroke deaths had declined by approximately 55 percent by 1984. Three years ago the NHLBI started the National Cholesterol Education Program, in hopes of achieving similar positive results in controlling serum cholesterol, which is strongly linked to heart disease.

Cigarette smoking is still the single most destructive preventable health risk. It is estimated to account for nearly a third of all deaths that occur as a result of cardiovascular disease, cancer, and respiratory diseases. As a result of an array of public and private efforts to educate the public about the health risks of smoking, the percentage of adults who smoke dropped from 42 percent in 1965 to 26 percent in 1987. Death rates for some of the illnesses associated with smoking, such as heart attacks and stroke, already show clear evidence of decline.

Injuries rank fourth among the leading causes of death, after heart disease, cancer, and stroke. They represent the leading cause of death for people between the ages of five and forty-four, and account for the most potential years of life lost to society for those under age sixty-five. Motor vehicle accidents are a prominent cause of preventable injuries. Failure to use seat belts, reckless driving, speeding, and substance abuse are the common and preventable risk factors. The fifty-five-mile-per-hour speed limit, the increased use of seat belts, and the campaigns to raise awareness about the dangers of drinking and driving—some initiated by students, mothers, and other concerned citizens—cut the motor vehicle death rate by nearly a fifth between 1978 and 1987.

Across the United States, public and private agencies attempting to control the spread of acquired immune deficiency syndrome, are in the midst of one of the most massive education efforts ever undertaken. It is too early to claim success, but because there is not yet a vaccine or cure for AIDS, prevention is the only weapon we have.

Obstacles to Paying for Preventive Services

Despite the potential, a leap forward in the ability to deliver preventive health services to individuals cannot happen without changes in the way Americans pay for health care. The pattern of a system dictated by large sums for disease treatment will not be altered until we remove the economic disincentives to prevention. Current reimbursement practices do not encourage doctors to offer preventive services. Inpatient services are reimbursed at a higher rate than those provided in ambulatory settings; technical procedures and diagnostic tests are assigned a higher dollar value per unit of time invested than services requiring cognitive and communications skills.

Reimbursement rules are discriminatory. Most treatment services must be shown only to be reasonably safe and possibly effective in addressing a given problem to qualify for reimbursement. Preventive services must be proven effective with a higher degree of certainty. What's more, Medicare and many other insurers often require clear evidence of cost savings before they will pay.

Typically, when insurers and employers consider covering preventive services ranging from immunization for influenza to screening for cancers, they compare the costs with the costs of treating disease after it occurs. Some health economists have even estimated the total cost of prevention by including the costs of routine (or catastrophic) medical costs, pensions, and Social Security for those individuals positively affected by prevention efforts. If payment policies for treatment followed this reasoning, we could imagine an insurer refusing to cover the victim of a heart attack or an automobile injury on the grounds that letting the victim die would save money.

Cost of care is a reasonable concern when resources are limited, but analyses compel decisions that will, in health terms, be inevitably inefficient. The double standard—one for treatment and another for prevention—is inimical to a rational health policy that bases health care investment decisions on expected relative returns to health. In the presence of unprecedented insight into the etiology and prevention of disease, society has investment rules that often present barriers to action based on those insights. The result is that the U.S. health care system misses few opportunities to treat diseases or injuries (even though the treatments may be unsuccessful), yet misses countless similar opportunities to seek their prevention. As a public consequence, the aggregate national decisions on investments for health are not made or acted upon in a way that yield the greatest amount of health returned for dollars invested.

Market research shows that consumers are interested in preventive coverage, are willing to pay extra for it, and would prefer preventive services benefits to some others traditionally provided. The insurance industry, however, has in the past responded somewhat hypocritically. A 1988 survey indicated that although almost half of the companies that offer individual medical insurance employ controllable risk factors in determining acceptance or rejection of applicants, their provision of preventive services varies widely from 20 percent to 80 percent (Gabel et al. 1989). Enrollment in health maintenance organizations (HMOs) committed to the delivery of comprehensive health services rose from 16 percent in 1987 to 18 percent of total group health plans in 1988. During the same period, enrollment in unmanaged fee-for-service plans dropped sharply from 41 percent to 28 percent (Gabel et al. 1989).

As part of an effort to promote the delivery of preventive services, the Public Health Service created the U.S. Preventive Services Task Force. Its report, the *Guide to Clinical Preventive Services,* was released in May 1989 and represents more than four years of effort by the task force. The *Guide* is the most comprehensive review of clinical preventive services to date; more than 300 expert reviewers examined the strength of the evidence for 169 preventive clinical interventions in 60 topic areas. The task force's four years of literature review, debate, and synthesis of critical comments from expert reviewers resulted in a broad range of age-specific and gender-specific recommendations for primary-care practice. These recommendations, including patient history and physical assessment, immunizations, laboratory and screening tests, and patient education and counseling, provide a framework upon which insurers might model preventive benefits packages. Estimates by the insurance industry itself suggest that such packages need not cost more than a small percentage of total premiums.

Of course, even when preventive services are adequately reimbursed, they are not always offered. Most clinical encounters are brief and designed for acute care. Doctors are not rewarded for spending time to counsel patients. Although doctors rarely disagree that health promotion and risk reduction are important, relatively few work with patients to change their habits. Surveys show that nutritional advice is rarely or never offered, and only 25 to 30 percent of smokers report ever having received a doctor's advice to quit. Some doctors feel that patient education and counseling are peripheral; they are diagnosticians and healers, not teachers. Some feel uncomfortable in the counselor role; others doubt its efficacy. Even when preventive services are offered, they are often merely tacked on to a regular office visit.

Many things can be done. Advances in biomedical knowledge and technology promise improved screening and more effective therapies for some chronic diseases. People inside and outside government are looking harder at the issues of financing and cost-effectiveness, at techniques for educating patients, and at opportunities to offer preventive services across a range of clinical settings and within a variety of specialties. Finally, any patient-physician encounter should be recognized as an opportunity for prevention.

Whatever the attitudes of insurers and doctors, people must accept more responsibility for their own health. Like consumers of other services, consumers of health care are becoming increasingly well informed. As medical and insurance charges rise and the share paid by consumers increases, people will be more adamant about getting the most for their money. It may be possible to improve the availability of preventive services by stimulating demand as well as supply.

With a more rational calculus on which to base decisions about investments in health, with better reimbursement of preventive services, and with a mode of medical practice more sensitive to consumer needs, this country may one day be able to move beyond its concentration on disease and adopt a health care system more truly reflective of its name.

A National Plan for Prevention

When opportunities and needs are great and resources are limited, as they are for the national disease prevention and health promotion agenda, we must choose our issues carefully, where efforts are most likely to yield results. A mechanism for doing so is already in place with the advent of the National Health Objectives for the Year 2000 and its predecessor effort for the year 1990.

In 1980 the Public Health Service (PHS) presented a ten-year strategy for setting and pursuing goals and for measuring progress: *Promoting Health/Preventing Disease: Objectives for the Nation.* This strategy grew out of an earlier study, *Healthy People: The Surgeon General's Report on Health Promotion and Disease Prevention,* published in 1979, which identified opportunities for prevention. The national objectives set by the PHS for 1990 fell into three categories: preventive services, health protection, and health promotion. The priorities within the category of preventive services included the control of high blood pressure, the control of sexually transmitted diseases, family planning, the health of pregnant women and infants, and immunization. The focus included services which health providers could deliver to individuals. The second category—health protection—focused on public and private agencies and industry. The priorities for this category were the control of toxic agents and radiation, occupational safety and health, prevention of accidents and injuries, fluoridation and dental health, and surveillance and control of infectious diseases. The third category—health promotion—emphasized what communities and individuals could do to promote healthy lifestyles and behaviors. The priorities included smoking, drug use, alcohol abuse, nutrition, physical fitness and exercise, and control of stress and violent behavior.

The 1990 campaign did more than codify goals. It set in motion an effort to achieve them. Each of the fifteen priorities was assigned to an appropriate agency within the PHS. These agencies in turn developed implementation plans that reach beyond the Department of Health and Human Services to include participants elsewhere in the federal government, at the state and local level, and in the private sector. The federal government has provided financial support, technical resources, and information, but the most critical activity has been occurring at the community level, where improvements in individual and collective health are essential to the achievement of the goals. For example, federal programs are in place to encourage good infant and maternal nutrition, fluoridation of water, and control of sexually transmitted diseases, but these programs can only succeed with local leadership.

Data to monitor progress have been gathered by a variety of means and analyzed by the responsible agencies and organizations. Each month the Public Health Service sponsors a meeting with lead agencies to evaluate progress toward achieving their assigned objectives and to discuss barriers that they have encountered or expect to experience. The PHS shares this information with health professionals and the public through a range of official, professional, and lay channels.

Policy makers and health providers at the state and local level have testified to the utility of having specific, measurable goals for their domains. As of 1990, all of the states had established objectives for at least some of the 1990 priority areas. The 1990 objectives effort provided precedents and initiated crucial networks for the year 2000 objectives. It has also generated lessons in how the objectives process can be improved. Though the approach taken in developing year 2000 objectives paralleled the 1990 objectives in the comprehensiveness of the issues it addresses, it was much broader in terms of the scope of participation. By working with the Institute of Medicine of the National Academy of Sciences, the Public Health Service led a three-year nationwide effort to elicit the opinions, expertise, and commitment of national professional and voluntary organizations, health care professionals, advocates, and consumers. These efforts began with regional public hearings held in 1988 in eight cities. The hearings were intended to clarify health care problems and opportunities around the country and to provide the PHS with a broad spectrum of detailed information about the special health care needs of racial, ethnic, and other population groups in America. Additionally, eighteen mini-hearings were held in conjunction with the national meetings of professional and voluntary organizations. This level of participation added a nonfederal perspective to the vast body of information generated by the hearings.

As a result of this input, the year 2000 priorities expand upon and revise those of the 1990 objectives, with the addition of areas focusing on topics such as HIV infection, food and drug safety, and mental health. The new objectives are also characterized by an increased emphasis on the prevention of disability and morbidity; greater attention to improvements in the health status of defined population groups at highest risk of premature death, disease, and disability; and inclusion of more screening interventions to detect asymptomatic disease and conditions early enough to prevent early death or chronic illness.

Further input was solicited when the draft objectives for the year 2000 were released for public review and comment. More than 13,000 copies of the draft were distributed, and approximately 600 sets of comments were received in response, many of which represented the input of twenty or thirty people in one organization. During the revision process, close attention was paid to addressing these comments.

The final document, *Healthy People 2000: National Health Promotion and Disease Prevention Objectives,* was released in September 1990 and set forth three broad goals for the year 2000:

- to increase the span of healthy life for Americans;
- to reduce health disparities among Americans; and
- to achieve access to preventive services for all Americans.

The number of priority areas established as important to these goals was increased from fifteen for 1990, to twenty-two for the year 2000 (table 1.3). A total of 300 year-2000 objectives were established across the twenty-two priority areas.

Follow-up to the goals and objectives of *Healthy People 2000* again emphasizes planning and implementation activities at the state and local levels as well as on the federal level. The PHS will work with the representatives of various population groups (American Indians/Alaska natives, Asians/Pacific Islanders, blacks, Hispanics, adolescents, older people, people with disabilities, children in schools, people at worksites, and people in clinical settings) to tailor programs to the specific risks that these groups face. This reliance upon a broad-based network of avenues for implementation is the crux of the year-2000 effort. It is also an effective means of achieving progress in an environment of constrained fiscal resources.

Through national objectives, a means of measuring national physical well-being, much like that used to assess material well-being, has been provided. This ability to document the state of the nation's health as we document consumer prices, the rate of unemployment, and the GNP brings with it an opportunity to create a public health index that should rank in importance and stature with leading economic indicators. After all, it is the health profile of the citizenry that ought to offer the most fundamental and direct measure of national vitality.

Table 1.3   Number of Objectives by Area

Area	Number of objectives
Health Promotion	
Physical activity and fitness	12
Nutrition	21
Tobacco	16
Alcohol and other drugs	19
Family planning	11
Mental health and mental disorders	14
Violent and abusive behavior	18
Educational and community-based programs	14
Health Protection	
Unintentional injuries	22
Occupational safety and health	15
Environmental health	16
Food and drug safety	6
Oral health	16
Preventive Services	
Maternal and infant health	16
Heart disease and stroke	17
Cancer	16
Diabetes and chronic disabling conditions	20
HIV infection	14
Sexually transmitted diseases	15
Immunization and infectious diseases	19
Clinical preventive services	8
Surveillance and Data Systems	7
Other	2
Total (including duplicates)	334
Discrete objectives	300

Looking to the Future

Over the last quarter-century, biomedical research has opened doors in the prevention of health threats such as heart disease, cancer, stroke, lung disease, and diabetes. Even greater progress is possible. Work in the genetic sciences and protein engineering points to the development of new vaccines, a deeper understanding of individual variation in susceptibility, and a host of new tools for early diagnosis. All have immense potential to prevent disease.

We need broader epidemiologic studies to fill in the gaps. Examples are abundant—chief among them is work to identify groups at high risk of developing heart disease and cancer on the basis of physiology and behavior as well as genetic predisposition. A better understanding of childhood risk factors for cardiovascular disease may offer a basis for appropriate intervention. At the other end of the age spectrum, research in exercise physiology is demonstrating how beneficial systematic physical training can be for most older men and women.

Nutrition is an area of research worth special mention. There is increasingly convincing evidence that dietary practices are important risk factors for the leading causes of death and disability mentioned earlier. Indeed, for Americans who do not smoke, use drugs, or abuse alcohol, diet is thought to be the crucial determinant of long-term health. Our total caloric intake (in relation to need), and our consumption of fat, cholesterol, salt, and alcohol all appear to be important, with fat—especially saturated fat—ranking first. Moreover, diet interacts with other genetic, environmental, and behavioral characteristics that affect health, albeit in ways that are not yet well understood.

The Surgeon General's Report on Nutrition and Health, released in July 1988, presents the scientific evidence linking specific dietary factors to specific diseases. For example, consuming too much saturated fat is clearly linked to high serum cholesterol and to heart disease. The report also authoritatively describes the contribution of obesity to heart disease, as well as to high blood pressure and stroke, some types of cancer, gallbladder disease, and to a generally increased risk of death.

The value of nutritional research will be lost unless the findings are translated into behavior, inspiring a shift away from alcohol and foods high in fat, cholesterol, sugar, and salt to vegetables, fruits, and whole grains. Such a shift will require more than individual will power. Public agencies and the food industry must respond to the evidence as well. The American diet is the product of habit—not just of consumers but also of producers—and lack of information. Only a little more than half of the products now on grocery store shelves carry nutrition information. In response, the Food and Drug Administration is presently drafting the new regulations for nutrition labeling.

Some of America's most intractable health problems—adolescent pregnancy, black infant mortality, drug abuse, and even heart disease and cancer—are exacerbated by poverty and lack of education, conditions beyond the reach of the public health apparatus. Restoring the vigor and integrity of schools is one of the most important steps we can take to improve health.

The public health system is by no means powerless, however. How well we deploy the resources that are available, the extent to which policies favoring preventive medicine can transform medical clinics from illness-care to health-care settings, and our efficiency in implementing scientific discoveries can make a big difference in the health profile of Americans. Meeting these challenges, in turn, depends on effective planning, appropriate reimbursement, and the timely application of the fruits of biomedical research.

If we are to be a society that makes steady improvements in the human condition, a fully educated citizenry is essential. If we are to be a nation of healthy people, there can be no tolerance for inequitable access to health care. Yet these ideals cannot be achieved without social commitment.

And so it is with prevention. Science and statistics can tell us much about the possibilities and priorities. Planners can chart a course. What determines the success of a policy, however, is the resolve to act. There are strong countervailing forces at play, whether the issue is clearly labeling the fat content of foods, protecting nonsmokers from the effects of environmental tobacco smoke, keeping handguns out of reach of criminals and minors, or enforcing measures to reduce the number of highway deaths that result from drinking and driving. Each of these is an example of issues crucial to the health of Americans—to the prevention of unnecessary social and personal disability—and of issues that must be addressed directly if our national health potential is to be achieved.

We have the knowledge and the means to become a healthier society. We need only exert the will to apply what we know systemically, in the interest of a truly vital nation.

References

Amler, Robert W., and H. Bruce Dull. 1987. *Closing the Gap: The Burden of Unnecessary Illness.* New York: Oxford University Press.

Centers for Disease Control (CDC). 1990. *Morbidity and Mortality Weekly Report* 39(2):21.

Gabel, Jon, Steven DiCarlo, Steven Fink, and Gregory de Lissovoy. 1989. "Employer-Sponsored Health Insurance in America." *Health Affairs* 8(2):116–128.

Health Care Financing Administration (HCFA), Office of the Actuary. 1990. Unpublished data.

Institute of Medicine (IOM). 1982. *Health and Behavior: Frontiers of Research in the Biobehavioral Sciences.* Edited by David A. Hamburg, Glen R. Elliot, and Delores L. Parron. Washington, D.C.: National Academy Press.

Kottke, Thomas E. 1986. "Disease and Risk Factor Clustering in the United States: The Implications for Public Policy." In *ODPHP Monograph Series: Integration of Risk Factor Interventions.* Washington, D.C.: Office of Disease Prevention and Health Promotion, Public Health Service, U.S. Department of Health and Human Services.

McGinnis, J. Michael. 1988. "National Priorities in Disease Prevention." *Issues in Science and Technology* 5(2):46–52.

McGinnis, J. Michael, and Margaret A. Hamburg. 1988. "Opportunities for Health Promotion and Disease Prevention in the Clinical Setting." *Western Journal of Medicine* 149(3):468–474.

National Center for Health Statistics (NCHS). 1990. *Health United States: 1989* (DHHS Publ. No. (PHS) 90–1232). Hyattsville, Md.: U.S. Department of Health and Human Services.

National Heart, Lung, and Blood Institute (NHLBI). 1989. *NHLBI Fact Book: Fiscal Year 1989.* Bethesda, Md.: U.S. Department of Health and Human Services.

Rice, Dorothy P., Ellen J. MacKenzie, and associates. 1989. *Cost of Injury in the United States: A Report to Congress, 1989.* San Francisco, Cal.: Institute for Health and Aging of the University of California-San Francisco and Injury Prevention Center, the Johns Hopkins University.

U.S. Department of Health, Education and Welfare. 1979. *Healthy People: The Surgeon General's Report on Health Promotion and Disease Prevention* (DHEW Publ. No. 79–55071). Washington, D.C.: U.S. Government Printing Office.

U.S. Department of Health and Human Services. 1980. *Promoting Health/Preventing Disease—Objectives for the Nation.* DHHS Publ. No. (PHS) 79–55071. Washington, D.C.: U.S. Government Printing Office.

U.S. Department of Health and Human Services. 1986. *The 1990 Health Objectives for the Nation: A Midcourse Review.* Washington, D.C.: U.S. Government Printing Office.

U.S. Department of Health and Human Services. 1988. *The Surgeon General's Report on Nutrition and Health.* DHHS Publ. No. (PHS) 88–50210. Washington, D.C.: U.S. Government Printing Office.

U.S. Department of Health and Human Services. 1990. *Healthy People 2000: National Health Promotion and Disease Prevention Objectives.* DHHS Publ. No. (PHS) 91–50212. Washington, D.C.: U.S. Government Printing Office.

U.S. Preventive Services Task Force. 1989. *Guide to Clinical Preventive Services: An Assessment of the Effectiveness of 169 Interventions.* Baltimore, Md.: Williams and Wilkins.

2

Healthy People 2000: National Priorities for Health?

Michael A. Stoto

On September 6, 1990, Secretary of Health and Human Services Louis W. Sullivan unveiled *Healthy People 2000: National Objectives for Health Promotion and Disease Prevention* (DHHS 1991). This report identifies three broad national goals: (1) to increase the span of healthy life, (2) to reduce health disparities among Americans, and (3) to achieve access to preventive services for all Americans. In support of these goals, the main body of the report details about three hundred objectives with specific quantitative targets to be achieved by the year 2000. As a whole, the report is a valuable compendium of professional and organizational views of health promotion and disease prevention for the 1990s.

The publication of this report follows by about a decade the publication of *Healthy People: The Surgeon General's Report on Health Promotion and Disease Prevention* (DHEW 1979), which proposed five broad quantitative national health goals to be achieved by 1990. A subsequent publication—*Promoting Health/Preventing Disease: Objectives for the Nation* (DHHS 1980)—identified 226 more specific quantitative objectives necessary for the attainment of the broad goals identified in *Healthy People*. As the latest and most developed report in the series, *Healthy People 2000* is the most clearly articulated statement of what might be regarded as *national health priorities* for the 1990s. The leap from goals and objectives to priorities is a major one, however. *Priorities* implies that some objectives are more important, in some sense, than others or that those stated are more important than those not stated. Thus two of the major questions that *Healthy People 2000* raises are whether the leap from objectives to priorities can be made, and if so, how can this best be done.

Some possible answers to these questions were discussed at a set of hearings sponsored by the Public Health Service (PHS) and the Institute of Medicine. Organized as an opportunity for cooperation among the diverse groups that play important roles in improving the nation's health, these hearings were held in seven cities across the country in 1988. Their purpose was to solicit testimony from a broad range of individuals and organizations about appropriate and attainable national health promotion and disease prevention objectives for the year 2000. Speakers at the hearings represented, among others, health care, education, highway safety, and workplace and environmental safety organizations; public and private health agencies at federal, state, and local levels; employers; schools; insurers; community organizations; and minority groups. More than 800 individuals and organizations spoke at one of the hearings or submitted written testimony (Stoto, Behrens, and Rosemont 1990).

Despite the strong response and range of views expressed at the hearings about how the objectives of *Healthy People 2000* could and should represent national health priorities, an analysis of the objectives, the structure of the report, and the process through which they were derived indicates that *Healthy People 2000* fails as a national health priority statement. The report does not convey a sense of what is important in health promotion and disease prevention or what needs to be done first. The ideas in the report and the momentum behind the process, however, offer opportunities for developing national or local health priorities.

The Year 2000 Objectives as National Health Priorities

As many individuals and organizations testified in the *Healthy People 2000* hearings, three issues arose in these discussions: whether *Healthy People 2000* should adopt a national or a federal perspective, whether the objectives should focus on health promotion and disease prevention or health more broadly defined, and whether they should be regarded as priorities.

National versus federal perspective

A group of state health officers, all of whom had worked to implement the 1990 objectives within their states, testified that the objectives should be for the nation, not just the federal government. They noted that although the federal government is providing leadership and a process for developing the objectives, federal, state, and local government officials; industry; educational institutions; and private, nonprofit organizations must all "take ownership" of the objectives and help implement them. The health officers also felt that establishing and achieving national health objectives is a process that will require the commitment of resources from all levels of government—federal and nonfederal—as well as from private sources. For the objectives to be realistic, however, the health officers felt that allowances must be made for local and regional variations so that communities can outline and address their independent needs within the national framework (Stoto, Behrens, and Rosemont 1990).

Representatives of the private sector agreed. According to Paul Entmacher, who represented the Business Roundtable at one hearing:

> The public sector should take the primary leadership role in establishing health objectives and providing surveillance over the nation's health, but the Business Roundtable endorses the concept of ongoing, nonpartisan, appropriate, public-private collaboration in setting and measuring the nation's health objectives. We naturally wish to contribute mainly to those objectives that could affect the employers and employees in the business community in the United States in the year 2000. There is a fundamental commonality, however, between the eventual national objectives and the nation's private sector work force because as citizens and taxpayers they either are or ought to be vitally concerned about the health of their environment. (Stoto, Behrens, and Rosemont 1990)

The federal government has accepted this perspective. *Healthy People 2000* notes,

> Alone, no one person, family, business, organization, or government has the resources to bring about the changes needed to implement this broad program, and yet the program cannot succeed unless each of us contributes individually. (DHHS 1991:88)

Roles for government, business, labor, education, professional groups, voluntary organizations, media, the family, and individuals are described in the report. Indeed, making the objectives national and not just federal is the primary reason that the PHS asked the Institute of Medicine to organize and cosponsor the hearings described above and to involve national organizations in the development of the objectives.

Prevention versus health

Although the provisions of *Healthy People 2000* are commonly referred to as "national health objectives," the report actually focuses on one approach to the improvement of health status: health promotion and disease prevention. The objectives specify health-promotion priorities to influence individual lifestyle factors, health-protection priorities for issues in which environmental or regulatory measures can provide protection to population groups, and preventive services priorities addressing contributions of the health care system. Only a few objectives call for the provision of clinical services. There is very little mention of health care costs or quality assurance, and the tradeoffs between access to high-tech procedures and basic primary care that are commonly discussed elsewhere are not emphasized in the report.

Some testifiers and reviewers called for a broadening of the definition of health and, implicitly, the focus of the national objectives, to that adopted by the World Health Organization: "a state of complete physical, mental and social well-being, and not merely the absence of disease and infirmity." Some who took this view would give more emphasis than *Healthy People 2000* currently does to the role of socioeconomic factors as determinants of health. In commenting on a draft of the objectives, the American Public Health Association (APHA) put socioeconomic factors at the top of its list of gaps in the objectives and called for objectives on improving housing, eliminating unemployment, and ending poverty (APHA 1989).

Other testifiers stressed the role of the health care system in health promotion and disease prevention and called for improved access. Milton Roemer of UCLA noted that "many, if not all, of the priorities of positive health activity on the national agenda can be substantially influenced by access to professional health care" (Stoto, Behrens, and Rosemont 1990:68).

Healthy People 2000 does not deny health as the ultimate outcome, and in fact the first two goals and many of the objectives center on health status improvements. The focus on health promotion and disease prevention, however, goes back to the original *Healthy People* report, which called for a "second public health revolution" going beyond the traditional curative interests of the health care community (DHEW 1979:vii).

While the tone of the new report is not as strident, the focus on prevention as a means to health remains clear.

Objectives versus priorities

Some testifiers suggested that the objectives could be more than a list of health problems on which progress was possible and of strategies for attaining goals. Instead, they suggested, the objectives in *Healthy People 2000* could convey some sense of what is most important in health promotion and disease prevention—in other words, they could serve as priorities.

Different meanings for the word *priority* exist, however, and seem to have been used during the course of the hearings. Many testifiers suggested that there should be fewer objectives for the year 2000 than the 226 set for 1990, or that priorities should be set among a large number of objectives. Their reasoning was that it is simply too difficult to assess progress on hundreds of different measures. Some testifiers clearly preferred that the objectives identify the most important health problems or the most important strategies for addressing them (Stoto, Behrens, and Rosemont 1990).

Witnesses testified that priorities are required to focus efforts and allocate resources. Robert Harmon, drawing on his experience in using state objectives as director of the Missouri Department of Health, said:

> When looking this far ahead, it helps to focus on priorities. Establishing a strategic vision or mission for the future not only helps to clarify desired achievements, it also helps eliminate those issues that may be very important but are not central to an agency's overall purpose. The nation should select priorities based on what is achievable by the year 2000, what represents a marked improvement over the status quo, what falls within the national public health mission, and what can be impacted directly or indirectly by a positive endorsement from the federal government. (Stoto, Behrens, and Rosemont 1990:12)

According to Bernard Turnock, Illinois Director of Public Health:

> Having clearly visible and repeatedly articulated priorities and broadly defining these priorities into categories is critically important. It allows all potential participants to better understand their

roles in addressing a collective health problem and serves to cata-
lyze inclusion and participation over exclusion and avoidance. It
focuses our efforts on the health outcomes and on the persons
affected or potentially affected by the problem, rather than on the
health care delivery system as so many of our past and current so-
called health priorities have done. It establishes a focal point for
integration and systemization of diverse efforts—including some
even outside the traditional notion of health strategies—and provides a rallying point for seeking and securing new and expanded
resources. (Stoto, Behrens, and Rosemont 1990:12)

Some private sector testifiers felt the same way. For example, Charles
Arnold, representing the Health Insurance Association of America, noted
that we cannot afford to specify an objective on every issue that needs
improvement. If the critical objectives are to be attained, he said, more
attention must be given to setting priorities (Stoto, Behrens, and Rosemont 1990).

Priority setting was discussed in a series of congressional hearings
held in early 1990. In two hearings on the year 2000 health objectives,
Senator Jeff Bingaman, chairman of the Subcommittee on Government
Information and Regulation, and many of his witnesses called for the
development of a short list of objectives that could be used for annual
health checkups at the national, state, and perhaps substate levels.
Robert Lawrence of Harvard Medical School and others called for
setting priorities among the objectives, and Bingaman agreed (NIH
1990).

The same issues also came up again in a bill that was introduced by
Senator Tom Harkin in the 101st Congress. The Health Objectives 2000
Act (S. 2056) would assist states and localities in setting up objectives
and carrying out activities intended to meet them. To receive funds, a
state would have to identify and monitor progress toward at least five
"national health priorities," including all of the "core national health
priorities." These priorities are to be established by the Secretary of
Health and Human Services, "taking into account the 'Year 2000 Health
Objectives.' "

The PHS is somewhat ambiguous about the objectives/priority question. Rather than identify priorities, the PHS has adopted a manage-
ment-by-objectives philosophy. J. Michael McGinnis, director of the office responsible for developing the objectives, sees the objectives as
"useful in clarifying opportunities, recording successes, fostering accountability for failures, providing a common language for communicat-

ing about *priorities*, providing a national validation for local initiatives, and for identifying gaps in data collection efforts" (1990:242). Expanding on the first point, McGinnis says, "Measurable objectives have proven useful in clarifying the nature of national prevention opportunities in concrete terms that give a sense of both possibilities and *priorities*" (1990:242). On the point about a common language, he says, "Having agreed-upon objectives has facilitated communication around programs and *priorities* [emphasis added]" (1990:243).

Thus *Healthy People 2000* does not claim that its objectives are priorities but does use the word *priority* frequently. The objectives are intended as a "statement of national opportunities" (DHHS 1991:iv) and the report is described as deliberately comprehensive so as to "allow local communities and States to choose from among its recommendations in addressing their own highest priority needs" (DHHS 1991:2).

Analysis of the Year 2000 Health Objectives

The publication of *Healthy People 2000* represents a milestone in public health. The PHS deserves credit for setting up a process to engage the participation of a broad cross-section of health professionals and other community leaders around the country in the development of the objectives. In addition to the testimony obtained through the hearings in 1988, a draft copy of the objectives was published for comment in 1989 (PHS 1989) and PHS made serious efforts to respond to concerns raised in response to that draft. By continuing an activity started a decade before under a different presidential administration, and by involving a spectrum of health-related interest groups, the PHS has institutionalized and legitimized health promotion and disease-prevention activities.

Healthy People 2000 is also noteworthy in that it represents in concrete statistical terms the potential health-status gains that can be expected from health-promotion and disease-prevention activities. Unlike the beneficiaries of curative care, the beneficiaries of prevention are known statistically but are never individually identified. The report presents a set of 300 specific, quantitative objectives arranged in twenty-two chapters or priority areas. The priority areas, with some sample objectives, are listed in table 2.1. By stating objectives for the future in quantitative terms now, the PHS has found a way to recognize the vast but hidden potential of health promotion and disease prevention.

As a list of public health issues and activities, the objectives are

Table 2.1   Healthy People 2000 Priorities for Health Promotion and Disease Prevention

1. Physical Activity and Fitness
   • Increase moderate daily physical activity to at least 30% of people.
   • Reduce sedentary lifestyles to no more than 15% of people.
2. Nutrition
   • Reduce overweight to a prevalence no more than 20% of people.
   • Reduce dietary fat intake to an average of 30% of calories.
3. Tobacco
   • Reduce cigarette smoking prevalence to below 15% of adults.
   • Reduce initiation of cigarette smoking to no more than 15% by age 20.
4. Alcohol and Other Drugs
   • Reduce alcohol-related motor vehicle crash deaths to no more than 8.5 per 100,000 people.
   • Reduce alcohol use by school children aged 12 to 17 to less than 13%; marijuana use by youth aged 18 to 25 to less than 8%; and cocaine use by youth aged 18 to 25 to less than 3%.
5. Family Planning
   • Reduce teenage pregnancies to no more than 50 per 1,000 girls 17 and younger.
   • Reduce unintended pregnancies to no more than 30% of pregnancies.
6. Mental Health and Mental Disorders
   • Reduce suicides to no more than 10.5 per 100,000 people.
   • Reduce adverse effects of stress to less than 35% of people.
7. Violent and Abusive Behavior
   • Reduce homicides to no more than 7.2 per 100,000 people.
   • Reduce assault injuries to no more than 10 per 1,000 people.
8. Educational and Community-Based Programs
   • Provide quality K-12 school health education in at least 75% of schools.
   • Provide employee health promotion activities in at least 85% of workplaces with 50 or more employees.
9. Unintentional Injuries
   • Reduce unintentional injury deaths to no more than 29.3 per 100,000 people.
   • Increase automobile safety restraint use to at least 85% of occupants.
10. Occupational Safety and Health
    • Reduce work-related injury deaths to no more than 4 per 100,000 workers.
    • Reduce work-related injuries to no more than 6 per 100 workers.
11. Environmental Health
    • Eliminate blood lead levels above 25 μg/dL in children under age 5.
    • Increase protection from air pollutants so that at least 85% of people live in counties that meet EPA standards.
    • Increase protection from radon so that at least 40% of people live in homes tested by homeowners and found to be/made safe.
12. Food and Drug Safety
    • Reduce salmonella infection outbreaks to fewer than 25 yearly.
13. Oral Health
    • Reduce the incidence of dental caries to no more than 35% of children by age 8.
    • Reduce edentulism to no more than 20% in people aged 65 and older.
14. Maternal and Infant Health
    • Reduce infant mortality to no more than 7 deaths per 1,000 births.
    • Reduce low birth weight to no more than 5% of live births.
    • Increase first trimester prenatal care to at least 90% of live births.
15. Heart Disease and Stroke
    • Reduce coronary heart disease deaths to no more than 100 per 100,000 people.
    • Reduce stroke deaths to no more than 20 per 100,000 people.

- Increase control of high blood pressure to at least 50% of people with high blood pressure.
- Reduce blood cholesterol to an average of no more than 200 mg/dL.
16. Cancer
    - Reverse the rise in cancer deaths to no more than 130 per 100,000 people.
    - Increase clinical breast exams and mammography every 2 years to at least 60% of women aged 50 and older.
    - Increase Pap tests every 1–3 years to at least 85% of women aged 18 and older.
    - Increase fecal occult blood testing every 1–2 years to at least 50% of people aged 50 and older.
17. Diabetes and Chronic Disabling Conditions
    - Reduce disability from chronic conditions to no more than 8% of people.
    - Reduce diabetes-related deaths to no more than 34 per 100,000 people.
18. HIV Infection
    - Confine HIV infection to no more than 800 per 100,000 people.
19. Sexually Transmitted Diseases
    - Reduce gonorrhea infections to no more than 225 per 100,000 people.
    - Reduce syphilis infections to no more than 10 per 100,000 people.
20. Immunization and Infectious Diseases
    - Eliminate measles.
    - Reduce epidemic-related pneumonia and influenza deaths to no more than 7.3 per 100,000 people aged 65 and older.
    - Increase childhood immunization levels to at least 90% of 2-year-olds.
21. Clinical Preventive Services
    - Eliminate financial barriers to clinical preventive services.
22. Surveillance and Data Systems
    - Develop and implement common health status indicators for use by federal/state/local health agencies.

SOURCE: *Healthy People 2000: Citizens Chart the Course* (DHHS 1991).

relatively complete and compelling. The list of priority areas and the objectives in them are comprehensive and they reflect major health problems and public health initiatives. It is instructive to have each of the many aspects of health promotion and disease prevention covered in a parallel fashion in a single document. Within each priority area the main issues that a public health official would want to monitor are identified.

The PHS made a serious effort in *Healthy People 2000* to focus attention on a full range of health outcomes, going beyond traditional mortality measures. Furthermore, it paid substantial attention to disparities in health status experienced by various minority groups and to specific interventions and targets intended to close these gaps. These undertakings, together with the enhanced efforts to involve the professional community in the development of the objectives, represent important advances in the formulation of national health objectives.

A number of features of *Healthy People 2000* and the objectives, however, that inhibit their use, especially for priority setting. These problematic features include gaps in coverage, the sheer number of objectives, and the way in which they are organized.

Gaps

Despite the intention that the objectives be national, and not just federal, *Healthy People 2000* was published by the federal government. As one would expect, the report does not conflict with established Bush administration policy or political views. One result of this conformity is that, from a public health perspective, important substantive gaps in coverage exist. American Public Health Association (APHA) president Myron Allukian, while calling *Healthy People 2000* "a landmark achievement," noted that it "falls short in some areas critical to the health of the American people" (APHA 1990).

For instance, the family planning objectives put little emphasis on contraceptive services and mention abortion only as something to be avoided. Rather, the focus is on abstinence. The objectives remain vague on the use of contraceptives by teenagers and on the provision of sex education. The main objective is phrased in terms of reducing the number of pregnancies rather than births, implicitly leaving out abortion as an option. This general approach contrasts with testimony and comments from many individuals and public health organizations. Contraceptive services and abortion are controversial issues, but a realistic assessment of the consequences of unintended childbearing on both mother and child, and the limited possibilities of reducing unintended fertility through abstinence alone, suggest that these controversial options need to be available.

Similarly, although "weapon-related violent deaths" are the focus of one objective in *Healthy People 2000*, no aspect of gun control is directly mentioned. The subject is only approached through two related issues: weapon carrying by adolescents and inappropriate storage of weapons. Data are not available to assess progress toward either of these two objectives, and guns are generally not distinguished from other weapons as a means of inflicting violence. Given the large number of objectives calling for legislation and government regulation of various sorts in other areas, handgun control is an obvious omission.

In fact, the objectives call for many actions on the part of state and local governments but none from the federal government. For example, some *Healthy People 2000* objectives call for state immunization and clean air laws, state exposure standards to prevent occupational lung diseases, state and local construction standards to minimize indoor radon exposure, state emergency medical services and trauma systems, and the establishment of general community health promotion programs and special community programs to promote exercise and prevent violence. Numerous objectives also call for the establishment of different kinds of school and worksite programs. No objectives explicitly call for federal action, however, presumably to avoid making *Healthy People 2000* into a "statement of federal standards or requirements" (DHHS 1991:i). Federal responsibilities are described only in general terms in one section. To function as a complete list of options for health promotion and disease prevention, *Healthy People 2000* needs a better balance between recommended federal and nonfederal actions.

The number and organization of objectives

Testifiers identified the large number of 1990 objectives as an impediment to effective assessment and implementation efforts. Yet *Healthy People 2000* contains 300 separately stated objectives, some of which have multiple parts, with almost 400 statistical series that will have to be monitored. With the more than 200 additional special population targets for high-risk groups, quantity alone will make monitoring the year 2000 objectives at the national, state, and local levels a formidable statistical challenge.

The detailed presentation may be helpful to specialists in particular areas charged with developing detailed action plans. The large number of objectives, however, diminishes the amount of attention that can be paid to any one objective. The large number of objectives also makes it difficult to understand the structure that ties them together. Furthermore, having so many objectives fails to focus attention on what is most important. Commenting on a draft, the APHA said that "the cogency of a limited number of measurable objectives is losing its strength by being drowned in the flood of materials coming forth" (APHA 1989). The rationale for presenting a comprehensive list of objectives from which other groups can choose in *Healthy People 2000* is legitimate, but 300 objectives is too many from which to make an informed choice.

Part I of Healthy People 2000 contains three lists that might be interpreted as national health priorities per se, or that might be expected to help in setting priorities among the many specific objectives, summarized below:

1. The three broad national goals (listed earlier in this chapter).
2. Twelve specific measures of progress toward those goals. The

discussion of the span of healthy life, for example, features four statistical series: life expectancy at birth, deaths before age seventy-five, healthy life expectancy, and percentage of the population experiencing limitation of major activity.

3. A list of forty-seven specific objectives in the chapter called "Priorities for Health Promotion and Disease Prevention," including at least one from each priority area (see table 2.1).

From their placement in the report, one might assume that these three lists are a summary of the longer list of specific objectives or a selection of the most important objectives.

The relationship between these three lists and the 300 specific objectives is very complicated and not clearly explained in the report. The introduction to the chapter on "Priorities for Health Promotion and Disease Prevention" is ambiguous about whether the priorities are the chapter titles from part II or the forty-seven objectives that appear within the same chapter. The forty-seven objectives seem intended to represent the others in the chapters from which they were selected, but the criteria used to choose them is not defined. There is no direct connection between the forty-seven objectives and the three national goals or the twelve measures of progress.

In contrast to the specific objectives, no public discussion of part I of *Healthy People 2000* took place before it was published. In particular, neither the rationale for the short list of objectives nor the criteria for choosing them was reviewed outside of the federal government. While this does not necessarily mean that the choices were poorly made, it does undercut the positioning of *Healthy People 2000* as a set of national, and not just federal, objectives.

The Potential Contribution of the Objectives to the Development of Health Priorities

As the preceding analysis suggests, *Healthy People 2000* falls short of being the statement of national health priorities that some observers have thought that it could be. The development of objectives, however, still offers an opportunity to develop national or local health priorities now and in the future. As a state-of-the-art synthesis of a welath of information on the entire field of health promotion and disease prevention, the report is directly relevant to priority setting. Particularly helpful are both the statement of relevant issues and the possibilities that experts see in those areas, as well as statistical specifications for measuring progress. The report presents opportunities, furthermore, for individual states to set priorities in developing their own health objectives, objectives that might contribute to the development of national health priorities in the future by some organization other than the federal government. To advance discussion about how this might be done, conceptual difficulties in setting priorities will need to be overcome and alternative approaches developed.

Conceptual difficulties

A number of inherent conceptual difficulties impede the development of health priorities that focus on health promotion and disease prevention. These include incorporating diverse values, structuring the objectives in a meaningful way, and evaluating costs and benefits.

Incorporating diverse values. Priority setting is an inherently political action and needs to be recognized as such. Economic theory suggests ways to use cost-benefit information in setting priorities, usually under assumptions about common values and joint resources. The pluralistic nature of the development of *Healthy People 2000*, however, belies such simplifying assumptions. Indeed, interest-group participation is a hallmark of the process. The problem is to construct a coherent national document that somehow takes into account a diverse set of individual and group values.

The many public and private-sector institutions involved in the process obviously have different interests. They reflect, in part, the varying health problems and concerns experienced in different parts of the country and in racial, ethnic, and socioeconomic population groups. Because the benefits of health promotion and disease prevention programs depend on the current risk profile and health status of these different groups, the benefits are not evenly distributed among the population. Decisions about which issues or programs be priorities implicitly determining which population groups benefit. Given these potentially unequal outcomes, the most appropriate role for the government might be to identify the options, the costs and benefits of change, and what we know about how to achieve certain goals, leaving communities and other organizations to decide for themselves which strategies to adopt.

On the resources side, to assume (as standard economic theory does) that there is a single national account for health promotion and disease prevention efforts or a single decision maker charged with allocating it is a mistake. In fact, interest-group participation inhibits efforts to reallocate resources. Any priorities need to be able to accommodate the efforts of groups willing to contribute to health promotion and disease prevention efforts, even if their contributions are narrowly focused on problems that may not be the most severe. Dental hygienists, for instance, are eager to find a role in health promotion and disease prevention, but their contributions cannot be expected to go much beyond oral health concerns.

Structure of the objectives. An analysis of *Healthy People 2000* reflects the inherent difficulty of setting up a structure to make informed tradeoffs among health promotion and disease prevention interventions. The objectives in each priority area are divided into three groups: health status, risk reduction, and services and protection. The inclusion of the second two categories presents two conceptual difficulties.

First, there is the danger of confusing ends and means. Risk-factor objectives are useful because they measure the impact of intervention programs more directly and immediately than any analysis of heart disease, cancer, or other diseases caused by smoking. In order to choose from among goals, a common scale is needed for comparing outcomes. The ultimate health effects, not the reduction in risk factors per se, provide such a scale.

Part of the confusion between ends and means is inherent in our understanding of health promotion and disease prevention. Mortality and disability reductions are clearly ends and intervention programs means, but risk factor changes are a combination of both. A reduction in the proportion of adults who smoke cigarettes seems like a victory in itself, but aside from improvements to indoor air quality, we value the reduction because of its implications for mortality and morbidity in the future. Some issues are both risk factors and outcomes. For instance, drug and alcohol abuse cause health problems in the long run but also have immediate social consequences.

Second, setting priorities among health status measures, risk factors, and intervention programs assumes that the causal relationships among them are well known. In fact, causal relationships in health promotion and disease prevention are quite complex, especially among chronic diseases. For example, hypertension and diabetes are both serious diseases in their own right, but both predispose individuals to a range of other chronic diseases and disabling conditions. The ends in question all have independent risk factors as well. In light of these complex relationships, it is difficult to make an accounting of the implications of meeting a single objective and compare it to the benefits of achieving other objectives.

Evaluating costs and benefits. An essential part of any priority-setting effort, the evaluation of costs and benefits is especially difficult for health-promotion and disease-prevention programs. First, the benefits of preventing a problem are not equal to the current burden of illness associated with that problem. For most diseases, even eliminating all risk factors will not totally eliminate the disease. Furthermore, no program aimed at behavior change can expect to eliminate the targeted risk factors in the population. On the other hand, some programs such as vaccination are clearly more valuable than the current burden of illness suggests, precisely because they have been successful.

Second, the benefits of many health-promotion and disease-prevention interventions occur far in the future. Changes in chronic-disease risk factors among adults, for instance, result in lower mortality and disability decades in the future. Altering behavior patterns in children might have a powerful effect, but mostly not until they reach middle age. Thus the benefits of any intervention have to be appropriately discounted.

Third, the costs of programs aimed at behavior changes are particularly difficult to estimate. A complete accounting would include not only program costs such as staff time, materials preparation, and advertising, but also the costs to individuals of forgoing a behavior that they enjoy. This issue is especially difficult if people come to like the new lifestyles they adopt. What is the cost, for instance, of avoiding red meat if some who do it discover that they like fish?

As the foregoing examples illustrate, the costs and benefits of an intervention generally cannot be estimated in the abstract; the details of the specific programs are important. The level of detail needed, however, is not generally appropriate for the national objectives.

The standards for comparison are also open to question. Many medical interventions are evaluated on the basis of medical effectiveness alone. Prevention programs, however, are often expected not only to achieve their health goals but to be cost-effective or cost-saving as well (Warner 1990). Few prevention programs reduce costs, but they can be cost-effective measures for decreasing mortality and improving the quality of life (Russell 1986).

Alternative approaches

Despite these difficulties, the ideas in and the momentum behind *Healthy People 2000* offer significant opportunities for health priority setting. States and local areas will adopt objectives of their own, using the national objectives as a starting point. They can take this opportunity to choose from among the many possibilities listed in the report, setting priorities according to local needs and opportunities. National groups might decide to develop priorities of their own, also using *Healthy People 2000* as input. And hopefully, there will be national health objectives for 2010.

The experience of developing the year 2000 health objectives and the prceding analysis suggests approaches to future priority setting activities, whether they are based on *Healthy People 2000* or developed independently. Such efforts should (1) focus on outcomes, not tactics, (2) develop a unifying framework for evaluating outcomes, (3) develop a short list of sentinel objectives, and (4) employ a staged process of identifying issues, developing statistical measures, and choosing target values. These guidelines can help clarify the complex relationships among health status, risk factors, and programs that influence them; and while they do not provide a recipe for setting priorities, they can help policymakers better understand the tradeoffs involved.

Focus on outcomes, not implementation steps. Setting priorities requires making tradeoffs. To make reasonable tradeoffs, potential targets must be compared on a common scale. Since all of the objectives and strategies are intended to increase the span of healthy life or to reduce disparities in health status, health-status outcomes provide a common scale to unite the many objectives and strategies in Healthy People 2000. To make the tradeoffs among objectives more straightforward, then, the focus should be on health-status measures. Furthermore, because of uncertainties about the effectiveness of programs and because of different concerns and professional perspectives, it is easier to achieve consensus on health status goals than the programs that will get us there.

Risk-related behaviors, the use of preventive services, and the availability of community health-protection programs should be monitored as intermediate outcomes and indicators of program success or failure but not as ends in themselves. Other supporting activities—surveillance systems, public and professional awareness efforts, organization and provision of services, and so on—could be described in detail, but labeled as "implementation steps" or "tactics."

Develop a unifying framework. To make the logical connections between health status improvements and the many strategies and implementation steps needed to bring them about, a unifying framework is needed. William Lassek, Regional Health Administrator for Public Health Service Region III in Philadelphia, for instance, called in his testimony for

> a significant change in the organization of the objectives to bring them in line with accepted principles of public health epidemiology, i.e., beginning with a negative health outcome, determining

its risk factors, and designing an intervention to reduce the risk factors. (Stoto, Behrens, and Rosemont 1990:7–8)

Lassek proposed that (1) goals be defined by age group, (2) for each age group, the leading causes of death and morbidity be enumerated and tracked by race and sex, (3) for each major cause of death or morbidity within each group, the major risk factors be enumerated, and (4) objectives set for interventions known to reduce these risk factors (Stoto, Behrens, and Rosemont 1990:8).

Paul Entmacher recommended the development of a "guiding conceptual framework" based on several aggregate measures of the public health to bind together disparate objectives toward a common goal of improving the public's health. Candidate objectives would be evaluated on this scale. For the aggregate measures, Entmacher suggests "preventable potential years of life lost" (based solely on mortality statistics) and "preventable productive work loss years" (years of life between eighteen and sixty-five discounted for health-related disability and productivity loss) (Stoto, Behrens, and Rosemont 1990:13). He and others have also suggested the possibility of using "quality-adjusted life-years" to integrate mortality and disability information into a single comprehensive health status measure (Erickson et al. 1989; Patrick and Bergner 1990; Kaplan 1990).

Currently available epidemiological risk-factor models that relate health outcomes to risk factors and to specific interventions for many diseases and health-related behaviors can help to clarify the relationships among different kinds of objectives and also provide insight into achievable health-status targets. For example, the CAN*TROL model developed by the National Cancer Institute was used in preparing the cancer objectives for *Healthy People 2000*. This model projects cancer incidence and mortality under various cancer control programs such as prevention programs, screening, and treatment (Eddy 1986; Levin et al. 1986). Similar models have been developed for cardiovascular disease, AIDS, and other diseases (Weinstein et al. 1987). Using such models as appropriate, *Closing the Gap* synthesizes much of what is known about the potential health effects of health promotion and disease prevention (Amler and Dull 1987).

Develop a short list of sentinel objectives. The three national goals in *Healthy People 2000* accurately sum up what is at stake in the process of developing objectives, but they lack specificity and accountability. The many specific objectives are critical to public health professionals trying to design programs in particular areas, but they are too numerous for the public and political leaders to follow on a regular basis. A short list of sentinel objectives that can be understood and followed on a regular basis is necessary to maintain public and professional attention.

The sentinel measures should strike a balance between comprehensiveness and conciseness. The list should be comprehensive in summing up progress on a much longer list of health status measures and relating them to the overall national goals. On the other hand, because the sentinel objectives should be understandable to the public and our elected leadership, and be measurable on a regular and timely basis at both national and subnational levels, they need to be few in number and to rely on readily available statistics. One possible strategy is to choose a combination of comprehensive and indicator measures.

Comprehensive measures such as death rates or general quality-of-life measures for specific age groups that evaluate comprehensive interventions for a range of problems are clearly needed. For instance, because of the interrelatedness of heart disease, cancer, stroke, and diabetes and their risk factors, the combined death rate from all four causes for the population under age sixty-five might be a good measure of preventable, premature chronic-disease mortality.

Other measures that are easily monitored and are indicators of progress in a variety of related issues can also be helpful. For instance, the incidence of one reportable sexually transmitted disease (STD) might be used as a measure of progress in fighting all STDs and in changing the underlying behaviors that cause their transmission. Similarly, a measure of the use of one preventive service such as mammography for a particular age group might indicate progress on the utilization of all preventive services and on removing the barriers to their further use.

Organizing the sentinel objectives by age has a number of advantages. First and foremost, many people organize their thinking about health issues in terms of age groups. This is apparent in the life-course approach to health promotion developed by Breslow and Somers (1977), as well as in the original *Healthy People* report (DHEW 1979). People concerned with children, say, will find it easier to understand what the overall objectives contain for them if a set of sentinel objectives for children is identified. Furthermore, thinking in terms of age groups makes it easier to identify the issues to include; looking at one age group at a time obviates the need for imponderable comparisons between reduction in teenage fertility and improvements in the quality of life for older people and the like.

Separate issue identification, measure development, and choice of target values. In the development of the year-2000 health objectives, three separate technical steps were carried out by a single group of people: (1) identifying issues for which there would be objectives, (2) developing statistical measures and proxies for those issues, and (3) choosing target values for the objectives. One result is that *Healthy People 2000* often does not distinguish between general health issues and operational measures of these issues. Objective 2.21, for instance, calls for 75 percent of primary care providers to "provide nutrition assessment and counseling and/or referral to qualified nutritionists or dietitians" but uses as baseline data "physicians provided diet counseling for an estimated 40 to 50 percent of patients." These statements of the service to be provided, who is to provide the service, and the population to which the percentage is applied are contradictory. Furthermore, most numerical target values were set intuitively because there was no opportunity to develop trend analyses or risk factor models to guide the choice of target values.

One possible way to avoid these problems is to organize the objective-setting process to accommodate the three separate technical steps described, assigning each to different kinds of experts. This would capitalize on the strengths of these experts: those who can identify the critical health issues, those who know the data bases necessary to monitor progress, and those with the analytic sophistication needed to determine what is feasible in each area. Interaction between the three types of expert during various stages of the process should lead to more practical decision making. On the most basic level, for instance, knowing what improvements are possible and the impact they will have upon health should influence the decision to include a measure. In this way, identifying the three steps as separate tasks might allow them to be done better.

Examples of similar processes already exist. According to Clark (1989), the state of Oregon successfully used a process similar to the one described above in setting its year 2000 health objectives. In a related field, a committee of the Institute of Medicine was able to develop national priorities for medical technology assessment by seeking suggestions for needed assessments from many interested organizations, evaluating the benefits to be gained from each assessment in a common analytical framework, using a broadly constituted committee to select twenty priorities, and presenting enough of the results so that other groups could choose for themselves among the targets selected and those eliminated in the last round (IOM 1990).

Although some testifiers called for the *Healthy People 2000* objectives to express national health priorities, *Healthy People 2000* does not represent priorities—and was not intended to. Although it expresses many important ideas well, it fails to convey a sense of what is important in health promotion and disease prevention. Given the pluralistic nature of the *Healthy People 2000* development process and inherent conceptual difficulties, it is probably unrealistic and perhaps inappropriate for a federal government document to attempt to set national priorities.

Although *Healthy People 2000* is a milestone in public health policy, more could have been done to facilitate its use in setting priorities at the national, state, or local level. A shorter, better organized list of objectives, for instance, would have made the scope of the report easier to comprehend and progress easier to monitor. Better organization might help to facilitate tradeoffs between targets in different areas. Also, more attention to the ultimate health effects achievable through each of the proposed strategies would have helped decision makers to choose between strategies.

Yet *Healthy People 2000* is a carefully crafted statement of what the nation wants to achieve in a wide range of public health arenas and could be the basis for priority setting activities at the federal, state, and local levels. Efforts to develop priorities based on the objectives ultimately should (1) focus on outcomes, not tactics, (2) develop a unifying framework for evaluating outcomes, (3) develop a short list of sentinel objectives, and (4) employ a staged process of identifying issues, developing statistical measures, and choosing target values.

References

American Public Health Association (APHA). 1989. "Comments on the Year 2000 Health Objectives." Unpublished document submitted to the Public Health Service.

American Public Health Association (APHA). 1990. "APHA Commends National Prevention Initiative." News release (September 6).

Amler, Robert W., and H. Bruce Dull, eds. 1987. *Closing the Gap: The Burden of Unnecessary Illness.* New York: Oxford University Press.

Breslow, Lester, and Anne R. Somers. 1977. "A Lifetime Health Monitoring Program: A Practical Approach to Preventive Medicine." *New England Journal of Medicine* 296:601–698.

Clark, Donna L. 1989. "Oregon's Health 2000 Project." *Proceedings of the 1989 Public Health Conference on Records and Statistics.* Washington, D.C.: National Center for Health Statistics.

Eddy, David M., 1986. "Setting Priorities for Cancer Control Programs." *Journal of the National Cancer Institute* 76:187–99.

Erickson, Pennifer, E. Allen Kendall, John P. Anderson, and Robert M. Kaplan. 1989. "Using Composite Health Status Measures to Assess the Nation's Health." *Medical Care* 27:S66–S76.

Institute of Medicine (IOM). 1990. *National Priorities for the Assessment of Clinical Conditions and Medical Technologies.* Washington, D.C.: National Academy Press.

Kaplan, Robert M., and John P. Anderson. 1990. "The General Health Policy Model." I S. Spilker, ed., *Quality of Life Assessments in Clinical Trials.* New York: Raven Press.

Levin, D.L. et al. 1986. "A Model for Projecting Cancer Incidence and Mortality in the Presence of Prevention, Screening, and Treatment Programs." In *Cancer Control Objectives for the Nation, 1985–2000.* NCI Monographs no. 2. Bethesda, Md.: National Cancer Institute.

McGinnis, J. Michael. 1990. "Setting Objectives for Public Health in the 1990s: Experience and Prospects." *Annual Review of Public Health* 11:231–249.

National Institutes of Health, Division of Legislative Analysis. 1990. "The Quality of U.S. Health Promotion Statistics to Review Year 2000 Objectives." *Highlights* 2:85–87.

Patrick, Donald L., and Marilyn Bergner 1990. "Measurement of Health Status in the 1990s." *Annual Review of Public Health* 11:165–83.

Russell, Louise B. 1986. *Is Prevention Better than Cure?* Washington, D.C.: Brookings Institution.

Stoto, Michael A., Ruth Behrens, and Connie Rosemont. 1990. *Healthy People 2000: Citizens Chart the Course.* Washington, D.C.: National Academy Press.

U.S. Department of Health, Education and Welfare. 1979. *Healthy People: The Surgeon General's Report on Health Promotion and Disease Prevention.* Washington, D.C.: U.S. Government Printing Office.

U.S. Department of Health and Human Services. 1980. *Promoting Health/Preventing Disease: Objectives for the Nation.* Washington, D.C.: U.S. Government Printing Office.

U.S. Department of Health and Human Services. 1991. *Healthy People 2000: National Objectives for Health Promotion and Disease Prevention* (Conference edition). Washington, D.C.: U.S. Government Printing Office.

U.S. Public Health Service (PHS). 1989. *Promoting Health/Preventing Disease: Year 2000 Objectives for the Nation.* Washington, D.C.: U.S. Department of Health and Human Services.

Warner, Kenneth E. 1990. "Wellness at the Worksite." *Health Affairs* 9:63–79.

Weinstein, Milton C. et al. 1987. "Forecasting Coronary Heart Disease Incidence, Mortality, and Cost: The Coronary Heart Disease Policy Model." *American Journal of Public Health* 77:1417–26.

3

Rationing Health Care: The Choice Before Us

❖

Henry Aaron and William B. Schwartz

Rising sales cause joy in most industries, but increasing outlays for health care are causing distress not only among those who must pay the bills but among health care providers themselves. After adjusting for inflation, total and per capita personal health care expenditures have risen at annual rates of 5.5 and 4.1 percent since 1950 (Letsch, Levy, and Waldo 1988; Feldstein 1988). The proportion of gross national product (GNP) devoted to personal health care has nearly tripled. Official forecasts project that the United States will be devoting 15 percent of total production to health care by the year 2000 (Blendon 1986). Successive administrations have proposed a variety of measures intended to contain medical costs, but the results have been so unsuccessful that some observers speculate that the United States may be forced to ration health care (Aaron and Schwartz 1984; Callahan 1987; Blank 1988).

The term *rationing* is used in two distinct senses. First, market economies persistently deny goods to those who cannot afford them. All goods, including health care, are rationed in this sense, especially for the poor and some others who face large expenses and lack insurance. Such price rationing of medical care has a long and, in our view, ignoble history in the United States. This problem affects about 15 percent of all Americans. Second, the term *rationing* is used to refer to the denial of commodities to those who have the money to buy them. In this sense sugar, gasoline, and meat were rationed during World War II. The question now being raised is whether health care should be rationed in this sense, whether its availability should be limited, even to those who can pay for it. This kind of rationing would affect the 85 percent of all Americans who currently have health insurance and any others who may later be added to their ranks. While the first question is urgently important, rationing in the second sense is the focus here.

Key questions surrounding rising health costs such as: Why have recent efforts at cost containment failed? Can the United States afford unlimited, high-quality care for everyone? If not, is rationing avoidable? And if so, how will it be carried out and what will be its effect on the health and lives of most Americans?

The Economic Basis of Rising Outlays for Health Care

Standard economic theory suggests that current spending on health care is excessive. According to this doctrine, when people pay less than the full cost of what they buy, they will consume more than is socially optimal unless their consumption benefits not only themselves but others. This line of argument suggests that insurance induces excessive health expenditures because people pay for only part of the cost of care.

Patients in 1987 paid, on the average, only about ten cents of each dollar devoted to hospital care, a share that has changed negligibly for two decades. And they pay about twenty-six cents of each dollar paid to physicians, a share that has fallen steadily. Although these averages conceal large differences among patients, the fully insured (or those who have exceeded ceilings on patient outlays) and physicians acting in the patients' interests have the incentive to seek any service, however costly, that provides any benefit at all. Because of insurance, these decisions impose large costs on others.

The Unavoidable Dilemma

The intersection of this payment system and three distinct features of the health care system leads inevitably to rising costs. The first and most important is technology. Diagnostic procedures and therapies that are now routine were unknown when most physicians now in practice began their training. Computed tomography, magnetic resonance imaging, nuclear medicine, organ transplants, many of the drugs for control of ulcers and the symptoms of coronary artery disease, open heart surgery, total parenteral nutrition, and a host of other diagnostic and therapeutic procedures have been introduced or become standard in the last two decades. Other technologies, described later, indicate that the rate of innovation is not abating. Nearly all of these innovations promise to increase the number and cost of beneficial interventions.

A second factor driving up costs is the tendency for the price of services characterized by low growth in productivity to rise relative to the price of commodities (Baumol 1967; Baumol and Bowen 1966). Although a day in the hospital today differs in many ways from a day in the hospital in, say, 1960, the hotel services of feeding and space rental and most services of nurses and orderlies are produced with little more efficiency than in the past.

The final factor is the aging of the population. Although the average annual cost of health care rises sharply with age, this factor accounts for only a minor proportion of the 651 percent growth of real personal health care outlays between 1950 and 1987 (Fisher 1980).

Each of these inflationary forces shows every sign of continuing for decades.

Many observers deny any imminent need to consider rationing. They argue instead that we can continue to provide whatever beneficial services are available if we eliminate inefficiencies and wasteful practices. But, as we shall show, such reforms, although potentially important in absolute size, promise one-shot savings and can only briefly defer the need to consider whether and how to ration medical care.

Why One-Time Savings Cannot Solve the Cost Problem

Various methods have been proposed for cutting costs and improving efficiency: elimination of redundant medical capacity, cessation of useless medical procedures, increased competition, better management, and reduced fees for certain physicians. Unless these are used to reduce the availability of beneficial services—in short, unless they are used to compel nonprice rationing—all promise to arrest or slow the growth of medical costs only temporarily.

The potential savings from eliminating chronically empty beds, now numbering some 300,000, are surprisingly small because the same number of patients presumably will be cared for whether or not the duplicated facilities are closed and because the marginal costs of alternative care are high relative to the marginal savings from closing excess facilities (Schwartz and Joskow 1980).

The potential savings from eliminating useless medical procedures, by contrast, could run into many billions of dollars. Health maintenance organizations (HMOs) claim that through superior efficiency and elimination of useless services (mostly excess hospital days) they deliver high-quality service at costs will below those of other providers. One study supported these claims (Manning et al. 1984), in that it was found that one HMO provided comprehensive care for approximately 25 percent less than did providers reimbursed on a fee-for-service basis for fully insured patients. However, the HMO was no less costly than fee-for-service care for patients who faced an annual deductible of $450 per family or 95 percent cost-sharing (Manning et al. 1984). If costs of all fee-for-service hospital and physician care were reduced by 15 percent, an estimate based on the difference between costs of HMOs and the mixture of other insurance plans, there would have been once-and-for-all reduction in expenditures of approximately $20 billion (Manning et al. 1984; Newhouse 1981; Schwartz 1987; Welch 1985).

Additional savings that entail no rationing will become possible as evaluation of established medical procedures identifies classes of patients in which selected procedures now in use produce no medical benefits (Winslow 1988a, b). Even a small percentage saving in an industry currently absorbing more than $500 billion per year is a high-stakes effort that should be vigorously pursued, but continuation of annual growth of real personal health care expenditures of 4.1 percent per capita would quickly dwarf the savings from increased efficiencies (Letsch, Levit, and Waldo 1988; Feldstein 1988).

For a variety of reasons, not all providers could become as efficient as the best-run HMOs, and economies would be realized over many years. As a result, savings would be achieved gradually and, therefore, would be hard to detect against the strongly rising trend in medical outlays. In short, the United States faces a choice between letting medical outlays claim an ever-rising share of output, while recognizing that some will go for services producing small but positive benefits, and trying to devise socially acceptable arrangements under which some patients who have the means to pay, directly or through insurance, are denied some beneficial care.

Policy Attempts to Control Spending on Health Care

The last two decades have seen repeated and highly touted efforts fail to slow the growth of spending on medical.

Regulation

Starting in 1974 Congress sought to curtail growth of investment in medical structures and equipment by requiring advance authorization (a certificate of need, or CON). Although potential penalties for noncompliance were severe, evaluations found that they were seldom invoked and that many hospitals allocated to other activities the resources not used in disapproved investments (Schwartz 1981).

President Richard Nixon's price-control program, begun in 1971, temporarily lowered the growth of spending on hospital services. The controls were so complex that they could not be sustained. When controls were removed, real hospital spending rose at an average annual rate of 6.9 percent in 1975 and 1976. President Jimmy Carter responded in 1977 by proposing a cap on growth of revenues per patient-day. Hospitals promised to slow spending growth voluntarily but, after brief success, the effort wilted following congressional rejection of President Carter's proposal.

In 1984 the Health Care Financing Administration (HCFA) began to reimburse hospitals fixed sums for Medicare patients based on primary and secondary diagnoses at the time of admission (the diagnosis-related group, or DRG, system). Under the prior system, HCFA had paid hospitals the audited cost of services covered by the Medicare program. Under the DRG system, hospitals receive the same amount whatever they spend, except in relatively rare outlier cases. Preliminary evidence suggests that the program has slowed growth of hospital spending under Medicare (Russell 1989). However, it is not clear how much of this slowdown is simply the realization in the Medicare program of economies being achieved throughout the health care system, how much entails shifting of costs outside the hospital setting, and how much represents the rationing of beneficial services.

Competition

Some analysts have claimed that competition among health care providers can greatly reduce growth of spending on health care without any loss in the quality of care or the imposition of rationing. In pursuit of this goal, some have supported a cap on the exclusion from the personal income tax of employer-financed health insurance premiums, development and dissemination of statistics on the quality of care rendered by various hospitals and physicians, solicitation of competitive bids by employers from various groups of providers, and a host of other measures to promote efficient provision of medical care and to narrow margins earned by hospitals and physicians (Enthoven 1986; McClure 1985). Increased cost consciousness, it is claimed, would encourage insurance plans in which patients directly pay for an increased share of the cost of their own health care. If, in addition, patients had reliable data on medical outcomes of various providers, patients and their employers

Table 3.1   Health Care Outlays as a Percentage of Gross
Domestic Product, 1960–1986

Country	Year		
	1965	1980	1986
Australia	4.9	6.6	7.2
Canada	6.1	7.4	8.5
Denmark	4.8	6.8	6.1
France	5.2	7.4	8.5
Germany (West)	5.1	7.9	8.1
Italy	4.0	6.8	6.7
Japan	4.5	6.6	6.7
The Netherlands	4.4	8.2	8.3
New Zealand	4.3	7.2	6.9
Norway	3.9	6.6	6.8
Sweden	5.6	9.5	9.1
Switzerland	3.8	7.2	8.0
United Kingdom	4.1	5.8	6.2
United States	6.0	9.2	11.1

SOURCE: George H. Schieber and Jean-Pierre Poullier, "International Health Spending and Utilization Trends," *Health Affairs* 7(4):105, 1988.

would be able to avoid high-cost hospitals and physicians who do not provide demonstrably superior care. Supporters claim such measures will not only improve the quality of care, but will also save enough money to forestall the need to ration medical care.

Even if increased competition achieves all that its advocates claim, the elimination of inefficiencies promises a one-time saving unless it slows the introduction of new medical technologies. If new technologies are introduced at an unchanged rate, the main underlying force that has driven up outlays for four decades would remain intact. In that event, the respite from rising outlays, however welcome, would be transitory.

Costs in Other Developed Countries

Many developed nations other than the United States provide seemingly high-quality care on a basis many regard as more equitable than our own and for much lower overall costs (table 3.1). Only Great Britain among advanced societies avowedly rations medical care. Since medical techniques disseminate rapidly, yet spending varies widely, a puzzle emerges. How can countries with per capita incomes approximating our own spend so much less on medical care than we do and yet avoid rationing?

Demography is not the answer. European countries, with per capita incomes comparable to our own, have older populations yet spend less on health care than we do. Alternative explanations are that the relative price of health care has risen faster in the United States than elsewhere or that growth of gross domestic product has been slower. In fact, economic growth in the United States in the last fifteen years has been about average among major industrial countries. Furthermore, reliable information from which to measure health care spending in constant prices is unavailable.

A contributory factor to high outlays in the United States seems to be that we spend more on billing and other such administrative costs as marketing than do other countries. Some estimates place the cost of administration at as much as 22 percent of national health care spending, perhaps two-fifths larger than would be necessary with a single payer. (Others estimate that the United States could have saved $29.2 billion to $38.4 billion of the $77.7 billion spent on health care administration in 1983 [Himmelstein and Woolhandler 1986].)

Indices such as life expectancy and infant mortality in other industrialized countries typically match or exceed our own (OECD 1987). This fact is often taken to mean that significant denial of services cannot be occurring in these countries. But rationing of such health services as measures to prevent blindness, relief of severe skin disorders, replacement of a damaged hip, and relief of the pain of coronary artery disease, which serve primarily to improve the quality of life, rather than to extend it, would not show up in mortality statistics. Furthermore, mortality rates are heavily dependent on lifestyle, diet, and income distribution, factors generally regarded as far more important than medical care as influences on mortality rates (Fuchs 1983).

What Rationing Entails

Americans are unfamiliar with nonprice rationing or its consequences. They have not thought about whether or not to implement it. Should we turn to rationing, which services will be denied to which patients, and how will the decisions be made?

The clearest answers to these questions come from Great Britain. Per capita spending on health care, in Britain about one-third of that in the United States, requires a rationing far beyond any that is conceivable here. But Britain and the United States share many important features—language, democratic values, and similar patterns of medical education and physician competence—as well as important political and social similarities. For this reason, British experience shows the kinds, if not the severity, of choices we shall face.

One of the most remarkable aspects of rationing in Britain is that some decisions that appear medically irrational are socially acceptable. For example, per capita spending on total parenteral nutrition, or TPN (an expensive form of intravenous feeding often of marginal value), was nearly as high in Britain as in the United States. At the same time, many tertiary-care university hospitals lacked a CT scanner.

Nonmedical values and circumstances appear to explain such situations, For example, services depending on specialized capital equipment are easier to ration than are those that rely on multiple-use inputs. Thus CT scanning, which requires specialized equipment and staff, is tightly controlled. TPN, in contrast, is difficult to control without directly infringing on each physician's clinical freedom.

Age and cost interact to influence allocation decisions. Until the early 1980s, most patients over the age of fifty-five or sixty with chronic kidney failure were allowed to die without hemodialysis, a costly procedure dependent on specialized equipment and dedicated clinic space. After continuous ambulatory peritoneal dialysis, a relatively low-cost procedure, became routine, the number of older dialyzed patients nearly doubled (Wood, Mallick, and Wing 1987). In contrast, the British have made full-scale treatment of hemophilia generally available through special clinics. Although per capita costs are high, aggregate costs are low because only about seventy-five new cases of hemophilia appear each year. Furthermore, the symptoms—severe bleeding and swollen joints—are highly visible. British physicians and administrators generally acknowledge that equally generous treatment would not be provided if there were seventy-five hundred new cases annually instead of seventy-five (Aaron and Schwartz 1984).

Still other considerations influence allocations to other diseases. A dread disease such as cancer elicits disproportionate support. The high costs of failure to treat patients with severe arthritis of the hip help explain the relatively generous allowances made for hip replacement. In contrast, funding for surgical treatment of coronary artery disease is meager because treatment with drugs is relatively inexpensive. These factors influence the availability of resources in a fashion independent of the expected medical benefits.

The Physician as Gatekeeper

The denial of useful or even lifesaving care is hard on both providers and patients. In Britain, primary care physicians, who are forced to act as gatekeepers for the system, bear this unpleasant responsibility.

Physicians make the denial of potentially beneficial care seem routine, or even optimal, by recasting a problem of medical scarcity in economic terms.

Some British physicians understand clearly that they are not providing all care that could be beneficial. As one doctor put it,

> The sense that I have is that there are many situations where resources are sufficiently short so that there must be decision made as to who is treated. Given that circumstance, the physician, in order to live with himself and to sleep well at night, has to look at the arguments for not treating a patient. And there are always some—social, medical, whatever. In many instances he heightens, sharpens or brings into focus the negative component in order to make himself and the patient comfortable about not going forward. (Aaron and Schwartz 1984:102)

Although rationing has been most dramatic in the treatment of chronic kidney failure, many senior British health officials and physicians long denied that any age cutoff existed. The explanation for this puzzling disparity lies in the referral patterns of primary care physicians. Recognizing that dialysis capacity was limited, these doctors routinely favored younger over older patients whenever some complicating illness such as diabetes was present. Even older patients without other medical problems were usually viewed as unsuitable for referral because, as one doctor put it, without trying to be arch, "everyone over the age of fifty-five is a bit crumbly."

Such rationalization is understandable. Continued referrals of "inappropriate" candidates would be pointless, forcing the nephrologist either to tell patients that care is unavailable or to contradict the clinical judgment of the referring doctor. The local physician responds by telling the patient that, given the overall medical picture, dialysis is not appropriate. In short, rationalization serves the function performed in ordinary markets by price: it equates the amounts demanded with the amounts supplied.

Acknowledging Appropriateness of Limits

Some British physicians acknowledge resource constraints but justify them because their country is just not wealthy enough to do all that might be medically beneficial. In the words of the head of the intensive care unit at one of London's major teaching hospitals,

[The number of intensive care beds has] to be appropriate to the surroundings. Now what we have by your standards is way short of the mark. It would be too small in America, but if you took this unit and put it down in Sri Lanka or India, it would stick out like a sore thumb. It would be an obscene waste of money. (Aaron and Schwartz 1984:102)

Against this background, a leading oncologist described his thoughts about the problems that might be caused by development of a costly cure for a common form of cancer, metastatic carcinoma of the colon:

It is something I wake up screaming about. I suspect that not everybody who might benefit from [therapy] would get it in practice. If you could cure every patient who has cancer of the colon, most of whom are going to be over sixty-five, over fifty-five anyway, I think we might find ourselves making value judgments about which to treat and which not to. (Aaron and Schwartz 1984:94)

Safety Valves for the Disaffected

The professional and managerial classes in Britain are less willing to accept no for an answer than are other social classes. Many routinely seek such elective care as hip replacement, elective abortions, or hernia repair outside the National Health Service (NHS) by paying for such care either directly or with private insurance, which about 10 percent of the British now have (*Britain 1989*).

Although blatant corruption is apparently rare, aggressive or influential patients can often secure referrals from general practitioners for a second opinion at specialized centers or by going directly to emergency rooms for services that local doctors deem "unsuitable." As a result, per capita expenditures by the National Health Service were reported to be 41 percent higher for members of the upper two socioeconomic groups (professionals, employers, and managers) than for members of the "lowest" two classes (LeGrand 1978). Such safety valves help explain the continued popularity of the NHS.

Rationing in the United States

Health care rationing in the United States has moved from the realm of academic speculation to practical reality during the 1980s. Its role is likely to grow in the future. The introduction of DRGs signaled that government would not reimburse hospitals for any and all costs they might incur for Medicare patients. While initial DRG reimbursements were generous and imposed onerous choices on few hospitals, annual adjustments have been insufficient to cover both inflation and the added costs of new technology. As a result, the margin between hospital income and expenditures has narrowed (CWM 1989). In addition, many private insurance companies have begun to require prior approval for reimbursement for various diagnostic and therapeutic procedures.

In perhaps the most dramatic instance of avowed rationing, the legislature of the state of Oregon announced in February 1988 that it would not pay for organ transplants for patients under the Medicaid program because, in the view of the legislature, the same funds would provide greater benefits if devoted to prenatal services and because the legislature was unprepared to pay for both. Following this announcement, the Oregon legislature sought the opinions of various groups on the relative priorities that should be attached to different medical interventions and of the cost of providing all care with priority scores above specified levels. With this information in hand, the legislature plans to decide how much it can spend per capita under the Medicaid program. It will then solicit bids at that cost from providers prepared to provide care under the Medicaid program for all eligible patients. The per capita allowance will require providers to limit services to those that fit within the predetermined spending level—in short, to ration care. The Oregon procedure underscores the fact that every other state already limits the range of services provided to Medicaid patients and denies reimbursement for all services to low-income households who are ineligible for Medicaid.

The strongest evidence that the United States will have to ration care if it wishes to slow growth of health care spending on a sustained basis comes from the creativity of medical scientists, who continue to develop new services that promise both significant benefits for large numbers of people and large added costs for public and private budgets. Indeed, the flow of technological innovation shows little sign of abating and may be accelerating. Some permit previously impossible interventions. Others reduce the discomfort or risk associated with previous procedures. Even if a given diagnostic service is less costly per patient, total outlays may rise because the noninvasive nature of such technologies frees the physician from the need to balance pain or risk to the patient against the value of information to be gained. Still other advances improve previously available therapies, sometimes at great cost. The following advances illustrate both the potential value and cost of emerging medical technologies.

Magnetic resonance imaging is the latest addition to the list of diagnostic devices that provide useful information noninvasively. But other expensive technologies, such as positron emission tomography and magnetic resonance spectroscopy, are already in limited use and can be expected to be applied with increasing frequency.

Other costly emerging technologies include erythropoietin, a hormone that stimulates production of red blood cells. This drug has become available for treatment of severe anemia associated with chronic renal failure. Given that roughly 80,000 of the 106,000 patients undergoing chronic dialysis are suitable for this treatment (HCFA 1988; NKF 1989), and that the estimated cost is $10,000 per patient-year, the annual cost from this new drug will approach three-quarters of $1 billion. Because it is also likely to be valuable in the treatment of anemia associated with AIDS and cancer, the total cost will eventually be much larger.

A second example is the automatic implantable cardiac defibrillator, a device that is activated when the heart develops life-threatening arrhythmia. Expert opinion suggests that given the likely diffusion of the technology, there will be about 20,000 potential candidates for this therapy annually. At a total cost per patient of about $46,000 ($16,000 for the device and $30,000 for the hospitalization and surgical implantation), the annual cost would be about $1 billion (Larsen et al. 1989).

The recent finding that AZT can delay the onset of AIDS in patients who test positive for human immunodeficiency virus opens up a new use for this drug. The estimated cost for this therapy is $5 billion annually (Arno et al. 1989).

Some advances bring demonstrable improvements in traditional procedures, but at great cost. Radiopaque contrast media are used in about 10 million X-ray examinations per year (Jacobsen and Rosenquist 1988). Fatal reactions to this material are rare, but perhaps 300 deaths per year could be prevented by the use of a new low-osmolar agent that is ten times as expensive as those now in use (Jacobsen and Rosenquist 1988). The cost of this switch would be about $1 billion, or more than $3 million per life saved (Jacobsen and Rosenquist 1988).

The successful development of an artificial heart promises to have an equally large impact. Some 30,000 potential recipients per year would add $3 billion to $4 billion to expenditures, and follow-up care would increase this estimate substantially (Evans 1986).

Other therapies, at an earlier stage of development than those just listed, also promise to boost costs. Such treatments include gene therapy, proton beam accelerators, tissue growth factors, and monoclonal antibodies. It is apparent that the advances now coming, together with those now in development, will quickly overwhelm any one-time savings that can be achieved by eliminating useless care.

In addition to higher costs that advancing technology will imply for the large majority of the U.S. population with insurance, measures to extend health insurance to the roughly 15 percent of the population currently without it would also add to the growth of total health spending. The increase in costs would be less than proportional, however, for two reasons. First, about 22.8 percent of the uninsured had incomes of at least $30,000 per year in 1986 (Chollet 1988). Such households no doubt directly pay for many health services already. Second, even those who are too poor to pay anything themselves now receive some care. The cost of this care is now covered in a variety of ways—through taxes, charitable contributions in cash or in kind, and through premiums for the insured that are inflated to cover the costs of uncompensated care.

Although nonprice rationing seems inevitable if the growth of health care spending is to be slowed, it is unlikely that the United States ever would impose limits as severe as those common Britain. Patients and physicians in the United States enjoy a well-merited reputation for demanding and supplying aggressive, high-quality treatment. Furthermore, cost containment is likely to increase the frequency of malpractice claims by discouraging physicians from providing some services that would otherwise be deemed appropriate. U.S. courts have explicitly stated that although cost consciousness has become an important feature of the U.S. health care system, both insurers and providers can be held responsible "when medically inappropriate decisions result from defects in the design or implementation of cost containment mechanisms . . ." (*Wickline v. State of California* 1986). In the conflict between cost containment and standards of care, the mandate for cost containment is likely to prevail, but not without turmoil.

Growth of medical costs will be contained on a sustained basis only if we are prepared to ration care to those who are insured and are able and willing to pay for services. If we choose this road, we shall have to face many of the issues with which the British have grappled.

Concern for fundamental values such as age, visibility of an illness, and aggregate costs of treatment will inevitably shape our decisions on resource allocation. Physicians and other providers will increasingly experience tension between their historic commitment to doing all that is medically beneficial and the limitations imposed on them by increasingly stringent cost limits. And we can almost certainly expect a substantial fraction of our society, much larger than in Britain, to use whatever means are available to get care that is in short supply. Whether we allow a separate hospital sector to develop outside the constrained system will be a key policy issue and a difficult political decision. We see the British experience not as a frightening deterrent to serious consideration of rationing. Rather, the British experience with rationing, particularly stark because of its severity, sharply delineates the kinds of choices we shall have to make. Understanding how the British made these decisions can help us find ways to make our less extreme but still painful choices acceptable. The current cost of excessive spending on services providing only small benefits is enormous and is certain to grow. The stakes in evolving politically and socially acceptable methods of curtailing such outlays are enormous.

References

Aaron, Henry J., and William B. Schwartz. 1984. *The Painful Prescription: Rationing Hospital Care*. Washington, D.C.: Brookings Institution.

Arno, Peter S., Douglas Shenson, Naomi F. Siegel, Pat Franks, and Philip R. Lee. 1989. "Economic and Policy Implications of Early Intervention in HIV Disease." *Journal of the American Medical Association* 262(11):1493–1498.

Baumol, William J. 1967. "Macroeconomics of Unbalanced Growth: The Anatomy of Urban Crisis." *American Economic Review* 57(3):415–426.

Baumol, William J., and W. G. Bowen. 1966. *Performing Arts: The Economic Dilemma*. New York: Twentieth Century Fund.

Blank, Robert H. 1988. *Rationing Medicine*. New York: Columbia University Press.

Blendon, Robert J. 1986. "Health Policy Choices for the 1990s." *Issues in Science and Technology* 2(4):65–73.

Britain 1989: An Official Handbook. 1989. London: Her Majesty's Stationery Office.

Callahan, Daniel. 1987. *Setting Limits: Medical Goals in an Aging Society*. New York: Simon & Schuster.

Chollet, Deborah J. 1988. *Uninsured in the United States: The Nonelderly Population without Health Insurance, 1986*. Washington, D.C.: Employee Benefit Research Institute.

Committee on Ways and Means (CWM), United States House of Representatives. 1989. "Background Material and Data on Programs within the Jurisdiction of the Committee on Ways and Means." Washington, D.C.: U.S. Government Printing Office.

Enthoven, Alain C. 1986. "Managed Competition in Health Care and the Unfinished Agenda." *Health Care Financing Review* (Annual Supplement):105–119.

Evans, Roger W. 1986. "The Heart Transplant Dilemma." *Issues in Science and Technology* 2(3):91–101.

Feldstein, Martin S. 1988. *Health Care Economics*. 3d ed. New York: Wiley.

Fisher, Charles R. 1980. "Differences by Age Groups in Health Care Spending." *Health Care Financing Review* 1(4):65–90.

Fuchs, Victor R. 1983. *Who Shall Live and Who Shall Die?* New York: Basic Books.

Health Care Financing Administration (HCFA). 1988. "The End Stage Renal Disease Program and Medical Information System." In *Facility Survey Tables as of December 31, 1988.* Washington, D.C.: Health Care Finance Administration.

Himmelstein, David G., and Steffie Woolhandler. 1986. "Cost without Benefit: Administrative Waste in U.S. Health Care." *New England Journal of Medicine* 314(7):441–445.

Jacobson, Peter D., and C. John Rosenquist. 1988. "The Introduction of Low-Osmolar Contrast Agents in Radiology." *Journal of the American Medical Association* 260(11):1586–1592.

Larsen G.C., et al. 1989. *Medical Decision Making* 9:324.

LeGrand, Julian. 1978. "The Distribution of Public Expenditures: The Case of Health Care." *Economica* 45(178):125–142.

Letsch, Suzanne W., Katharine R. Levit, and Daniel R. Waldo. 1988. "National Health Expenditures, 1987." *Health Care Financing Review* 10(2):109–122.

McClure, William. 1985. "Buying Right: How to Do It." *Business and Health* 2(10):41–44.

Manning, Willard G., Arleen Leibowitz, George A. Goldberg, William H. Rogers, and Joseph P. Newhouse. 1984. "A Controlled Trial of the Effect of a Prepaid Group Practice on Use of Services." *New England Journal of Medicine* 310(23):1505–1510.

National Kidney Foundation (NKF), Ad Hoc Committee. 1989. "Report." *American Journal of Kidney Disease* 14:163.

Newhouse, Joseph P., Willard G. Manning, Carl N. Morris, Larry L. Orr, Naihua Duan, Emmett B. Keeler, Arleen Leibowitz, Kent H. Marquis, M. Susan Marquis, Charles Phelps, and Robert H. Brook. 1981. "Some Interim Results from a Controlled Trial of Cost Sharing in Health Insurance." *New England Journal of Medicine* 305(25):1501–1507.

Organization for Economic Cooperation and Development (OECD). 1987. *Financing and Delivering Health Care: A Comparative Analysis of OECD Countries.* Paris: Organization for Economic Cooperation and Development.

Russell, Louise B. 1989. *Medicare's New Payment System: Is It Working?* Washington, D.C.: Brookings Institution.

Schieber, George J., and Jean-Pierre Poullier. 1988. "International Health Spending and Utilization Trends." *Health Affairs* 7(4):105–112.

Schwartz, William B. 1981. "The Regulation Strategy for Controlling Health Costs." *New England Journal of Medicine* 305(21):1249–1255.

Schwartz, William B. 1987. "The Inevitable Failure of Current Cost-Containment Strategies." *Journal of the American Medical Association* 257(2):220–224.

Schwartz, William B., and Paul L. Joskow. 1980. "Duplicated Hospital Facilities: How Much Can We Save by Consolidating Them?" *New England Journal of Medicine* 303(25):1449–1457.

Welch, W. P. 1985. "Medicare Capitation Payments to HMOs in Light of Regression toward the Mean in Health Care Costs." *Journal of Health Economics* 4:293–299.

Wickline v. State of California, 192 Cal. App. 3d 1630, 1647 (1986).

Winslow, Constance M., Jacqueline B. Kosecoff, Mark Chassin, David E. Kanouse, and Robert H. Brook. 1988a. "The Appropriateness of Performing Coronary Artery Bypass Surgery." *Journal of the American Medical Association* 260(4):505–509.

Winslow, Constance M., David H. Soloman, Mark R. Chassin, Jacqueline Kosecoff, Nancy J. Merrick, and Robert H. Brook. 1988b. "The Appropriateness of Carotid Endarterectomy." *New England Journal of Medicine* 318(12):721–727.

Wood, I. T., N. P. Mallick, and A. J. Wing. 1987. "Prediction of Resources Needed to Achieve the National Target for Treatment of Renal Failure." *British Medical Journal* 294:1467–1470.

4

The LORAN Commission: A Report to the Community

Harvard Community Health Plan

Founded in 1969, the Harvard Community Health Plan (HCHP) is New England's oldest health maintenance organization (HMO); with over 400,000 enrollees, it is also the region's largest.

Consistent with its mission of "serv[ing] people in all segments of the community with excellent prepaid, integrated health care at a reasonable cost," the HCHP Foundation invited an esteemed group of citizens* to advise HCHP on how to evaluate new medical technology. The group, known as the LORAN Commission, took its name from a method of navigation used by ships and planes: long-range navigation. Some members of the commission were experts in medical technology and its evaluation; all possessed an abundance of wisdom, creativity, and independence.

The need for the commission became apparent in the wake of HCHP's decision to cover heart and liver transplants. The increasing sophistication and cost of new technology poses a dilemma for all HMOs and health insurers: the HMO or insurer must balance the welfare of the individual patient against the welfare of all the people who pay premi-

*The commission members included David Banta, M.D., Robert Cushman, Douglas Fraser, Robert Freeman, Betty Friedan, Benjamin Kaplan, Frederick Mosteller, David Nathan, M.D., Albert Rees, Hays Rockwell, Robert Sproull, and Marshall Wolf, M.D. The Rev. John Paris served the commission as a consultant in medical ethics.

ums into the fund. A similar dilemma confronts government officials who are the custodians of tax-funded public insurance programs. Expensive technology often saves lives, as in the case of heart and liver transplants. But not all advances are a matter of life and death; some expensive innovations improve the lives of otherwise stable patients. It is possible, for example, to contemplate prosthetic devices with capabilities far outstripping today's devices but at a cost of hundreds of thousands of dollars. Nor is the problem always the cost per unit of service. Sometimes it is the cumulative cost, resulting from frequent use of a moderately-priced service. However the costs accrue, the complexity of the issues is compounded when the success rate is low or when there is an alternative therapy that is almost as effective but at a lower cost.

HCHP asked the LORAN Commission to develop a framework for analyzing these complex issues. To add realism and a sense of urgency to the deliberations, the Commission was asked to adopt the perspective of HCHP, not that of society. The focus on HCHP had important implications. The commission had to consider, for example, how the adoption of a new technology might affect HCHP's competitive position. On the other hand, the focus on HCHP diminished the need for broad discussions about the societal importance of health care as compared to other goods and services—for example, education, nutrition, housing, and national defense.

Even so, the broader community's attitude about new technology was never far from the commissioners' minds. HCHP does not operate in a vacuum. To a degree, all HMOs, insurers, and providers are in the same boat. The ability of any one of us to adopt new processes and standards for making coverage decisions is determined, in part, by the policies of the others.

Framing the Issues

The LORAN Commission's first task was to define the issues and to develop a common base of information. It drew from a wide range of sources, including discussions, testimony from experts, studies, and case histories.

It quickly became evident that new technology was not necessarily a piece of equipment. The commission elected to define *medical technology* broadly to include a wide range of goods and services, including surgical techniques and drugs.

A review of cost trends convinced the commission that the health care sector's demands on the economy could not continue growing at the current rate. Yet, there is no end in sight. Indeed, the growth in health care's share of gross national product (now almost 12 percent of GNP) continues to accelerate. To put the U.S. investment in perspective, no other nation spends as much as 10 percent of GNP on health care (most spend far less), even though other industrialized democracies provide universal health insurance; 35 to 40 million Americans are uninsured.

"It became clear to us," the commission noted, "that, although greater efficiency is needed in the health care system, difficult choices are going to have to be made among competing technologies, since even greater efficiency will not leave the system with unlimited resources." The commission concluded, "Ultimately, no health plan will be able to cover it all." When that happens, "All insurers will be forced to confront the ethical dilemma presented when the rights of an individual, hoping to call upon more and more of a group's resources, conflict with the needs of that group as a whole."

How Choices are Being Made Now

Once health plans—and their enrollees—conclude they cannot afford everything, they must compare the value of each new technology against other alternatives for spending the funds. The LORAN Commission criticized as obsolete the ad hoc assessment of new technologies now done by most insurers and providers: "If no framework exists to evaluate new technologies prospectively, decisions about whether to adopt them are likely to be . . . put off until times of crisis [and then] are more likely to be influenced by emotions or political expedience than by medical efficacy. Not only might undeserving technologies be approved, but the most deserving technologies may be overlooked."

The commission cited the federal government's decision to insure patients with end-stage renal (kidney) disease "as an example of what can happen when no plan exists" to ensure resources are used effectively. In 1972, when kidney patients were added to the Medicare rolls, Congress predicted that it would cost taxpayers no more than $400 million in any year. By 1987, the annual tab had exceeded $2.3 billion, or $33,000 per patient. "Even many of those on dialysis agree that some of those resources might, in some cases, be better used elsewhere," the commission members wrote. "Although dialysis increases the life expectancy of its users an average of five years, the quality of that life is sometimes so diminished by mental disorientation, fatigue, discomfort, and depression that one in six elderly dialysis patients elects to stop treatment."

Not everyone would agree, of course, with the commission's assessment of Medicare's dialysis program. It is a wonderful achievement to extend the lives of patients with severe kidney disease. Unlike some other expensive practices, dialysis has at least been proven effective. Whatever one's views about the dialysis program, however, there is no escaping the commission's basic point: not even the federal government, which can run continuing deficits, can fund every worthwhile program. Many federal officials would like to spend more on improving maternal and child health, since the U.S. infant mortality rate is one of the highest among industrialized nations. They are constrained, however, by "budget pressures." What should give way? Treatment of end-stage renal disease or maternal and child health? The answer may not be self-evident. Perhaps the answer is neither. What is clear is that resources are limited, and choices are already being made.

Assessing Medical Value

Newer, more expensive interventions are often adopted without systematic effort to determine whether the new technology is better than existing alternatives. When assessments are done, moreover, they vary significantly in quality.

David Eddy, a physician and mathematician at Duke University's Center for Health Policy, contends that the medical literature is rife with unfocused or poorly designed research protocols. He cites, for example, studies of two widely used treatments to increase blood flow to the lower leg; restricted circulation may cause cramping and, in severe cases, lead to complications requiring amputation. In one procedure, called percutaneous transluminal angioplasty (PTA), a balloon is inserted down the vessel to the blockage. The balloon is then inflated, pushing the plaque against the vessel walls and widening the passage. In a more expensive procedure, bypass surgery, an alternate vessel is sewn around the blockage. Which procedure is best, and for whom? Eddy and a colleague, Raphael Adar, studied the literature and found that, though 39 studies of PTA had been performed, none compared angioplasty with bypass surgery. Not one study was controlled, much less randomized. Finally, none of the studies answers the questions most important to patients who must decide which, if any, procedure to undergo: Did it relieve the pain? Improve the ability to walk?

Summarizing this research in *Health Affairs*, Eddy and John Billings concluded: "There is no way to determine with any degree of accuracy the relative merits of the two approaches. . . . Some practice standards are created without knowledge of the actual impact of the practice on health and economic outcomes and without knowledge of how people would compare the benefit and harm. . . . The logic appears to be that a practice will be considered appropriate if it *might* have benefit. This criterion translates easily into 'when in doubt, do it.' "

According to Eddy and Billings, "the criterion of potential benefit" works well when the benefit is so obvious and the potential harm so small that no formal trials are needed. Rabies vaccine is a good example. But the dangers of applying such a criterion are many:

- When the potential harm is great, focusing on potential benefit is a disservice. "To the extent that we are promoting practices for which the benefit is small (or nonexistent) compared to the harm, we are doing harm," Eddy and Billings wrote.
- The criterion of potential benefit is also of little help when we must choose between competing practices, as in the case of PTA and bypass.
- Perhaps the most insidious danger is that the criterion of potential benefit can lead us to overestimate our knowledge.

Testimony by Eddy and others led the LORAN Commission to recommend against covering a new, more expensive therapy unless it has been "deemed superior . . . for at least some cases, to the one it replaces."

In fact, most medical practices have never been assessed carefully. The Food and Drug Administration (FDA) did not have the authority to require that medical devices be proved safe and effective until 1976. The FDA still does not have the authority to regulate many other innovations—for example, new surgical procedures. Whether further government regulation of new medical procedures is either desirable or feasible was beyond the scope of the commission's charge. The commission did conclude, however, that HCHP and other providers and insurers should subject innovations to more scrutiny before accepting them into everyday practice. According to the Congressional Office of Technology Assessment, only 10 to 20 percent of medical practices are supported by results from randomized controlled trials. Such trials are the scientist's proof that a procedure works.

Why aren't new technologies more rigorously assessed? There seems to be an unspoken, yet strong, presumption in favor of adopting new procedures, even in the absence of proof that they are better than old ones. The rapid adoption of tissue plasminogen activator (TPA) may prove to be just such a case.

TPA is a genetically engineered drug for dissolving the blood clots that cause heart attacks. The good news is that TPA and other clot-dissolving drugs may well reduce mortality when administered soon after the onset of symptoms (for example, chest pain and shortness of breath). But the magnitude of the benefit remains uncertain. The existence of several so-called thrombolytic agents further complicates matters. TPA costs about $2,000 per dose, while streptokinase, a competing drug, costs under $200 per dose. Streptokinase may be as effective as TPA—at least when administered in combination with that old pharmaceutical standard, aspirin. Large-scale clinical trials are now underway to determine which of the drugs is really better, but definitive results may not be available for some months. And by then, newer, and possibly better, drugs may be on the horizon.

Another example is the almost universal acceptance of transurethral resection for the removal of the prostate (also known as TURP). The procedure has replaced open resection in 98 percent of cases in this country, yet a recent analysis by John Wennberg and others suggests that, for at least some subgroups, TURP may be associated with worse outcomes than the older procedure. In their study, Wennberg and colleagues also compared TURP to a strategy of "watchful waiting" for patients with symptomatic prostatism. Their analysis indicated that TURP "does not prevent death in men without chronic obstruction. In fact, because of the risk of postoperative death, [TURP] results in a decrease in average life expectancy, and the net benefits of surgery derive from improvement in the quality of life associated with symptom reduction."

Studies that determine whether a new technology is better than an old one, and at what cost, are often difficult to design and expensive to carry out. They may require, for example, tracking patient outcomes for years at multiple institutions. The funds currently available for such research, from both public and private sources, are inadequate. The nation's total investment, public and private, on technology assessment has been estimated as less than one-half of 1 percent of our expenditure on health care services. And the bulk of that spending is on premarketing tests of drugs for safety and efficacy.

Who should pay for better assessments? While recognizing the important work of private organizations (including medical and disease-related societies), the LORAN Commission concluded that the need exceeded their means, let alone those of any individual HMO or insurer. The commission members would agree with William Roper, chief of the U.S. Health Care Financing Administration, that the government should bear a substantial portion of the cost. As Dr. Roper and colleagues wrote in the *New England Journal of Medicine,* "information about the effectiveness of particular services provides a public good, both in the every day sense and in the specialized sense used by economists. . . . [B]ecause the benefit of better information accrues to the public at large, not just to those collecting it, the market system may not ensure adequate investment. . . . [G]overnment should help fill this gap."

But the onus should not be solely on the government. The commission also recommended that "HCHP should encourage and support the creation of a consortium [of insurers and health care providers] to participate in such assessments. Such a collaboration would share data and experiences about the selection of procedures and their best utilization. These findings would be made available to the medical community."

New technologies are not the only ones that may need to be assessed. The LORAN Commission concluded that older technologies ought to be evaluated periodically as well. The commission cited the practice of circumcision, routinely performed in most hospitals in this country. "It was once thought that the minimal dangers of circumcision were far outweighed by health benefits to the child, and so the practice was commonly covered by insurers. Recent findings have led many in the medical community to question whether the procedure provides any health benefit. As a result, some insurers now consider continued coverage of the procedure to be a misapplication of resources." (Since the commission issued its report, the American Academy of Pediatrics has concluded that circumcision "has potential medical benefits and advantages." The Academy stops short of recommending the procedure, however.)

Assessing the Costs

The LORAN Commission emphasized that assessing the effectiveness of services is essential, but not sufficient. After a new technology "has been shown to be superior, its cost must be assessed. If it is cost-saving, there is no problem. . . . But in most cases, new technology raises costs."

Even when it is established that a new, more expensive therapy is better than the existing alternatives, one must question whether the added benefit is worth the added cost. The LORAN Commission illustrated this point with an apocryphal example: the $10,000 Band-Aid. No matter how much better such a Band-Aid might be, it could not be worth the added cost. The example brought the commission to one of its most important recommendations: insurers ought to "avoid treatments that cost far more than any benefits they might bring about are worth." This recommendation, read literally, would seem to be a truism. Who would defend paying for services that "cost far more than they are worth?" Read in context, however, the recommendation has profound implications. It reflects the commission's conclusion that cost is a legitimate consideration in making coverage decisions. Though that may seem axiomatic to people who must work within budgets, few, if any, health plans now acknowledge considering cost in their coverage decisions. The result is that cost-effectiveness is rarely analyzed in any rigorous way, and there is little pressure on the proponents of new therapies to establish their relative effectiveness.

The commission also recommended that "those technologies that offer the greatest incremental gain for the incremental cost ought to be adopted first." Furthermore, "new technologies . . . that benefit the largest number of members [should be selected] before . . . those whose benefits would be limited to a few members."

Even for technologies of proven value, the LORAN Commission suggested that "perhaps an upper limit should be set in the relative cost of a new technology." The limit could be based, for example, on "how many years' worth of earnings ought to be devoted to extending a member's life for one year." The commission was unwilling to adopt a rigid formula, saying only that "as more and more resources are devoted to extending a life for a short time, it becomes clear that choices must be made between competing goods. At the very least," they urged, some figure ought to be used "as a signal for special attention."

Coverage of "life-enhancing" technologies poses different issues than "life-extending" practices. The commission discussed in vitro fertilization (IVF) as an example of a procedure that may greatly enhance lives. Some women who would otherwise be infertile are able, through IVF, to have children. IVF is expensive, though, about $6,000 per attempt. Estimates of the success rate per attempt range from 10 to 20 percent.

Although this case is now moot (Massachusetts has since mandated coverage of IVF), the commission's reasoning is valuable. They attempted to find a way that a life-enhancing procedure might be made available without placing an unfair financial burden either on HCHP (which would risk attracting a disproportionate number of members who join primarily to receive the benefit) or on those members who do not benefit. The commission recommended that HCHP "consider introducing waiting periods, deductibles, and copayments for some life-enhancing technologies that could not otherwise be offered to members." IVF, if it is offered, "ought to be made available to older people facing their final opportunities to have a family before it is made available to younger, otherwise healthy people who are also experiencing difficulties in conceiving." Finally, special resources ought to be made available to families who would otherwise be unable to afford the copayment, the commission wrote.

Making Fair Decisions

Decisions about what should be covered might ideally be made through a "town meeting of the well." Unable to predict their individual medical needs, healthy members of a community—for example, the members, clinicians, and managers of HCHP—would collectively decide which interventions to cover. Once made, these decisions would be final.

The concept, proposed by Eddy, is appealing. It removes the choice from the bedside, where patient and physician are apt to misjudge the benefits and risks. Furthermore, the costs of alternatives may be discussed without assigning a dollar value to the well-being of an identifiable patient. The "town meeting" would also guarantee members a voice in the selection of benefits.

Not surprisingly, the commission concluded that holding such a "town meeting" would be impractical. But the basic point is still valid. Insuring organizations, including HMOs, face a unique set of challenges. "All insurers will be forced to grapple with the question of whether any constraints should be imposed on individuals whose medical demands, if unreasonable or unwise, threaten the common good," the commission wrote. In the process of spreading risk, there is inevitably tension between the needs of the claimant and those of the group. Health plans must serve those in need, without forsaking their obligations as custodians of a common fund. To formulate sensible policy, the values of members, not just physicians and plan managers, should be represented.

To explore this issue further, the commission analyzed three experimental, yet promising, technologies—laser angioplasty to clear out diseased arteries, pancreatic transplants to delay the complications associated with diabetes, and monoclonal antibodies for the treatment of some forms of cancer. For purposes of discussion, the commission assumed that HCHP's medical director proposed funding of all three, but that HCHP could only afford two of the three if it wished to have a fair, and competitive, premium for all members.

The commission decided that each new technology should be compared to the one it is replacing and that the technologies offering "the greatest incremental gain for the incremental cost ought to be adopted first. In comparing technologies with roughly equivalent benefit-cost ratios, the commission recommends that new technologies be selected that benefit the largest number of Plan members."

Because of the many variables involved, the commission recognized that no rigid formula could be constructed to systematize comparisons of technologies. The comparison of different benefits (e.g., relief from suffering for a child versus a few months of extended life for an eighty-five-year-old) poses profoundly difficult choices. "The value of technology cannot be determined by cookbook methods," the commission members wrote.

The commission took a hard line against covering experimental therapies which have not been proved beneficial, unless the patient is participating in an approved clinical trial: "Experimental [therapies] may seem to represent the 'last hope' for people devastated by a debilitating or fatal disease, and they may request such interventions under the assumption that nothing can worsen their plight. They are sometimes wrong. Desperate efforts using untested regimens can prove not only ineffective, but harmful to the patient. Their cost can go beyond finances to include equipment, laboratory work, and personnel. Experimental treatments often cause side effects that require subsequent treatment. Lurking among these unproved products may be another thalidomide, the drug that caused thousands of birth defects abroad before it was banned."

From Coverage to Care

Deciding whether to cover a new technology is only one part of the challenge facing health plans and health care providers. Equally important are decisions about how and when to apply a therapy or course of treatment once it is covered.

During the LORAN Commission's early meetings, several members expressed the belief that "everything medically possible must always be provided." Several case studies suggested, however, such a principle could lead to "the misuse of technology and poor care for the patient."

One case concerned Baby L, then twenty-four months old. During birth, she had been deprived of oxygen and suffered profound brain damage. She was blind and deaf and had no control of her arms or legs. She was able to breathe only occasionally on her own. There was no hope that her condition would improve. She responded only to deep pain.

Shortly after she was born, Baby L's physicians questioned whether she should be resuscitated. At the mother's insistence, the infant was mechanically ventilated. Most of her first year of life was spent in a major pediatric hospital where she underwent repeated surgical procedures and multiple resuscitations. Her mother continued to insist that everything possible be done to preserve the baby's life.

Baby L was eventually discharged home, where she still required around-the-clock nursing care and suffered recurrent bouts of pneumonia. During one of those bouts, the director of the hospital's intensive care unit, who had often cared for her, refused the mother's demand that the child be mechanically ventilated. The physician believed ventilation would, in this case, be cruel and inhumane.

Despite calls to several other hospitals, no other pediatric ICU would accept Baby L on transfer. The mother then hired an attorney, who threatened legal action against the hospital and the child's physicians if they did not accede to the mother's requests.

Again, the treating physician refused, with the concurrence of the senior medical staff and others involved in the child's care. The hospital administrator and the hospital's ethics committee supported the attending physician. At a predawn court hearing hastily assembled at the hospital, the judge asked the physicians what they would do if he ordered that Baby L be ventilated. The physicians responded that they would defy the order: to comply would violate their standards of medical care and ethics. The situation was defused the next day, when a physician at another institution's intensive care unit agreed to accept Baby L into her care. The transfer occurred, and the child continued to be treated, her condition unchanged.

The medical expenses of Baby L were fully covered. In two years, her care had cost more than $1 million; her home nursing bill was $7,000 a month. At the time of the commission's report, there was no expectation that the child's condition would ever improve.

The LORAN Commission agreed that the case was an example of the misuse of technology. "The belief that 'everything possible must always be done' is not supportable," they concluded. "Attempts to do so can result in misplaced treatment priorities, unnecessary suffering, and an unfair allocation of resources. . . . At times, death must be accepted as an inevitability instead of an enemy." Sound medical judgment, they wrote, "sometimes requires that physicians *not* use all the technologies in their armamentarium."

"We're fighting two battles," commented the director of one intensive care unit. "One is to stand at the bedside and take care of the patient, doing what we think is right even if it means accepting that there are some things we cannot do. The other battlefield is asking: 'When should we quit? When do these enormous intrusions become unjustifiable?' "

A report from Congress' Office of Technology Assessment reflects similar concerns. "As once 'extraordinary' measures become common-place and as ever more powerful technologies emerge, it becomes increasingly important to understand the problems as well as the potential associated with the use of these technologies and to devise policies that reflect this understanding."

Medical resources are most likely to be misused at the extremes of life, the commission noted, "times when enormous resources are some-times devoted to futile treatments undertaken with no expectation of a cure." The LORAN Commission concluded from its discussion of the Baby L case that the care due a dying patient "is comfort and company, not pretended remedies or futile interventions inspired by unrealistic expectations and false hopes." They added that "individuals are thus permitted to live their final days with as much dignity, freedom, and independence as their conditions permit. They ought to be allowed to experience those waning moments unencumbered by high tech devices that serve only to impede their capacity for human interaction. Here it is the patient's comfort, not the caregiver's need 'to do something,' that should prevail."

The commission also addressed misuse of therapies in more common situations. The increasing numbers of deliveries by cesarean section provide an example. While cesarean sections are clearly appropriate in some cases, most experts agree the technique, employed in about one in four deliveries in the United States, is used more than necessary. That contention was supported by a study published recently in the *New England Journal of Medicine*. The obstetrics department at Mt. Sinai Hospital in Chicago reduced the incidence of cesarean section from almost 18 percent to almost 11 percent "without changing the outcome for the mother or the infant." The researchers noted that high cesarean rates were not linked to a lower rate of newborn death. On a national basis, it is estimated that we spend $1 billion performing unneeded cesarean sections. The cost to patients is higher: 25,000 infections and two to four times increased risk of maternal death.

By investing in more research on the effectiveness of services, we may be able to develop practice guidelines so compelling as to reduce inap-propriate care. But better information is not a panacea. As highlighted by Wennberg's research on prostatectomy, even rigorous technology assessment may not yield simple answers about the appropriate course of treatment. Wennberg found that transurethral resection of the pros-tate (TURP) does not prevent death in men without chronic obstruction;

in fact, it seems to reduce life expectancy. The surgery may improve the quality of life, however, by relieving symptoms. Only the patient can decide whether the improvement is worth the risk. Such choices will become more and more prevalent as more money is spent on life-enhancing services.

Patients

Service to patients is the preeminent goal of any health care organization. The commission believed, nevertheless, that patients should not be the final arbiter of the care they will receive. The commission wrote that "the autonomy of patients should be valued highly, but not worshipped. There may be times when the interests of the common good should be weighed in making individual treatment decisions."

The commission stressed "that the highest degree of respect ought to be accorded the patient's right to accept or reject proposed therapies. Nevertheless, neither the patient nor his or her family has the right to mandate exactly what care should be provided." According to the commission, a physician might be justified in refusing a family's request that a patient be kept in an intensive care unit. To accede might clash with the physician's responsibilities to other patients. The Baby L case, described earlier, illustrates the same point. "Whereas patients may reject proposed interventions, it is neither possible nor wise to allow patients to determine specific treatments."

The commission relied heavily on the report of the President's Commission for the Study of Ethical Problems in Medicine, "Deciding to Forgo Life Sustaining Treatment" (1980). In that report, two principles stood out:

- The autonomy and responsibility of the individual ought to be maximized.
- Decisions about individual patients should not be permitted to jeopardize the welfare of the group.

"Within the tension of these principles," the LORAN Commission sought to support individual autonomy and dignity as much as possible. The commission suggested that HCHP encourage the use of advance directives, also called living wills. Physicians need to be "informed of patient desires on treatment issues before a critical situation arises. [HCHP] should also provide members with information on health care proxy forms so that patients can designate someone who knows their values and interests to make medical decisions on their behalf, without the need for legal intervention, should they become incapable of making such decisions themselves."

The LORAN Commission encouraged HCHP and other health plans to cover alternatives to traditional forms of treatment—for example, home care and other forms of noninstitutional care, especially in the cases of AIDS patients and other terminally ill patients and the elderly. These recommendations will become ever more relevant, as aging members of the baby boom generation consume more health care resources.

To better understand public attitudes, the LORAN Commission, with financial support from the HCHP Foundation, commissioned a national public opinion survey by Louis Harris and Associates in 1987. The poll revealed that the views of commission members were not always consistent with those of the general public. A majority of the public (51 percent) refused to set any monetary limit—even up to $5 million—on what should be spent in the attempt to save a life. Ninety-one percent thought that "everyone should have the right to the best possible medical care— as good as the treatment a millionaire gets."

Leadership groups, however, felt differently. Only 6 percent of the representatives of large employers and 18 percent of the political leaders thought it would be unreasonable not to provide all available treatment.

When first questioned, only a third of the general public considered it reasonable that "health plans cover the cost of some treatments and medical procedures and do not cover others." Yet three out of four people agreed that "by 1990 there will be so many new and so many expensive ways of treating sick people that all health insurance plans will have to make tough choices about what they will and will not pay for."

Most of the people surveyed said that desperately ill infants should be cared for differently from elderly patients in similar situations. If forced to choose between a treatment that would cure fifty dying children or one that would give three or more years of life to each of 1,000 seventy-five-year-olds, the overwhelming majority (81 percent) of adult Americans would opt to save the children. Half of the general public thought that doctors should "do everything in their power" to preserve the life of a newborn infant, "even if it is very seriously deformed and will never be able to live a normal life." At the same time, 70 percent of the public would concur if parents of a child born with serious brain damage decided not to take any special steps, such as surgery, to preserve the baby's life.

These findings, combined with the fact that the public believes "cost is the least important health care consideration," illustrate why the Baby

L case is difficult for society. Nonetheless, the commission wrote, "when these problems are placed in the context of the principle that futile or ineffective technologies ought not to be employed, and the realization that, as a society, we cannot provide everyone with everything, the commission believes the recommendation on the nonprovision of ineffective interventions . . . will . . . be supported by the general public." They noted that it already has the backing of all the leadership groups, except political leaders.

On most other issues, the general public, as well as the leadership groups, expressed preferences corresponding to the commission's recommendations. For example, the public supported limiting access to experimental procedures, encouraging the use of living wills and health care proxies, consulting members in establishing priorities for coverage, and setting a low priority for coverage of in vitro fertilization.

The commission's own fallibility did not go unnoticed, however. The commission concluded that "as an antidote to any false sense of self-importance the commission might have, it should be noted that the Harris poll revealed that 'a committee of distinguished citizens' ranked with insurance companies and the federal government as the groups least nominated to make coverage selections."

Physicians

The commission took pains to emphasize that HCHP should decide prospectively which new technologies to adopt; so far as possible, decisions should not be made in the context of a medical crisis. Even more important, HCHP, not the attending physician, should assume responsibility for establishing whatever limits are necessary on the resources available to individual patients.

The LORAN Commission felt strongly that physicians ought not to be required to bear the brunt of societal pressures to control costs. Physicians should, of course, participate in HCHP deliberations about coverage policy, including how to achieve the maximum benefit for patients within the available resources. So far as possible, however, the physician at the patient's bedside should be free "to serve as an advocate for the patient and to seek, within the limits of institutional policy and the means available, what is best for the patient," the members wrote.

Doing what is best for the patient does not mean trying anything that just might work or doing whatever the patient wants. "Physicians should recommend treatment to patients only when there is a realistic expectation of significant and necessary benefit." This recommendation con-

trasts with Eddy's assessment of current practice. All too often, according to Eddy, physicians seem to follow the guideline "When in doubt,
do it."

The commission also emphasized the importance of *how* information
is presented to the patient and the patient's family. According to the
commission, "the physician who has the best overview should coordi-
nate the exams, interpret for the patient the chances of benefit and risk,
and make the treatment recommendations to the patient. Generally, that
person will be the patient's primary care physician." The commission
illustrated this point with a case involving an outstanding surgeon. A
pregnant woman was carrying a fetus that ultrasound had shown would
be born with massive, numerous birth defects. The surgeon encouraged
the parents to believe he could save the baby. On the strength of the
doctor's prognosis, the mother decided to carry the fetus to term. Yet
the prognosis was incomplete. The specialist had neglected to mention
that the infant's chances for survival were less than 10 percent; that only
1 percent of such fetuses are born neurologically intact; and that the child
would surely require many surgeries and be severely disabled.

Tragically, the infant was born profoundly brain-damaged, underwent three months of intensive treatment, and died. "In this case, it was
clear that the child was not helped by all the medical interventions it had
endured," wrote the commission. What is not clear is whether the specialist understood or communicated the totality of the baby's problems—
or indeed, whether the final decision reflected the surgeon's values or
those of the parents.

The commission also noted that there exists no legal impediment to
halting treatment once it begins. Initiating care "is not an irreversible
commitment to its continuation in the face of too little hope or the
realization that it is exacting too great a price in pain and suffering."
Admitting that initiating a therapy sometimes "creates expectations,"
the commission proposed that the "physician and patient [might] agree
on a time-limited trial for a particular intervention, with the understanding that, unless the therapy achieves certain goals, it will be halted. Such
agreements are already common regarding chemotherapy and should be
extended to other interventions."

Finally, the commission expressed concern that too few physicians
have received training in case analysis and decision making "so that they
may appreciate the social and ethical ramifications of the issues they may
be called upon to address." Refined technical skills no longer suffice to
make a complete physician. "[T]he concept of quality care does not
always demand that death be regarded as an enemy to be fought with
every weapon at the physician's disposal," the commission wrote. "An

obsession with quantity of life can adversely affect its quality. . . . [T]here are instances when the vast array of medical technological interventions . . . ought to be limited; there are times when graceful death with dignity is preferable to living torment."

A Final Word

Early in its discussions, the LORAN Commission concluded that the "combined cost [of medical innovations] will soon exceed the ability of any competitive insurer to pay. . . . [I]mproved efficiency in serving the health care needs of [people], although desirable, will not allow all the technological interventions rolling out of inventors' labs to be covered." Health plans, therefore, should require more thorough analyses of the risks and benefits of new technologies before adopting them. Physicians, moreover, should commit themselves to using therapies or diagnostic tools only where there is a reasonable expectation of benefit for the patient. It is not enough, in the commission's view, that something "just might work."

Even while issuing a challenge to HCHP, the commission recognized that its recommended course would require community-wide discipline. No individual insurer or provider can afford to depart dramatically from community standards. Nor can individual insurers and providers fund the necessary research. Consistent with its responsibility for providing "public goods," government must invest more money in discovering what works in medical practice.

The crucial question is how to change public attitudes about medicine. Such a change is essential if insurers, providers, and government are to fulfill their respective missions. It is unpleasant for people to confront their mortality by contemplating the limits of technology, and the limits of society's resources. Yet, confront them we must. The alternative is initial paralysis, followed by a spasm of action—action marked by arbitrary restrictions on access, since the analytic, organizational, and philosophical groundwork for a more sensible policy would be missing.

The challenge before us is daunting, but not insurmountable. The Harris poll found that people are willing to reconsider their views when forced to think about the problems—even in a brief public opinion survey. According to the pollsters, "Widespread debate of these issues . . . is likely to substantially change public and leadership positions. At the end of the survey, the proportion of the public who thought it reasonable that all health insurance plans do not cover the cost of all treatments and medical procedures had increased from 37 percent to 56 percent. It is a reasonable assumption that widespread public debate of these issues would move public opinion in the same direction."

References

Eddy, David M., and John Billings. 1988. "The Quality of Medical Evidence." *Health Affairs* 7(1):19–32.

Myers, Stephen A., and Norbert Gleicher. 1988. "A Successful Program to Lower Cesarean-Section Rates." *New England Journal of Medicine* 319:1511–1516.

Roper, William L., William Winkenwerder, Glenn M. Hackbarth, and Henry Krakauer. 1988. "Effectiveness in Health Care: An Initiative to Evaluate and Improve Medical Practice." *New England Journal of Medicine* 319:1197–1202.

5

Problems in Ethical Rationing: The Elderly, Hidden Costs, and Infants

Paul T. Menzel

Rationing and the Maintenance of Moral Fidelity to Patients

The escalating cost of health care has forced us to confront the issue of rationing. In rationing, beneficial care for patients is forgone in order to use the resources either to care for others or for other things in life entirely. Usually rationing is thought to pose a moral dilemma between meeting the needs of the individual patient and attending to the welfare of the larger society. The choices seem to be, on the one hand, don't ration—and deliver all medically appropriate care portending net benefit for the patient. Or on the other hand, do ration—and reserve resources for other things more important in the larger social order.

With the issue framed this way, it will be a long and difficult time indeed before American society comes to any kind of reasonably secure and ethical satisfaction with selectively restricting medically beneficial care. Rationing care will be called, plausibly, a moral assault on the nation's most vulnerable citizens, the sick and disabled.

The entire matter may be viewed in a very different way, however. Suppose the welfare-of-society side of the conflict represented an individual's hard judgment about the kind of society in which, on balance and in the long term, he or she wishes to live, even when implementation of that considered judgment later results in withholding something of immediate value. And suppose that commitment to individuals were seen as involving much more than maximizing the individual's welfare *as a patient.* A promising line of analysis lies precisely in this direction. The point that provides the actual reconciliation of respect for individual patients with the larger welfare of society is then essentially simple: if individual patients have beforehand consented to substantive and procedural rationing policies, the appeal of those policies when implemented will rest not merely on attachment to the morally controversial goal of increasing aggregate societal welfare, but on respect for the patients' own will (Menzel 1990:3–21, 45–53).

A straightforward instance of this is when subscribers to insurance plans actually consent to restrictions to save financial resources. If people in situations of scarcity decide to omit coverage, for example, of $500,000 adult liver transplants from the policies they purchase, they can hardly complain when their livers fail later, and no transplants come to the rescue. Another instance occurs in political settings in which the financing of health care has been pulled into the public arena (let us assume for good reason). If an individual has participated in that political decision and community representatives approve restrictions on care to preserve public monies for valid competing purposes, then, though personally that individual may later be shortchanged by those restrictions, the public plan has not assaulted his or her individual worth or dignity as long as its restrictions are not arbitrary or inherently discriminatory.

A third sort of case is perhaps morally more complicated, though finally the central point holds here too. Suppose an individual has given no actual prior consent either to the rationing policies or to the representative process through which those policies were adopted. Nevertheless, under these circumstances, it is clear that *if* the individual *had* had to choose earlier whether or not to invest available resources into the broader or leaner coverage in question, he or she undoubtedly would have chosen the leaner option. Such hypothetical, presumed consent, though the conditions that legitimize its invocation are tricky, can reconcile a later withholding of beneficial care with respect for the individual person who is now a patient (Menzel 1990:22–36). A good example may be care for patients in persistent vegetative state (PVS). The real individuals of our society, *if* they really had to judge how to use a limited set of resources for themselves, probably would regard $30,000–per-year nursing home care and life-extending artificial nutrition and hydration for PVS patients as below the line of expense per benefit worth spending (Brock 1988:89–91). When this is the case, withdrawing or withholding such care is no insult to such patients, even though it may be their (or the public's) best guess that life in these circumstances still constitutes some slight benefit.

To be sure, though American society might in such fashion legitimately restrict care, the practical road toward effective rationing will still be difficult and delayed. For one thing, defensive medicine stimulated by malpractice suits threatens to undo providers' intention to actually implement the rationing of care. If the society increasingly comes to see the rationing of care as morally legitimate, though, eventually malpractice law will follow. Americans might choose to view such a development as returning to use of the legal defense of the plaintiff patient's assumption of risk. Regardless of the particular legal structure the defendant's argument takes, its fundamental driving force here is moral: if a physician or hospital has acted on a defensible perception that restricting the care in question stems ultimately from the patient's own will, then withholding that possibly beneficial care because it costs too much is not breaking faith with commitment to the patient (Menzel 1990:150–168).

Perhaps the most obvious and powerful sort of case where prior consent legitimates the rationing of care—namely, private subscriber choice of comparatively lean insurance coverage—will become increasingly irrelevant. Basic problems of justice such as the cream-skimming of healthier clients by insurance companies and the rejection of the neediest applicants could inevitably push Americans toward some more national, governmentally organized system of care. Even then, however, the nation will still face the nasty moral question of how providers can approach patients denied care under the rationing's restrictions. Will patients be told the truth, or instead the excuse (lie?) that they are "too crumbly" to benefit (Aaron and Schwartz 1984:35)? The latter not only deceives the patient but constitutes a major point of instability on the professional side of any rationing arrangement. Clinicians of integrity will refuse to believe the deception, and some of them will work hard and with conviction to skirt the rationing criteria and get their patients treated. If, however, they realize that they can respect their commitment to individual patients while selectively restricting beneficial care, they will be less likely to undercut rationing. For providers to see how to resolve the alleged moral conflict between society welfare and fidelity to patients is as important in a nationally organized health system, even a national health service, as it is in a private, competitive market.

Suppose that with such an approach American society increasingly sees its way through to a morally justified rationing of care. Even so, three interesting and difficult matters will remain particularly contentious: (1) so-called age-rationing, (2) whether to include in the total actual costs of lifesaving several disturbing hidden factors, and (3) whether to restrict the aggressive beneficial care of newborn infants who cannot in any sense be seen as hypothetically consenting to the rationing policies.

Age-Rationing

One of the first targets for rationing will be life-extending care for those who have little life left no matter how aggressively they are treated. Using the full range of cardiac resuscitation and stabilization techniques on an eighty-year old with other health problems, for example, can be one of the lowest benefit-per-cost procedures in our medical armamentarium. As with the means of sustaining the lives of PVS patients, these procedures in such circumstances will be some of the first to be forgone if Americans ever get down to thinking through allocation policies for their lives. Because many of the measures that clear-headed rationing of health care will end up withholding are those used on elderly patients with relatively little life left even if the measures succeed, citizens might easily form the impression that a concerted attempt to ration medical care will embark the nation on a strategy of rationing according to age.

It is important to see that this is not necessarily the case. Of course, true age-rationing strategies are possible. One particular version has been urged by Daniel Callahan: after a "natural life span," life-extending care (though not palliative care) should not be provided at public expense. Callahan argues that elderly people can themselves come to see considerable value in not using societal resources to stay alive when they have already had their fair chance at a good life over a natural life span (1987). By his argument, it is not unfair to deny life-extending care, even if an elderly person takes quite a different view and sees great benefit in living even a short while longer. At work in his view is a lifetime equality principle: the eighty-year-old has a weaker claim simply because, being eighty, he or she has already had a shot at the good things of life. This principle generates an argument for true age-rationing: care is rationed not essentially because it provides a relatively low benefit per cost, but because the patient has passed the age where he or she can justifiably claim this form of society's support.

Not surprisingly, Americans resist such proposals, most important because we recognize that a segment of life bought after a certain old age can be both long enough and personally appreciated enough to be extremely valuable. Even from the earlier perspective of trying to make tough savings and allocation decisions for the resources available for whole lives, Americans are not likely to throw all life-extending care after a given age into the same low-priority bag. "If I get there," the thinking goes, "maybe it'll be the most appreciated time in my life." If care is to be rationed at all in old age, most Americans would prefer to ration it by the relevant characteristics of care *in* old age, not by age itself.

An appearance of rationing by age itself is probably what strikes many people as objectionable about British kidney dialysis policy: no one over sixty-five, Americans hear, gets that treatment in Britain (Halper 1989:125–126). The question, though, is whether the British practice is really intended to exclude prospectively stable, long-term dialysis patients. If it is, and if dialysis for those patients is not just seen to be more expensive per benefit achieved than care already forgone in other parts of the system, British practice would be an example of real age-rationing.

But is it? Dialysis for such patients might be seen as virtually always drawing a low-priority ranking because of its quasi-terminal character (it might work, but only, say, for a few years), or because of the real drop in the quality of life it brings, given the complications that frequently occur. If either of these factors is present in the bulk of actual cases, denial of dialysis is hardly just a stigmatizing affront to patients who are considered old and dispensable, for with these two factors in mind, people very likely would consent beforehand to such policies of denial.

The assumption that the life dialysis adds is diminished in quality might itself be considered biased against patients on dialysis. There is, though, some objective basis for this assumption: a significant number of patients themselves reject dialysis (Neu and Kjellstrand 1986:17). Apparently these patients believe that the added life dialysis could bring is either so short or so low in quality that its net value to them is essentially zero. If this is really the basis for their rejection of dialysis, and if those who thus reject treatment are already of significant numbers, a still larger group of kidney-failure patients undoubtedly get small enough benefit from dialysis that, though they do not now reject it themselves, dialysis would clearly become a first-order candidate for rationing. After all, in-center dialysis is a $30,000 per year therapy.

We should also be frank about the value of certain other sorts of life with which old age may confront us, though the situations may not be terminal. Extending severely demented and senescent patients' lives should have lower priority, even if their lives have no predictable limit. Severe dementia may not be morally significant if a patient has never been competent. But when dementia falls at the end of a long and richer sort of existence, most people, when trying to think out how to use a limited set of resources, would see the relative importance of such life as lower. Individual Americans, *if* they really had to make such a judgment for themselves, would almost certainly regard life-extending care for the severely demented as of very low priority indeed (Brock 1988:89–91; Buchanan 1988:299). Most would think it crazy to pass up life-extending care for other kinds and stages of life before cutting out life-prolonging care for the severely demented.

Thus like low-benefit terminal care, life-extending care of the severely demented becomes a first-order candidate for restriction if we take seriously the task of matching rationing policies with people's actual values. Both, however, are very different from long-term chronic care of elderly people who are not severely demented. If Americans think at all clearly about the allocation of resources for our lives, we will give chronic palliative care for the elderly high priority in any trade-off context; we will not end up abandoning them to waste away in misery.

The issue, then, is not age-rationing but the general rationing of care that is of low benefit per cost. True age rationing is very problematic, but the rationing of relatively low-benefit-per-cost care in old age is a natural part of any rational policy. The only way to reject this is for Americans to deny in general that health care should be thought of as a matter of hard tradeoffs between relative priorities. Clearly the nation had already decided to engage in that difficult game when it adopted a public program like Medicare to cover the bulk of medical care for the aged. With that decision, the whole cultural context of considerations about medical care for the elderly has necessarily become what might be called "congressional": seeing ourselves as responsible legislators. If Americans are going to stick with the basic decision that most old-age care be publicly funded, to ignore tradeoffs between all the various problems to which public monies might be applied is plainly irresponsible.

Hidden Costs: Later Health Care, Added Pension Payouts

If low-benefit-per-cost care is to be the main target of reflections on medical rationing choices, Americans need to know the true costs of care. Costs need to be conceptually as well as empirically clear if this whole business of trying seriously to decide what to spend is to make any sense. For example, if Medicare funds flu vaccinations for nursing home residents, the matter of cost is much more complex than just the money laid out for the lifesaving vaccine.

A somewhat different case provides an initial comparative example. When funding a lifesaving anti-smoking program, the public tends to think of the direct cost of paying for it. Perhaps the program also saves some money: it allows people to live further money-earning years, and it obviates the need for tobacco itself, for repairing the fires that smokers cause, and for the medical care that would have been needed for their smoking-related diseases. The anti-smoking program begins to look like a real bargain, even a money-saving way of saving lives.

But along comes a shrewder cost analyst. In the long haul, he or she will say, reducing the incidence of smoking in the population doesn't save the government or other people anything at all. There are two huge compensating costs of lengthening the lives we've saved: later, unrelated health care expenditures and longer pension payouts. The typical non-smoker hardly lives in perfect health to age eighty and then gets killed instantly; he or she experiences the typical and often costly illnesses of older age and draws additional years of Social Security benefits. In the long run smoking, it turns out, doesn't really cost much money at all, and stopping it, while lifesaving, doesn't save money (Manning 1989; Warner 1987).

Such a factual analysis may surprise many people, but it hardly poses a serious objection to noncoercive, reasonably designed anti-smoking programs. We may realize that anti-smoking programs do not save money, but whatever small net expense incurred seems well justified by the quality of the life that gets prolonged. The matter can be disturbingly different, however, with other health measures, particularly those for elderly people that occur both at the end of their earning years and when they are about to begin running up the bigger expenses of the more common diseases of old age. Go back to the nursing home influenza immunization program mentioned first, or to other simple and apparently inexpensive health care measures for elderly populations. Using penicillin to stop a case of pneumonia, for example, ultimately costs not only the $50 for the penicillin shot and its administration, but all the additional medical and long-term-care expenses and pension payouts incurred in the years of life saved by the penicillin shot. Unless Americans decide that resource tradeoffs are irrelevant and effective health-producing care ought never be limited, shouldn't we know what we really will be paying before we decide to save lives?

Whether these two often unacknowledged costs of lifesaving—later pension payouts and unrelated medical expenses—in fact are actual costs is an issue that deserves critical exploration. And if we decide that they are real costs, should they be counted in Americans' conception of what we will pay to save a life?

Later health care expenditures

Future health care expenditures incurred by extending the lives of the elderly seem to be real costs. Though two objections to thinking that they are readily come to mind, neither is telling:

1. The economist Louise Russell has refused to count such expenses in her economic analyses of various preventive health measures because, she says, they "are one of the indirect consequences of the health gains

from a program. . . . They are not an addition to health effects" (1986:35–36).

But Russell fails to explain why the distinction between "health effects" and "indirect consequences" should matter. Are indirect costs that come as a consequence of a decision any less real? Her decision to ignore the indirect consequences in an economic analysis might rest on a hidden assumption about which of the admittedly real costs we should count: the moral distinction between intended and merely foreknown effects. This well-known "doctrine of double effect" says that, though we foresee the later, unrelated health care expenses of added life, when we save a person from pneumonia with penicillin, we surely do not intend to create those expenses. We do not even intend them as a means to our aim (longer life). They are only side effects.

If this is Russell's unstated argument, it doesn't help much. We still would have to admit that these later health care expenditures are real costs. And even if we admit this but only want to claim that morally they shouldn't be counted, we would still be on slippery ground: the moral significance of the difference between intended and merely foreknown effects is itself notoriously debatable (Bennett 1985; Nagel 1985).

2. Alternatively, one might argue that though later health care expenditures are real costs, now, in the current decision about whether to administer penicillin to a eighty-year-old, for example, is not the time to count them. They should and will be counted when later decisions are made about whether to use the measures that incur these later expenses. People will decide then whether the human benefit of those measures justifies their cost.

This may seem to make sense, but excluding these later, statistically predictable medical expenses from assessments of lifesaving programs would require unusual and incredibly cumbersome cost-accounting procedures. To be consistent, we would have to exclude from the benefit side of our current assessment all the life and health benefits of the later care, counting only the benefits achieved between now and then. In statistical estimates of the life a particular program buys, how could we separate out these two temporal categories of benefit? To assume that any later health care will buy sufficient benefits to be worth its cost then, and consequently count now both the costs and benefits of that later care, seems much more sensible.

Added pension payouts

With added pension payouts the problem is more complex. A virtually standard assumption among economists is that pension benefits to the elderly are transfer payments, and therefore are not overall costs from any society-wide point of view. Assume that a social security tax transfer scheme does not create any serious disincentives to work and invest and does not incur significant administrative costs. Then, though someone through taxes or premiums pays such benefits to someone else, society—everyone, all of us together—incurs no net cost at all. When older people die, they lose a pension benefit, but the rest of us have saved a roughly equal expense; when the lives of older people are saved, we incur the expense of later pension payouts, but they receive that payout as an equivalent benefit. Either way, this contrasts with consumption, which involves real uses of goods and services.

This assumption is correct if the two courses of events compared occur among populations that are numerically the same. Either one individual transfers to another and the other gains as much in value as the first individual might have kept, or one individual keeps what he or she has and the other individual gets along without, though here too, the second individual is still around. This traditional economic explanation of why pensions are virtually costless serves very well for the typical set of circumstances which it assumes: people are staying alive whether or not a transfer is made. But things look very different when the comparison is between courses of events in which the number of people changes.

This is exactly what happens in lifesaving programs. The comparison is between (1) a course of events in which an individual is alive to receive a payment from others, and (2) a course in which the others save that expense, but not because the individual is doing without—the individual is just not around at all. Compared to (2), is (1) a cost? To the others, of course, it is (so it is clearly what economists call an external cost), but is it a cost from the wider, total, social point of view? In an obvious sense the cost of (1) is neutralized by being a benefit to one individual, yet this is only a sense. In the second course of events, (2), in which an individual dies, goods and services will be spread among fewer people. Someone, somewhere down the economic line, is going to have more in the second situation than in the first, without anyone in the second getting less. In this respect, (2) is a gain compared to (1), and (1) is a cost compared to (2).

The easiest way to describe this crucial respect is probably to say that per capita net income is lower in (1). This does not refer to a given individual's own per capita income per se, or to another's, but to per capita income generally. The frame of reference is still society-wide, so in one genuinely societal sense, pensions are real costs. Whether it is per capita or aggregate income that ought to be considered is then itself the important and open question. Many economists focus more on aggregate than per capita benefit, perhaps because of the impersonal sense of value with which they typically work. Most people, however, think with more of a per capita perspective. Particularly in a resource tradeoff situation, people try to decide whether their lives will be better or worse if they incur or do not incur this or that lifesaving expense. It is the likely benefit per person, not some more abstract total good, that they try to keep in focus. For purposes of making resource-allocation decisions, therefore, later pension payouts do seem to be a real cost.

People might try another way in which to save the costless transfer-payment view, even if they are focusing on per capita costs. Suppose the missing person in the course of events (2) would have injected additional goods and services into the society had he lived (as in case (1)): some distinctive "labor" in old age—cheering up children, for example, or teaching others the subtle lessons of gracious appreciation. That person would indeed have pulled out more pension benefits with added years of life, but would also have created fully compensating, equivalent goods.

But that's a tall order—*equivalent* goods. By the hypothesis, these goods are not created through paid economic productivity, nor are they hidden in the "value of life" for added years that will be counted on the intangible-benefit side when we subsequently decide whether or not the cost of prolonging life is worth paying. These goods have to reside in some other kind of value in the pensioner's longer life. Without them, the pension payouts of added years of life still emerge as real costs.

Thus future pension payouts as well as later unrelated health care expenditures appear to be real costs of lifesaving. The nursing home flu vaccine case, for example, incurs much greater costs than the nominal amount of money society pays for the vaccine and its administration. Modest estimates of costs per year of life prolonged might easily be another $2,000 of unrelated medical expenditures, $7,000 of Social Security payments, and $20,000 in nursing home fees. Costs could easily approach $30,000 for every year of life saved with the flu vaccine—a total bill that puts flu vaccination for the elderly in the same ballpark with such obviously cost-controversial candidates for rationing as dialysis and heart and liver transplants.

Ought we to count all real costs?

Still, a number of arguments and intuitions tell us that no matter how real these two kinds of costs, we should not count them as we go about considering what to spend to save lives. Russell's distinction between "health effects" and "indirect consequences" that rests on the debatable traditional principle of double effect is one argument against counting admittedly real later health care costs that fails. But a different, more widely shared argument remains to be considered.

Suppose someone proposed counting future food and clothing costs in deciding whether to save a life. Wouldn't people's reaction be, "You can't count those, they're just part of what anybody needs to live!"? This response does not deny that food and clothing are actual costs. It only makes a moral claim about them: when people continue to live, they should not in any way be held accountable for using up financial resources for the bare essentials of life.

Put the matter this way for analogous health care expenditures: suppose an elderly person lives longer. Thus alive, that person certainly cannot be expected to reduce or eliminate the consumption of bare essentials. But later medical care is just as much a necessity as food or clothing, so if an individual should not be "charged" for the food and clothing he or she uses in living longer, so also he or she should never have to justify later use of medical resources.

Some such argument is probably at the core of common reactions to this larger cost-counting issue, but it is beset with problems. Admittedly, individuals have a right to minimal food, clothing, shelter, and health care in the time during which they are *already living*. But why must we therefore ignore these items' cost when the matter at issue is explicitly the *extension* of life? Admittedly, food is a necessity to which people have rights partly or even largely because it is essential to their living longer, not merely to enjoying the life they would have had in any case. Still, there is a difference between having rights to certain things when being alive is assumed as a background condition, and having rights to those things when life extension is the issue. If we had a distinct shortage of food, for example, wouldn't we see to it first that people who were going to live a considerable time anyway got sufficient food to avoid lingering and debilitating malnutrition? Wouldn't we think it crucial to count food consumed in figuring the cost of saving people's lives?

So the argument equating medical care with food and clothing, while cogent, is sharply limited in two ways: (1) The more scarce basic necessities are, the weaker the food-and-clothing argument gets. If sufficient resources exist to provide everyone with minimal food and clothing, even those who might live longer, perhaps we should not consider the cost of such essentials. On the other hand, if we already regard such essentials as scarce, we are hardly attracted to the argument at all. (2) Morever, we are already beginning to see the life extension that results from deliberate decisions to adopt lifesaving programs as significantly different from the natural continuance of people's lives. In fact, the whole business of finding ourselves in a resource scarcity situation, when we are really making priority decisions between lifesaving measures and other good things in life, constitutes a situation in which we single out decisions to extend life from decisions in which, either way, the affected people are going to be alive. Any serious economic inquiry in a larger rationing context causes us to perceive a difference between mere continuance of life and deliberate lifesaving.

How does the food-and-clothing objection then finally stack up? It falters as we come to view health care resources as scarce, and as we begin to see deliberate life extension as different from life's natural continuance. Especially because of the latter, the parallel between medical care and food and clothing in arguments for excluding later health care expenditures loses its force in our current historical context. While the objection is bothersome, it is hardly persuasive.

In the case of added pension payouts, the food-and-clothing objection is similarly weak. Here the argument is made when people say that pensions are the elderly's basic right. If society sets up a non-annuity pension scheme because it thinks older people have a right to be assured such a base of support regardless of their private arrangements, why should it "charge" pension costs against them when they live longer and draw out what they have a right to draw out?

But we quickly come back to the same problems in the argument. An individual may have a right to a pension benefit for the time when he or she is alive, but that hardly commits society to saying that the individual has a right to have his or her life extended without regard to the impact an individual has on others by drawing the benefit. We may not see much of a difference between these two degrees of rights in the case of food, clothing, and basic medical care. Insofar as pensions have been set up in order to provide for such equally basic needs as these, they may carry with them some of the force of the analogy with food and clothing. The parallel will deteriorate, however, to the degree that a pension program's benefits are not unconditionally "needed" by its recipients. Currently in the U.S., in fact, that consideration is very much at issue; Social Security benefits are often no longer regarded as going primarily to those strictly in need.

Thus, while both later health care expenditures and pension payouts might be in some sense older people's right, it is doubtful they should be excluded as we count up costs to decide whether lifesaving is worth what it costs. In the absence of any clear, reasonably persuasive argument against counting what we have already admitted is a real cost, we should count all these items.

There is, of course, no general or abstract way to decide whether

$30,000 per year of life saved at age eighty, for example, is too high a cost to pay for penicillin for pneumonia or vaccine for influenza. Everything will depend on all the other things society wants to do with its resources. What is clear is that people of integrity, appreciating all the ages they might live to, will not hide their heads in the sand about the real costs of lifesaving. There is seldom a free lunch, and lifesaving care in old age certainly isn't one of them.

Severely Handicapped Infants

At the other end of life, whether to treat aggressively a very ill and handicapped infant may be the most excruciating health care decision of all. These patients are so utterly, transparently dependent on us, pushed into life with huge burdens already.

Generally we haven't complicated these already torturous decisions with explicit consideration of financial cost. In the middle of their otherwise heated conflict in the famous Baby Doe cases of the mid-1980s, for example, both right-to-life organizations and pediatricians could publically announce their agreement on one thing: cost and scarcity of resources "must not determine . . . decisions" (*Seattle Times*, November 30, 1983:A8; Menzel 1990:97n2). Furthermore, though cost may affect some parental refusals of consent to aggressive treatment, in American law the issue is then one of parental rights, not cost per se.

The ultimate issue of rationing arises when lives are exchanged for money—when we decide not to devote the resources in question to lifesaving at all. This is already occurring with infants when, for example, we decide not to establish or expand an intensive care nursery with what would be new dollars for health care. Even in such a genuine rationing decision as this, however, we do not want to see rationing for what it is: our unwillingness to spend so much to save a baby's life. We try almost any other explanation. We may turn to the allegedly insufficient quality of their lives—insufficient quality to them, the infants. Yet if this is the only life they have, is its quality really insufficient? If this reason does not work, we still want to resort to something like it as a moral safeguard: if only our decisions can be made for the sake of the infant.

In the current economic and cultural situation, such well-meant moral caution is unlikely to keep the costs of care completely out of our decisions. One reason is simply the actual expense of caring for certain newborns. In the worst cases of spina bifida with meningomyelocele, $200,000 is not unprecedented for the first year of care. Our increasing ability to save newborns of lower and lower birth weight comes generally at great expense (Menzel 1990:98*nn*5–7). Staff at my local children's hospital speak of several million-dollar-plus cases in the last few years.

In any event, cost figures by themselves are only part of the story. Other fundamental factors contribute to our doubts about how incumbent saving the lives of newborns is. For one thing, some aggressive infant care may improve survival rates without improving quality of life. Perhaps more important, when an infant dies, it seems to suffer little of the despair of an older child or adult, and death is no affront to its nonexistent expectations. If, for a newborn, death and dying are simply not as bad an eventuality or process as they are for most of the rest of us, then apparently, without any discrimination against newborns whatsoever, we could spend less on them per survivor than we do on others. We would only be considering impartially all the various people we might save.

Yet what about the original feelings we had—feelings of special reluctance to pass up *anything* of benefit we can do for an imperiled infant? A disturbing and persuasive consent-based argument reveals that these feelings reflect real moral logic, and that puts us in a box: either we will have to accept this argument's conclusion that there is virtually no defensible limit on what we should spend to treat imperiled newborns, or we will have to deny them the status of moral personhood the argument assumes. Alternatively, another argument provides an avenue of escape via the concept of consent.

Unimaginable Bargains

Look at the moral argument for denying lifesaving care in the analogous case of adults. Suppose each person in a community of a thousand faces a one in a thousand annual risk of dying from some particular disease. The likely one person per year who gets the disease can be cured with million-dollar care. People agree that they are all willing—barely willing—to pay $500 a year to protect against such risks; they are not willing to pay $1,000. The total annual revenue thus available for the expensive treatment is $500,000, not $1 million. Why should people spend more than $500,000 to rescue one of their own who gets the million-dollar disease? If we said that they should, we would be saying they should not take a one in a thousand risk of dying in order to avoid spending more than $500 in extra premiums. But why should they not?

Right here is the rub when we get to infants. If imperiled newborns themselves can in no sense be thought to have chosen savings over safety, no arguments against care like "They should have respect for their own choices" can apply. The problem is not that defective infants haven't *actually* chosen savings over safety; adults, too, may not actually have chosen between these two. But if we have good reason both for not having asked them and for thinking that they would have so chosen if we had, we may presume their consent and proceed (Menzel 1990:22–36). The problem of justifying monetary limits on care in the case of seriously ill infants is much more exasperating: no even hypothetical prior consent to limitations on care on their part is possible for us to imagine.

Suppose we see infants as making some kind of mythical prenatal bargain for treating their future congenital anomalies. As long as the life saved or improvement accomplished is worthwhile to the child (considering, of course, what it must go through to get the improvement), at what point can we ever say that it had a significant chance of benefitting from tough cost-containment savings? Never, not even before birth; in its straits, what more important uses of the money does it have to save for? Any morally conscionable pricing of life is thus cut loose from its anchor in consent. (If, of course, the child would be better off without the treatment in question than with it, we certainly should not spend resources to treat. But then cost considerations become superfluous: we should not treat anyhow.)

Handicap Insurance

Ronald Dworkin has suggested a way of avoiding this implication (1981:297–299). The crucial condition of at some time having been in a situation of equality, with a choice before illness of whether or not to endorse a policy of later restraint is not actually met in the newborn case. But there is a way to imagine its having been met. Imagine that we all, before our births, see ourselves as having an equal chance of being born seriously ill and handicapped. Back then, prenatally, for what level of compensation or treatment for congenital defects would we insure? Let's call this the "handicap insurance question."

Unlike our previous attempts to imagine what choice of savings over safety imperiled newborns would make, this query erases any of their knowledge that they will be born unlucky. If prenatal "people" are thus looking ahead only to the possibility of being cursed with birth defects, their choices will probably not be radically different from insurance decisions at later ages where people consider the treatment of conditions that can incapacitate them for major portions of their lives. Undoubtedly they will insure for somewhat more if they honestly and vividly imagine starting off whole lives with tremendous burdens and diminished opportunities, but that will only marginally increase the upper limits on the cost and scope of care. The important point is that *if* the handicap insurance question is the proper one to ask, people will bind themselves to some limits.

The question itself, however, is terribly problematic. Dworkin himself worries about the indeterminacy of choices that it calls upon hypothetical insurers to make (1981:298–299), but there is a much more fundamental problem: the question totally fails to capture the injustice of handicapped infants' brute bad luck. To be sure, it brings all of us, handicapped and "normal" alike, under equal conditions. But for the child, the prenatal context in which Dworkin thus places the decision is not its real life of congenital illness, the only real life it will ever have. In more typical and justifiable cases of presuming people's consent we also refer to hypothetical choices, but they must be the predicted choices of actual persons in perfectly realistic prior situations. Therefore the answers bind *them.* By contrast, any prenatal version of Dworkin's hypothetical insurance question seems not to take real, impaired, handicapped children seriously. "You claim to be letting 'me' 'choose' from a position of equal chance and equal opportunity," the unlucky infant could complain, but "that's a purely mythical me and a totally fanciful choice. Why should I, the real me, be bound by it?" The handicap insurance question thus finally does little to assuage our doubts about placing on newborns the spending limits we impose on ourselves.

Should we have to refer to consent at all?

The more the implications of our inability to presume any sort of consent by defective infants to cost limitations sink in, the more frustrated we are likely to get. Seemingly we must spend whatever is possible in treating newborns who may benefit relatively little. How can that possibly be correct while we cut other patients off from less expensive care with greater marginal benefits? How, in fact, did we even get started on this line of argument? If infants aren't consenting agents, why should we have to go through all this business of individually prognosticating their best interest and inferring something about their consent (here, its absence)?

Our options have been sharply narrowed. We want to respect each defective infant, but then there are only two alternatives: either we must work within the rubric of prior consent and accept the disconcerting conclusion that there are virtually no justified limits on the cost of their care, or we will have to see their basic moral status as essentially different from other, not-so-young patients.

The second option admittedly is controversial, but it cleanly gets us out of our bind. As our society confronts questions of rationing beneficial health care more and more openly, we will have to explore it seriously: if newborns really just don't have the same moral status as people, maybe we have no obligation to "consult" them for their actual or presumed consent. And there is an obvious reason why in fact they are not people with such moral status whose will we need to consult: with them we are missing even the rudiments of consent.

The convention of proxy consent may seem to require us to consult the child's will, but when we probe deeper we can see that it does not. Precisely because the child does not have the capacity to give or withhold consent, someone else is required to make decisions on its behalf. On what is probably proxy consent's most favored interpretation, this involves the so-called "best interests" test: we are entrusted to give or withhold consent for the child on the basis of *its* best interests. This test's most distinctive characteristic is to give the interests of a single particular newborn the moral power to hold off much larger aggregates of competing welfare; a baby's proxies ought to consent for it solely on the basis of its interests, not their own, society's, or huge number of other people's.

That power of the individual infant is quite remarkable (though no more remarkable than the power of any person in a nonaggregating ethic). How can each infant have such incredible moral leverage without the special elements of personhood such as minimal decision-making capacity that drive our notions of equal justice and human rights? Why shouldn't we see the best-interests standard, then, as parasitic upon background characteristics of personhood? When those characteristics are missing, shouldn't the strict respect-each-person, best-interests test fade away?

Most people overlook how resourceful and unoffensive to the protection of infants this nonpersonhood view of the status of infants is (Menzel 1990:104–105). Though no infants are yet persons, the vast majority of newborns in any case will be; because of the current potential for damage to themselves as later persons, they must even now be treated as if they are individual persons with rights against the aggregate welfare of the larger society. Mixed in, however, are those who will not be persons, and as a matter of human reactions it is extremely difficult to keep them separate from the rest of the human community. It would then seem natural to spend on these infants up to the same cost-benefit limits we derive for adults from their consent. We are out of our disruptive earlier conclusion that we could put no moral limits on the costs of severely handicapped infants' care.

We must still, of course, confront an enormous point of alarm about this view. If severely ill newborns are not actual persons, normal infants do not seem to be either. Any normal infant, too, will have rights of personhood *if* it really is going to become a person, but what if it isn't? And suppose it isn't, precisely because we are in the very process of letting it die? Wouldn't the view that infants aren't actually persons then allow us to let even perfectly normal, full-term babies die?

The literal nonpersonhood of infants, however, entails no such drastic consequence. Actual potential to become a person is not the only vehicle by which nonperson infants can accrue the rights of persons. Another is the spinoff effects on others of denying the right to life to any normal infant—for example, the emotional threat to parent-child bonds in general. Just think of what letting a normal baby die would say about its parents' motivations and how threatening they would be for child welfare in general! People tend to think that any such "derived rights"— derived from characteristics of the situation not inherent in infants themselves—are flimsy, but that is simply a confusion. Our belief that emotional damage will inevitably result from violating such rights is much more secure than any belief of ours that infants have inherent rights.

Thus the view that infants aren't persons, as incendiary as it may be to some, does not throw open doors to abuse, neglect, and discrimination. It will, of course, allow us to let imperiled infants die whom we might conclude we have to save at virtually any expense were they already persons, but we can still treat them with the same cost-benefit standard we use for older patients whose prior consent generates spending limits.

Fortunately, though, we may not ultimately find it necessary to embrace the controversial nonpersonhood view to escape the earlier (tentative) conclusion that we can derive no morally acceptable economic limits to handicapped infants' care. There is another less controversial alternative. Even to autonomous persons, some kinds of death and nonexistence are not very disvaluable. One way to see this is through what has been called the asymmetry of our attitudes toward nonexistence: while we think it bad that we will die when we do and not later, we do not think it a shame that we were born only when we were and not earlier. That is, we do not regret the prenatal as much as the postmortem variety of our own nonexistence; our attitudes toward our own nonexistence are temporally asymmetric (Brueckner and Fisher 1986; Parfit 1984:149–186).

Why is death bad in a way that prenatal nonexistence is not? Both, after all, are nonexperiences. Someone might suggest the explanation that there is nothing we can do about having been born late, but there is something we can do about dying early. That, however, won't work. Apparently we have the same asymmetric response to the purely accidental deaths that we can't do anything more about than we can about our not-earlier births. There is a better explanation: death is bad in a way that not-earlier birth is not because it is a deprivation of *goods that we anticipate* (Brueckner and Fisher 1986:219–220).

Now, if this is the persuasive way to defend the extremely widespread difference in attitude that we hold toward not-later death and not-earlier birth, then in all consistency death itself should vary in its badness by how much its person-victim looks forward to the life it cuts short. But then, since an infant clearly does not look forward to the life cut off by early death like older children or adults do, infant deaths just are not as bad as other ones, even if infants are persons. Maybe in fact, the death of an infant who does not yet look forward to its life is not much worse to it than our not-earlier births are to us—namely, not very bad at all. Then it would seem all the more absurd to devote unlimitable expenditures to saving infants while we significantly restrict what we spend to save others. It is not just the lives that we value which we must take into account in prioritizing health care measures in relation to their cost; it is also deaths with their varying disvalue that we must consider.

Note, however, one important caveat to all this. If, regardless of aggressive treatment or nontreatment, the newborns for whom we are caring will live to become people anyhow, we probably should either look to their later preferences for how to allocate resources in their lives or apply a best-interests standard. We would then either try to prognosticate what their consent to cost-containment limits would be or assess their best interests. If treatment would improve their lives in the long run more than would other uses of the financial resources the treatment consumes, we should treat; if it would not, we should not.

Rationing is strong medicine. Americans will swallow its restrictions in as much as we see them to be ultimately what we ourselves, and not just doctors or administrators, have ordered. We will increasingly come to grips with the need for rationing not just as the cost pressures from modern medicine build, but as we gain maturity and integrity and take a longer temporal perspective on the shape of our lives. There will be innumerable points of hard moral controversy and bitter dispute along the way, but it is not impossible for people to work toward reasonable conclusions on even some of the most difficult disputes.

References

Aaron, Henry J., and William B. Schwartz. 1984. *The Painful Prescription: Rationing Hospital Care*. Washington, D.C.: Brookings Institution.

Bennett, Jonathan. 1985. "Morality and Consequences." In James P. Sterba, ed., *The Ethics of War and Nuclear Detterence*, pp. 23–29. Belmont, Cal.: Wadsworth.

Brock, Daniel W. 1988. "Justice and the Severely Demented." *Journal of Medicine and Philosophy* (February) 13:73–100.

Brueckner, Anthony L., and John Martin Fischer. 1986. "Why Is Death Bad?" *Philosophical Studies* (September) 50:213–221.

Buchanan, Allen E. 1988. "Advance Directives and the Personal Identity Problem." *Philosophy and Public Affairs* (Fall) 17:277–302.

Callahan, Daniel. 1987. *Setting Limits: Medical Goals in an Aging Society*. New York: Simon & Schuster.

Dworkin, Ronald M. 1981. "What Is Equality? Part II: Equality of Resources." *Philosophy and Public Affairs* (Summer) 10:283–345.

Halper, Thomas. 1989. *The Misfortunes of Others: End-Stage Renal Disease in the United Kingdom*. Cambridge: Cambridge University Press.

Manning, Willard G., Emmett B. Keeler, Joseph P. Newhouse, Elizabeth M. Sloss, and Jeffrey Wasserman. 1989. "The Taxes of Sin: Do Smokers and Drinkers Pay Their Way?" *Journal of the American Medical Association* 261:1604–1609.

Menzel, Paul T. 1990. *Strong Medicine: The Ethical Rationing of Health Care*. New York: Oxford University Press.

Nagel, Thomas. 1985. "Agent-Relative Morality." In James P. Sterba, ed., *The Ethics of War and Nuclear Deterrence*, pp. 15–22. Belmont, Cal.: Wadsworth.

Neu, Steven, and Carl M. Kjellstrand. 1986. "Stopping Long-Term Dialysis: An Empirical Study of Withdrawal of Life-Supporting Treatment." *New England Journal of Medicine* 314:14–20.

Parfit, Derek. 1984. *Reasons and Persons*. Oxford: Oxford University Press.

Russell, Louise B. 1986. *Is Prevention Better Than Cure?* Washington, D.C.: Brookings Institution.

Warner, Kenneth E. 1987. "Health and Economic Implications of a Tobacco-Free Society." *Journal of the American Medical Association* 258:2080–2086.

6

Confronting Health Care Rationing[*]

John C. Moskop

Beginning with *The Painful Prescription: Rationing Hospital Care*, Aaron and Schwartz' widely discussed 1984 examination of the British National Health Service, a number of books have appeared which directly address the moral and policy problems of rationing health care (Churchill 1987; Blank 1988; Callahan 1990; Menzel 1990). Two of these recent volumes share a similar sense of urgency regarding the problems of financing the American health care system. On the first page of his *Rationing Medicine*, Robert Blank asserts,

> It is becoming increasingly clear that major alterations in the health care system of the United States will be necessary in the coming decades if we are to avert a crisis of immense proportions. . . . The aging population, the proliferation of high cost biomedical technologies designed primarily to extend life, conventional schemes of retroactive reimbursement by third-party payers, and the realization that health care costs are outstripping society's perceived ability to pay, all lead to pressures for expanded public action. (1988:1)

In the Preface to *What Kind of Life: The Limits of Medical Progress*, Daniel Callahan writes,

*Portions of this paper are adapted from "Challenging the Current Health Care System: A Review of *Rationing Medicine* by Robert H. Blank," published in *Bioethics Books* 1:38–44, 1989.

I do not share the inveterate optimism that seems a kind of virus in much discussion of health care, and certainly in its politics. . . . I look instead at the projections of future health care costs, all of which are enormous, and take them seriously. I see no reason to believe in magic fixes, whether scientific, bureaucratic, or financial. The projections tell me that we are going to have to change, and change not just the mechanics of our system, but our way of thinking about and understanding illness, life, health, and death. I see no reason why we cannot have a perfectly adequate system if we are prepared to do that. It will just have to be very different. (1990:11)

Both Blank and Callahan offer various reasons why the problem of escalating health care costs is so serious, both offer a number of suggestions for changing the system, and their different approaches to this problem are worthy of further analysis.

Reasons for Rationing

Is the impending crisis in financing our health care system predicted by Callahan and Blank real, or just an economist's illusion? Despite their dire predictions, both Callahan and Blank acknowledge that most Americans do not perceive health care as a major national problem. Why, then, do these authors insist on the gravity of the problem and the need to confront it without delay?

The underlying problem, simply stated, is this: over the last quarter-century, the cost of health care in the United States has risen rapidly and steadily, consistently outstripping the general rate of inflation and demanding a larger and larger percentage of the nation's resources. National health expenditures have grown from 5.9 percent of the gross national product (GNP) in 1965 to a projected 12 percent of GNP in 1990 and 15 percent in the year 2000 (HCFA 1987:2). Despite similar trends in other industrialized countries, no other country matches the United States in the level of health care spending or the rate of its growth over the last ten years (Wing 1985–86:622). Though there is no fixed upper limit to the amount of resources a society can devote to health care, it is becoming increasingly difficult for Americans as individuals and as a society to afford our health care system.

Callahan and Blank identify a number of the same factors—government programs, technological innovation, and the cost of medical care for an aging population—as major reasons for the continuing increase in health costs. Both also call attention to underlying social values which shape the health care system and encourage its steady expansion. Let us briefly consider how each of these has contributed to the cost of health care.

Congress' 1965 establishment of the Medicare and Medicaid programs extended to the elderly and the poor the benefits of health care already enjoyed by most working Americans. Though they gave many more citizens access to care, their rapidly escalating costs have greatly increased the federal government's contribution to national health expenditures as well as the proportion of the federal budget devoted to health care (Wing 1985–86:655–660).

Steadily increasing federal support for biomedical research since World War II has contributed significantly to a second reason for cost increases emphasized by Blank and Callahan, namely the rapid pace of technological innovation and dissemination in medicine. Examples of the technological explosion in medicine over the last twenty-five years are ubiquitous. Among the most dramatic are the development and wide diffusion of specialized intensive care units for critically ill neonatal, pediatric and adult patients, and of new diagnostic imaging technologies including computerized axial tomography (CAT), magnetic resonance imaging (MRI), and positron emission tomography (PET).

Medical technology's dramatic successes have won for it the strong support of both providers and the public, while its costs, often emotional and physical as well as financial, are often not well recognized. The result has been a general increase in the intensity of health care, as patients receive more and higher technology services at higher costs. Callahan notes that with increasing control over infectious diseases, medical technology in more recent years has focused on treating the chronic and degenerative diseases of the elderly, thereby seeking to extend their lives indefinitely.

The successes of medicine in prolonging life have contributed, in their turn, to the third major factor in health care cost increases identified by Blank and Callahan, namely, the aging of the U.S. population. In an appendix to his book *Setting Limits: Medical Goals in an Aging Society*, Callahan cites projections of continuing rapid growth of all age groups over sixty-five, especially those over eighty-five (Callahan 1987:225–228). Because they make greater use of health care services, an increasing proportion of elderly citizens should further accelerate the rate of growth of health care costs.

Kenneth Wing emphasizes one additional factor in health care cost increases mentioned only briefly by Callahan and not at all by Blank, namely price inflation (Wing 1985–86:624–628). Wing argues that price inflation—that is, price increases for essentially the same goods and services, and not intensity of care or population growth—has been the leading causal factor in the growth of national health expenditures. Wing cites U.S. Department of Health and Human Services statistics to support his claim that rates of price inflation were consistently higher for health care than for any other item in the economy over the last two decades. This health-specific price inflation is, I presume, due to the fact that health care for many years was, and largely still is, a very attractive seller's market. That is, health care is a service for which there is high demand, high levels of third party reimbursement with little direct financial sacrifice by most consumers, and relatively weak competitive or regulatory forces constraining providers. There is, in other words, relatively little to prevent providers and suppliers from maximizing their own financial interests. Despite his emphasis on price inflation, however, Wing cautions that it may sometimes be difficult to distinguish price increases for the same health services from price increases due to changes in the intensity of services provided.

Blank mentions, and Callahan emphasizes, that several basic social values underlie Americans' long-standing willingness to accept higher prices for health care. Perhaps most important is a steady and strong public demand for health care. Americans place a very high value on health and the curative powers of medicine; they tend to view health, according to Callahan, as an end in itself, not merely a means to a good life (1990:113). This emphasis on health is coupled with a faith in the unlimited potential for progress of high-technology medicine. We expect medical research to find a cure for every disease and, indeed, to prolong our lives indefinitely. (Callahan explores the problems of relying on medicine to stave off death indefinitely in *Setting Limits*.) Finally, as medicine progresses, we expect its benefits to be available to us; we claim a right to the best that medicine has to offer.

These values and beliefs have combined to produce the steady and rapid growth in health care services and costs recorded over the last twenty-five years. Knowing this, however, must we conclude that our health care system faces a crisis or an impending crisis, as Blank and Callahan suggest? To justify assertion of an impending crisis in health care, I believe two further conditions should be met: (1) we must have no effective method for controlling additional health care cost increases, and (2) we must be reaching the limits of our ability to absorb further cost increases. Can both of these conditions be met?

Regarding methods of cost containment, Callahan points out that for two decades, we have made unsuccessful attempts to provide health care more efficiently (1990:69). The most recent major cost containment initiative was Congress' 1983 enactment of a prospective reimbursement system for Medicare. This system bases reimbursement not on services rendered, but on classification of the patient's condition according to a set of diagnosis-related groups, or DRGs. It is designed to give hospitals a financial incentive for withholding, not providing, additional services for each patient. The DRG-based prospective payment system did lower the rate of hospital cost increases in the mid-1980s, and a few officials hailed it as a solution to the problem of rising hospital costs (Schwartz 1987). As William B. Schwartz has argued, however, mechanisms like HMOs and DRGs are probably able to provide only temporary relief from rapidly rising health care costs. Schwartz claims that these methods cut costs by encouraging physicians and hospitals to eliminate unnecessary services (1987). Eliminating such services can provide a significant, but one-time-only reduction in spending; once the services have been eliminated, the underlying rate of increase, driven by factors such as population growth, higher-technology treatments, and price inflation, will recur. Callahan notes that by 1986, when the general rate of inflation was only 1.1 percent, health care costs increased 7.7 percent (1990:74). More permanent cost control, then, will depend on reining in the underlying forces of increasing intensity of care and price inflation, for which task no clear strategy has emerged. To attack these forces, Callahan adds, we must abandon the vain hope that greater efficiency can make available all the high-quality, high-tech care anyone may need.

Regarding the second condition, namely that we are approaching the limits of our ability to absorb further cost increases, the situation is perhaps less clear-cut. There are some obvious warning signs, however. Finding some way to reduce record federal budget deficits became the most serious recurring problem confronting Congress in the 1980s. In its continuing struggle with these budget deficits, the federal government has been less and less willing to accept increases in its health care programs. Instead, a growing number of Americans, estimated at 37 million or 15.5 percent of our total population (Friedman 1988:33), lack health insurance, often as a result of cuts in government programs. Moreover, large new increases in Medicare funding, or cuts in the program, will be necessary to prevent the predicted depletion of its hospital insurance trust fund within the next decade (Wing 1985–86:663). Prospects for relief from the deficit in the 1990s have recently been dealt heavy blows by the cost of the savings and loan bailout, the Gulf war, and an economic recession. In view of these fiscal pressures, our legislators might, of course, decide overtly, or more likely covertly, to continue to back away from the existing commitment to financing health care for elderly and disadvantaged citizens, but both Callahan and Blank find any greater inequality in access to health care morally unacceptable. Corporations and individuals as well as government have in recent years experienced repeated sharp increases in health insurance costs, forcing some to reduce or abandon coverage for their employees or themselves. Whether an individual views the current situation as a crisis may therefore depend on how disturbed he or she is about the fact that cost increases are making health care less accessible for a large and growing number of Americans. Like Blank and Callahan, I view this as a very serious problem.

Emphasizing Prevention: Robert Blank

Both Blank and Callahan offer a number of proposals for correcting the flaws of the U.S. health care system. After his strong statements about the need for rationing, Blank's major proposals are surprisingly bland. I can discern only three: first, that the public must drastically alter its expectations and demands concerning health care; second, that we must shift from emphasis on high-technology, curative medicine to a broad, preventive approach; and third, that our preventive efforts should emphasize individual responsibility for maintaining health (Blank 1988:189, 195).

A recurring theme of *Rationing Medicine* is that the public and health care providers both must lower their expectations regarding health care. This seems unavoidable, if Blank is correct about the problem of rising costs. If we can no longer afford the health care we want, and there is no way to make that care more affordable, then we must moderate our desires. Blank's call for lowered expectations, though important to recognize, does little more than restate the problem. To move toward a solution, we must address the more difficult question of *how* we should lower our expectations. What kinds of health care, in other words, should we be willing to give up, either for ourselves or as a matter of public entitlement?

Despite his review of several different kinds of high-cost health care, however, Blank does not directly address these latter questions. Instead, he strongly recommends that we do more in the area of prevention, presumably on the grounds that increasing prevention will decrease the need for curative health services, thus lowering costs and perhaps obviating the necessity to ration services.

Three obvious questions can be raised about the role of prevention in Blank's overall scheme: first, how effectively can prevention control health care costs? Second, how strongly should we emphasize individual responsibility for health? Third, does Blank's focus on prevention ultimately distract our attention from the problem of rationing?

To restate the first question, then, can prevention accomplish the admittedly difficult task of controlling costs Blank sets for it? The record of prevention, as Blank himself seems to admit in places, is very mixed. There is strong evidence that better food, housing, sanitation, hygiene, and population control have had a significant effect on health in the developed world (McKeown 1979). Since these measures by and large have already been implemented in the United States, Blank looks to other preventive efforts, including pollution control, workplace safety, health education, early detection programs, and, especially, measures designed to alter unhealthy behaviors (1988:36). The effectiveness of these latter measures is much more questionable, however. A few, such as routine prenatal care, appear to be effective and to save money in treatment costs (Firshein 1985). In contrast, Freudenberg argues that "the record of health education in getting people to stop smoking, lose weight, drive carefully, avoid unwanted pregnancies or exercise more is extremely disappointing. If well-designed, carefully executed studies have difficulty changing small groups of volunteers, the potential impact of such strategies on the general population is minimal" (1979). Blank recognizes this problem, citing Jennett's arguments for the ineffectiveness of efforts designed to prevent smoking (1988:241).

Even if a program is able to prevent disease, it cannot do so without costs and risks of its own. The costs of routine vaccination, health screening, workplace inspection, public education, and wellness programs can be considerable. Moreover, since none of us is immortal, preventing a disease we would have had only postpones the need for additional medical care that we will likely experience sometime later in our lives. Callahan calls this the "twice cured, once dead" phenomenon (1990:101). Like the elimination of nonbeneficial health care, then, even effective prevention may only temporarily slow the rate of increase in health care costs. Again, Blank seems to recognize this problem; he makes reference to Louise Russell's extended argument in a recent book that "even after allowing for savings in treatment, prevention usually adds to the costs of health care, contrary to the popular view that it reduces them" (Blank 1988:239). Blank does not attempt to refute this conclusion, but if Russell is right, then even though prevention may give us better health, it cannot by itself solve the problem of controlling health care costs. Why, then, does Blank so strongly embrace the need for prevention?

One possible answer to this question is suggested by Callahan, who, despite his stated skepticism about its ability to save money, also gives a high priority to preventive medicine in his proposed goals for the health care system. Callahan appears to value prevention not for its ability to save money, but for its ability to promote greater *equity* in the distribution of health care and in health status. He points out that basic preventive measures, such as nutrition, sanitation, and vaccination, are directed toward entire populations and address needs common to all. This distinguishes prevention from expensive therapies that benefit single individuals with more idiosyncratic needs (1990:136–137). Callahan also endorses arguments by James Fries that greater investment in preventive medicine will result in the "compression of morbidity," that is, it will allow more people to avoid the morbidity of chronic illness until later in life (Callahan 1990:173–175). This result is more equitable, Callahan argues, than the use of technology to indefinitely prolong a few lives accompanied by significant morbidity.

Though few will question the value of continuing basic preventive efforts such as sanitation and vaccination, programs designed to promote individual responsibility for health, as recommended by Blank, raise a number of practical and moral problems. Such measures include purely voluntary educational programs, increased taxes on unhealthy products, increased insurance premiums for noncompliant individuals, legal prohibition of risky activities or products, and denial of health care for persons with self-induced diseases. Each of these measures has its special problems, however. Health education, as already noted, is often notoriously ineffective, as our current difficulties with alcohol, drugs, and smoking amply illustrate. Increased taxes on unhealthy items are regressive, since they penalize and constrain individuals according to their inability to afford the taxed item. Pegging insurance premiums to healthy lifestyles poses difficult problems of identification and monitoring. Since most of us engage in some risky behaviors, which ones should be counted? How pervasive and invasive will efforts to identify behaviors and ensure compliance have to be? Think of those who have many sex partners, for example! Is the more coercive measure of behavior prohibition justified? If so, is it likely to be more effective than our past experience with alcohol prohibition or our current experience with illegal drugs?

Blank does not shrink from defending even the severe policy of denying health care to those who contributed significantly to their disease (1988:233). Once again, however, serious difficulties stand in the way of determining that particular behaviors did contribute to the disease, since some nonsmokers and teetotalers contract lung cancer and cirrhosis. Moreover, even if a person's behavioral contribution to a disease were clear, how could we establish, in view of social pressures or genetic predispositions, that that person could have abstained from the unhealthy behavior? Even if these problems could be solved, would it be wise public policy to require health care providers to investigate a patient's behavioral history before making a commitment to treat him or her? Would it be sound policy to leave helmetless motorcycle accident victims lying by the side of the road in view of their reckless choice to ride without helmets? Joel Feinberg (1986:139–141), for one, sees the latter example as an unacceptable social cost. There are, in sum, an array of problems confronting increased reliance on individual responsibility for health. Blank mentions a number of these but does not say specifically how he would enforce individual responsibility for health or how these problems could be overcome.

Finally, does prevention ultimately distract us from the problem of rationing? My conclusion about prevention should be obvious by now. Though the promotion of health and prevention of disease are worthwhile goals, they are not, in my view, the key to controlling health care costs. Thus the title of Blank's book, though engaging, is slightly misleading. Blank tells us why rationing is necessary and why it is so difficult, but he never tells us who—which groups or individuals—should be denied which specific kinds of care under which circumstances. Because Blank never addresses specific cuts in health care, he never convinces us that his proposals can orchestrate the big dollar cuts or tax increases needed to save Medicare or the structural changes needed to control health care price inflation. The more difficult but, I believe, ultimately more realistic approach to containing health care costs must confront these issues head on.

The Limits of Health and Medicine: Daniel Callahan

In contrast to Blank, Callahan makes bold to propose not only wholesale changes in the goals of the U.S. health care system, but also basic changes in Americans' attitudes toward life, health, old age, illness and death. This is clearly a tall order, but nothing less will do, Callahan argues, if we are to succeed in our efforts to make our health care system both equitable and affordable. Callahan echos Blank's call for fundamental changes in the system; he goes beyond Blank in his attempt to sketch out, even if only in broad outlines, what that restructured system should accomplish.

Throughout *What Kind of Life*, Callahan examines the American health care system as a whole and the basic values and beliefs which shape it. The underlying problem, Callahan suggests, is a kind of intemperance— Americans want better health and more health care than they can afford, and their efforts to satisfy this desire are endangering the health of the society. High demand drives up the cost of care and diverts resources from other areas. Within health care, demand for high-technology cure and life support diverts resources from basic primary care and preventive medicine. Thus, Callahan argues, we are faced with the dual problems of increasing costs of care for all and increasing gaps in access to care between rich and poor.

Solving these problems, Callahan maintains, will require changes in basic values. The desire for individual cure and faith in technological progress must give way to an acceptance of limits to medicine and to the prolongation of life. In place of the current demand for quality care and individual choice, Callahan proposes an emphasis on equity in basic services and on caring, understood as the relief of pain and a comforting presence to the sick person. Callahan would restructure the health care system to reflect these value changes, giving priority to caring, preventive medicine, and basic emergency and primary care over advanced curative and restorative therapies (1990:176–177). Such restructuring could, Callahan suggests, be accomplished in a three-tier system: first, expanded government-sponsored programs for the poor; second, employer-sponsored programs for most Americans; and third, a market system for purchasing additional care not provided in the first two tiers (1990:200).

Callahan's book offers a broad and penetrating analysis of the problems besetting the U.S. health care system as well as his own vision of a better alternative. It has the distinct advantages of a general account, allowing us to make connections and get some grasp of the whole. It also has the disadvantages of such an account, glossing over most of the difficult details. Callahan says, for example, that a government must have a major role in implementing his recommendations, but says very little about what kind of government regulation would be necessary to change our current three-tier system into one which emphasized primary and preventive care over high-technology medicine. Callahan's vision of an improved system will be most persuasive to those who share his value priorities, such as social over individual health and equity over autonomy. Although he invites the reader to embrace his vision, he does not attempt to defend those value priorities against other scholars. He does not address, for example, those with more libertarian leanings, like Engelhardt, who have proposed a very different ordering of moral principles (Engelhardt 1986:85–87).

Since Callahan acknowledges that current social values must change in order to implement the reforms he proposes, we may wonder how those changes will occur. In a chapter titled "Devising a Political Strategy: Can We Get There from Here?," Callahan lists some of the cultural and political changes that would allow his system to be implemented. Despite the chapter's title, however, he does not really examine *how* those changes could occur. In fact, Blank offers a closer examination of the prospects for government action on health care in *Rationing Medicine* (1988:135–187). Blank's observations provide little ground for optimism regarding change, however. Instead, his review of the various branches of the federal government only emphasizes how unsuited each one is for assuming leadership in reforming the health care system. He points out the extreme reluctance of Congress to tackle controversial issues in the absence of an overt crisis. He also notes that responsibility for health care is widely diffused throughout the federal bureaucracy, many of whose agencies are strongly influenced by the interest groups they serve. Moreover, even if Congress or federal agencies should enact significant health care legislation or regulations which adversely affect individual interests, they are likely to be challenged by courts intent on protecting individual rights.

In another article, Andreas Schneider (1985–86) elaborates on the obstacles to congressional leadership in health policy. He notes that few of our congressional representatives currently devote much of their personal or staff resources to health-care issues, since health care is viewed as a "take-away" area likely only to alienate potential supporters. Schneider also describes how congressional action on health care programs in recent years has been narrowly and exclusively focused on a single objective—lowering budget deficits to conform to Gramm-Rudman-mandated deficit-reduction targets. This focus, which has emphasized specific, concrete, short-term program cuts, not long-range comprehensive planning, is likely to persist for the next several years at least.

Callahan recognizes that unless Americans' values can be transformed along the lines he proposes, his vision will remain just that. Its chances of becoming more than a vision will depend on several unanswered questions. Who, or what, will focus public attention on the long term problems of the health care system? Will we respond to anything short of a breakdown in the system? If it should come to that, what would it take to rebuild the system? Who would lead the way? Until we can do more than speculate on the answers to these questions, the prospects for realizing Callahan's vision will remain uncertain.

References

Aaron, Henry J., and William B. Schwartz. 1984. *The Painful Prescription: Rationing Hospital Care*. Washington, D.C.: Brookings Institution.

Blank, Robert. 1988. *Rationing Medicine*. New York: Columbia University Press.

Callahan, Daniel. 1987. *Setting Limits: Medical Goals in an Aging Society*. New York: Simon & Schuster.

Callahan, Daniel. 1990. *What Kind of Life: The Limits of Medical Progress*. New York: Simon & Schuster.

Churchill, Larry. 1987. *Rationing Health Care in America: Perceptions and Principles of Justice*. Notre Dame, Ind.: University of Notre Dame Press.

Health Care Financing Administration, Division of National Cost Estimates, Office of the Actuary. 1987. "National Health Expenditures, 1986–2000." *Health Care Financing Review* 8(4):1–35.

Engelhardt, H. Tristram. 1986. *The Foundations of Bioethics*. New York: Oxford University Press.

Feinberg, Joel. 1986. *Harm to Self*. New York: Oxford University Press.

Firshein, J. 1985. "Preventive Health Programs Found to Be Cost-effective." *Hospitals* 59 (18):37–38.

Freudenberg, N. 1979. "Shaping the Future of Health Education: From Behavior Change to Social Change." *Health Education Monographs* 6:372–377.

Friedman, Emily. 1988. "38 percent Jump in Uninsured, Even Among Working Adults." *Medical World News* 29(24) (December 26):33.

McKeown, Thomas. 1979. *The Role of Medicine: Dream, Mirage, or Nemesis?* 2d ed. Princeton: Princeton University Press.

Menzel, Paul T. 1990. *Strong Medicine: The Ethical Rationing of Health Care*. New York: Oxford University Press.

Schneider, Andreas G. 1985–86. "Commentary: Legal and Political Pressures on Health Care Cost Containment." *Case Western Reserve Law Review* 36:693–707.

Schwartz, William B. 1987. "The Inevitable Failure of Current Cost-Containment Strategies." *Journal of the American Medical Association* 257:220–224.

Wing, Kenneth R. 1985–86. "American Health Policy in the 1980s." *Case Western Reserve Law Review* 36:608–685.

7

A Healthier Approach to Health Care

John Kitzhaber

Medicaid was created by Congress in 1965 to provide health care to poor people, with the federal and state governments sharing the costs. But the program is failing—it now serves a much smaller percentage of the poor than when originally enacted, and the states are buckling under the financial burden.

The economic crunch is due in part to the requirement that, in order to qualify for federal matching dollars, states must comply with a steady stream of federal Medicaid mandates to provide specific services or include certain populations. The resulting escalation of health care costs is forcing state legislatures across the country either to raise taxes or to limit investments in environmental protection, education, housing, law enforcement, economic development, and a host of other essential social programs.

This was the situation in Oregon in 1987 when the state legislature, faced with over $48 million in immediate social program needs and only $21 million available in the budget, voted to discontinue funding for most organ transplants for people on Medicaid. It was argued that these were high-cost procedures that would benefit only about thirty individuals during the next two years. The money was used instead to fund, among other things, basic preventive care for nearly 3,000 people with no health insurance coverage at all.

The legislature's decision received little attention at first. But in late

1987 a young boy with leukemia, unable to receive state funds to pay for a bone morrow transplant, died while his parents sought public contributions to finance the operation. The case prompted an effort in January 1988 to partially refund the transplant program for eight individuals in immediate need. This took the form of a motion before the Legislative Emergency Board, comprised of seventeen legislators, which has the authority to appropriate money from an emergency fund when the legislature is not in session. After an emotional two-day debate, the motion was narrowly defeated.

The debate did not turn on the question of whether organ transplants have merit—clearly they often do. Nor was the question whether the state at that point had sufficient resources to make that particular appropriation. It did. Rather, the question was simply this: if the state was going to invest more money in its health care budget, where should the next dollar go? What was the policy that would lead us to fund transplants as opposed to further expanding the availability of prenatal care? What was the policy that would lead us to offer transplants to eight individuals as opposed to nine—or to nineteen? Where was the equity in giving sophisticated and costly services to a few Oregonians covered under Medicaid before providing basic health care services to other equally needy citizens, including many of the "working poor," who lacked any public or private coverage?

What became readily apparent was that Oregon had no health care policy. We were responding to a highly emotional issue and had no way whatsoever to evaluate whether funding transplants was the best place to invest state health care dollars. By appropriating the money, we in the legislature would know that another eight transplants could be performed. Yet we had no way of knowing—or being held accountable for—the consequences of not using that money to expand access to other individuals who were currently excluded from the system altogether.

This realization—that we were making decisions unguided by any specific policy and untempered by accountability—made the legislature step back and take a look at the national health care delivery system and the role states play in it. What we discovered was that there was no clear policy at the federal level either.

Leadership Needed

Faced with the lack of any clear federal leadership, we in Oregon came to realize that by default we had to assume responsibility for health care reform. This led us to develop the Oregon Basic Health Services Act, adopted in 1989 after an intensive legislative effort. The act was motivated by the desire to build a new system that recognizes the reality of fiscal limits, carefully defines the public policy objectives, and, most important, includes a mechanism to establish accountability for resource allocation decisions and for their consequences. Let us consider each of these points in turn:

The reality of limits

Unlike the federal government, states are constitutionally required to operate within a balanced budget. Yet Congress has passed the buck to the states to raise substantial amounts of new revenue for Medicaid. In the Omnibus Budget Reconciliation Act of 1989, new mandates require states to provide Medicaid coverage for pregnant women and children up to the age of six who have family incomes below 133 percent of the federal poverty level. Furthermore, states must provide these clients nearly all "medically necessary" services—virtually everything our high-tech health care system has to offer—no matter the cost. Ironically, these new requirements were handed down just two months after the National Governors' Association, citing what it considered an imminent health care fiscal crisis, asked Congress for a two-year moratorium on Medicaid mandates. And in 1990, during the seemingly endless struggle to agree on its own budget, the federal government enacted a host of new mandates for the states, including the requirement that Medicaid cover all children born after 1983 until they turn nineteen.

The new mandates may seem laudable at first glance. But because they are not part of a comprehensive policy to deal with the problems of access for the poor, they have triggered unfortunate consequences. To support new mandates, states unwilling or unable to raise taxes or cut other social programs are often forced to change Medicaid eligibility standards for those individuals not specifically covered. This amounts to nothing more than "redefining the poor," throwing some people off the program to balance the budget.

To meet the 1989 mandates, nearly all states have restricted eligibility for women who are not pregnant and for children over the age of six. Alabama provides Medicaid coverage only to those families with incomes of less than 14 percent of the federal poverty level; California, which has the broadest coverage, includes those with incomes up to 79 percent of the poverty level. Yet, even in California, 5 million people are uninsured, and a measles epidemic rages among its more than 400,000 unimmunized children. Nationally, the average eligibility standard is under 50 percent of the poverty level, which means that a family of three with an annual income over $5,500 is regarded as too wealthy to qualify for Medicaid coverage in many parts of this nation.

Another action that states have sometimes taken to pay for new mandates is to cut provider reimbursement rates—that is, reduce the amount paid for medical services. But since some providers refuse to participate in the Medicaid program as rates drop, this can create yet another barrier to access. A recent Supreme Court ruling allowing hospitals to sue states for what they consider inadequate Medicaid reimbursement makes it less likely that states will take this approach and more likely that they will restrict eligibility further to control costs. The 1990 mandates exacerbate the cost squeeze by prohibiting reductions in reimbursement to pharmacists.

The current Medicaid program also runs afoul of fiscal reality in its assumption that all medical services and procedures are equally valuable and effective, an assumption directly contradicted by a growing body of information on medical outcomes. Although the latest federal Medicaid mandates require that all "medically necessary" services be provided, there is absolutely nothing in the system to measure which services are in fact necessary, or even effective. For example, Medicaid must pay for all services, including some of questionable or unproven benefit, for children five years of age and under, but it is not required to cover services of proven effectiveness for children six years and over.

The need for a clear policy

Unlike federal officials, Oregon's citizens and legislators believe that the policy objective is not simply to guarantee all state citizens access to health care, but rather to keep all of them healthy. The federal Medicaid program is based on the assumption that providing health care is the most important way to improve health. But we are convinced that health care is not necessarily synonymous with health. Indeed, it is clearly evident that the nation's enormous and increasing expenditure for health care has not actually made us healthier as a people. In 1988, for example, the United States led the world in health care spending with $1,926 per capita—far more than Canada (the second biggest spender at $1,370) and three times Great Britain's $711. Yet nineteen countries have lower infant mortality rates and twenty-six have better cardiovascular statistics. An American woman ranks seventh worldwide in life expectancy and an American males stands tenth.

These statistics are often explained by noting that 35 million Americans, many of them the working poor, lack public or private health coverage. The reality is that the statistics reflect not so much a problem of access to health care as a failure to allocate sufficient resources to a variety of other social conditions that also affect health in important ways.

Women fail to get prenatal care, for example, not just because they lack health insurance, but also because of transportation problems, communication barriers, and the lack of day care. Infant mortality reflects more than just a lack of prenatal care; it also reflects poor housing, environmental pollution, teenage pregnancies, and the growing problem of substance abuse. We cannot improve the health of our state or nation if, for example, we continue to focus expenditures on the medical complications of substance abuse while ignoring the social conditions that lead to addiction. That means dealing with issues such as education, income maintenance, and economic opportunity. Yet when health care costs go up, these programs are jeopardized.

The need for accountability

If we accept the fact that the health care budget is ultimately finite, then it follows that an explicit decision to allocate money for one set of services means that an implicit decision has also been made not to spend money on other services. That, in essence, constitutes rationing of health care, and legislative bodies do it every budget cycle. But they do it implicitly, with no real accountability for the whole of their actions.

This issue is graphically illustrated by the national debate over costly high-technology medical interventions for a few individuals versus preventive care for large numbers of people. The struggle in Oregon over funding of transplants is a case in point, but examples abound across the country. In 1985, Illinois passed legislation guaranteeing up to $200,000 in state funds for any citizen needing an organ transplant and lacking health insurance. By making this huge fiscal commitment, the legislature engaged in implicit rationing by ignoring the fact that 60 percent of the state's black preschoolers were not even immunized against polio and that inner-city health clinics in Chicago were being closed because of a lack of revenue.

In Florida—a state that sets its Medicaid eligibility at a mere 35 percent of the federal poverty level—former Governor Bob Martinez in 1989 approved spending $100,000 in an attempt to save the life of a two-year-old boy who had nearly drowned after falling into a neighbor's swimming pool. Lung infection set in and coma followed. The child was transferred to a Minnesota hospital and put on a sophisticated lung bypass machine, even though medical experts admitted he would probably remain in a vegetative state or, at best, be severely impaired.

Policymakers in both states were able to take credit for highly visible operations that "save lives," but did not have to assume any accountability for the consequences of what they implicitly chose not to fund. "How are you supposed to put a price on saving one child?" said an aide to the Florida governor. "You can't look at it as all this money for one kid. The truth is, when you have a two-year-old boy who is about to die, you don't have a hell of a lot of choice."

And it does seem, of course, that there isn't a choice, because the child is right in front of us. But each year in the United States approximately 40,000 children die before their first birthday—with no national uproar because they are not in front of us. Many of these deaths—the result of implicit social and legislative decisions for which there is no accountability—are preventable.

The moral here is not that we should abandon high technology or cast away human compassion. Rather, we must recognize that today's system allows us to make crucial allocation decisions in a vacuum, to take the easy and popular way out and avoid having to weigh the overall social costs and benefits.

Determining What to Cover

The Oregon Basic Health Services Act extends Medicaid eligibility to all persons with incomes below the federal poverty level, as the original legislation intended, thus establishing a definition of the poor based strictly on need—not on the complex and sometimes contradictory maze of federal "categories" and changing Medicaid mandates. It also requires comparable employment-based coverage for those with a family income above the federal poverty level, which brings the working poor into the system. By guaranteeing that virtually everyone in the state will have access to health care, the act fundamentally changes the issue from who is covered to what is covered.

In determining what services to cover, judgment should be made based on medical efficacy and cost-effectiveness of the services being purchased. The process we are using to accomplish this differs markedly from the current pattern of random federal mandates and piecemeal state insurance mandates, which are often based on the relative power of special interests. Rather, we are prioritizing health services according to the degree of benefit each service can be expected to have on the health of the entire population.

Responsibility for prioritizing health services is assigned to the Oregon Health Services Commission, an eleven-member body appointed by the governor and confirmed by the State Senate after public hearings. To establish priorities, the commission developed a formula that considers the benefit likely to result from each procedure, the duration of that benefit, and the cost involved. Panels of physicians and an extensive review of medical literature were used to provide information on the appropriateness, efficiency, and outcomes of specific procedures. In addition to its evaluation of cost-effectiveness, the commission took into consideration social values such as quality of life, equity, and community compassion, which were ascertained through forty-seven public meetings held around the state.

In May 1990 the commission conducted an initial computer run to test the methodology. As expected, this revealed a number of problems. Unfortunately, the media and some critics of the act seized upon the results and widely represented them as the final Oregon "priority list," leaving the impression that the effort was fatally flawed. In fact, the computer run was but a necessary part of an orderly process to develop a credible ranking system, an effort that was never before attempted. It was hoped that the exercise would not only reveal problems, but also shed some light on how they might be rectified.

This proved to be the case. The problems identified included disagreement about how to define the "duration of benefit" for various types of diseases and treatments, the lack of standards on how to group similar diagnoses, and incomplete or inaccurate data on costs. These issues were effectively addressed and the final priority list was substantially different.

The final document was released on February 21, 1991 and consists of seventeen categories, themselves prioritized on the basis of the commission's interpretation of the social values developed from the forty-seven community meetings mentioned earlier. Within each category are a series of condition/treatment pairs prioritized according to the benefit-cost formula. At the top of the list are: (1) acute fatal conditions where treatment prevents death with full recovery (e.g., appendicitis); (2) maternity care (e.g., prenatal, natal, postnatal); (3) treatment for chronic fatal conditions where treatment improves life span and quality of life (e.g., diabetes); (4) preventive care for children (e.g., immunizations); and (5) comfort care (e.g., hospice care). At the bottom of the list are conditions for which treatment does not significantly improve life span or quality of life.

The final priority list was given to an independent actuarial firm which determined the cost of delivering each element on the list through managed care. The list, along with the actuarial data, was given to the legislature on May 1. In May and June of 1991 the legislature will determine how many benefits on the priority list can be funded with existing revenue and how much additional revenue will be required to fund what the legislature considers an acceptable basic package. Because an estimated 120,000 citizens will be added to the Medicaid rolls, the legislature will unquestionably increase the total Medicaid appropriation.

We believe that the legislature will provide the extra funds for two reasons. First, legislators will know—for the first time—not only which services are being purchased with the new revenue, but also the effectiveness of the services and the value society places on them. Second, since preventive services are likely to be ranked highly, the investment will provide long-term cost savings by reducing the need for medical care later on.

Toward a Better System

Certainly the Oregon Basic Health Services Act constitutes a major departure from traditional approaches to solving problems of access and cost, and therefore should be scrutinized closely. No policy reform of this magnitude can avoid opposition, and our proposal has met with three main criticisms.

The most frequent, and most emotional, is that the act discriminates against women and children. This charge arises from the fact that only about one-third of all Medicaid dollars spent in Oregon go for services to aid families with dependent children, whereas the rest go to purchase services for the aged, blind, and disabled—groups excluded from the prioritization process. Thus it is argued that only women and children will suffer any benefit reductions that might result.

The argument ignores a critical distinction. Virtually all medical services for the elderly, the blind, and the disabled are funded by the federally administered Medicare program, not Medicaid. Most of the services provided for these groups under Medicaid are not medical treatments but social services, such as assistance in eating, bathing, and mobility. These services do not lend themselves to the medical services prioritization model and can be provided outside an institutional setting.

In fact, Oregon was the first state to be granted a federal waiver to use Medicaid funds for such services in home and community-based care, which we see as a less expensive and more humane alternative to institutionalization.

When these dollars are removed from the Medicaid pot, most of the remaining money is in fact spent on families with dependent children and, under the new act, on poor women and men without children. Also, the criticism confuses prioritization with resource allocation. Although social services were not prioritized, there is nothing in the legislation to prevent us from shifting some of these funds into the medical budget, if the public agrees that this is the best way to improve general well-being. Finally, this criticism ignores the thousands of women and children who are not now eligible for Medicaid but will be brought into the health care system through the employer participation required by the act.

The second criticism is that before we resort to rationing, we should eliminate waste from the current system. This assumes that we are not rationing health care now, which of course we are. And although the concern about eliminating waste is certainly valid, the Oregon proposal is one of the first to offer a systematic net-benefit analysis by which such waste can be identified and attacked.

Third, some critics suggest that if we must ration health care, the rationing should apply to all members of society, not just the poor. We agree in principle but believe that progress toward that policy objective will have to occur in several steps. Moreover, the criticism is more applicable to the status quo than to the Oregon proposal. For one thing, Medicaid now covers fewer than half of the people living below the poverty level, whereas our act provides assistance to all needy people.

In addition, the federal system offers public health care subsidies to virtually everyone in the United States except those who have no private insurance coverage and who are not eligible for either Medicaid or Medicare. In 1990 the government spent about $45 billion on Medicaid (states contributed another $33 billion) and $105 billion on Medicare; and because employer contributions to health insurance premiums are not taxable, the government provided a subsidy of well over $50 billion to the middle class.

Neither the Medicare subsidy nor that offered through the tax exclusion considers financial need—you get the subsidy regardless of your personal wealth. The irony—indeed, the hypocrisy—is that there are about 16 million working but uninsured Americans (plus their dependents) whose taxes help underwrite Medicaid, Medicare, and the tax exclusion but who are not eligible for any public subsidy themselves and cannot afford to pay private premiums.

Congress should correct the inequities in the current federal system of health benefits. In the meantime, we believe that Oregon is doing what a state can do to address today's implicit rationing of health care.

Federal Permission Needed

Oregon's proposal, passed by large bipartisan majorities in both houses of the state legislature and enjoying widespread public support, deserves the chance to move forward. What is needed is to have the federal government grant Oregon a waiver allowing the state to redesign the current package of mandated benefits. The waiver can be granted administratively by the Health Care Financing Administration (HCFA)—the agency that manages Medicaid—or granted statutorily by Congress. Because of the importance of this effort, and since HCFA has never awarded a waiver of this scope before, we are pursuing both routes.

Although the administrative waiver has not yet been submitted formally, HCFA officials have reviewed our draft proposal and offered technical recommendations that will be incorporated into the final request. Agency administrator Gail Wilensky, who generally favors allowing states to set up demonstration projects, has indicated that she will recommend approval of the waiver if it meets the agency's technical review.

HCFA has asked that the formal waiver request not be submitted until the Oregon Health Services Commission has completed its priority list and the legislature has established funding levels. Since the legislature will make its appropriation in late May or early June, the waiver process should be underway by early summer.

Once the waiver is submitted, HCFA will convene a panel of health care experts to pass judgment. The agency expects the review process to take about six months, which means that if HCFA approves the request Oregon would be able to implement the new program on July 1, 1992, Oregon's next fiscal year.

At roughly the same time our request is sent to HCFA, we will ask Congress formally to grant approval for the Secretary of Health and Human Services to issue the necessary waiver. It is important to note that our suggested waiver language asks for a waiver only if the secretary "determines that the standard of health benefits meets the basic health needs of the eligible population." We also are requesting a public comment period prior to any action by the secretary to allow our critics to examine the proposed benefit package before a waiver is granted.

Although the entire Oregon congressional delegation is supporting the waiver, two individuals are particularly well placed for the upcoming debate. Senator Bob Packwood is the ranking Republican on the Senate Finance Committee, which has jurisdiction over the Medicaid program in the Senate, and Congressman Ron Wyden, a Democrat, sits on the House Subcommittee on Health and the Environment, which oversees Medicaid in the House. In addition, support has been expressed by Senator Bob Kerry (D-Nebr.), Congressman Jim McDermott (D-Wash.), and Congressman Roy Rowland (D-Ga.).

Other states will be watching how Oregon's proposal fares at HCFA and in Congress. Colorado, Michigan, Iowa, Nebraska, Arizona, Massachusetts, Oklahoma, Alaska, and California have expressed considerable interest in our approach. Two states, Colorado and Michigan, have actually drafted similar legislation. In Colorado the legislation was introduced in early 1990; although the bill ultimately failed in committee, it precipitated valuable debate on the question of resource allocation. Most of the other states are waiting to see if Oregon is granted a waiver before beginning the difficult work of developing their own plans.

We believe it is clearly in the national interest to let Oregon put its plan into operation. Whether we are right or our critics are right cannot be known unless the plan is tried. At a minimum the experience will provide information that will be invaluable in addressing the health care crisis in America. If the plan succeeds, it can serve as a pattern for other states and, we hope, lead eventually to the kind of realistic and comprehensive federal action that the nation so sorely needs.

In June 1991 the Oregon Legislature appropriated $33 million in new revenue to this program. As expected, the availability of the priority list, the clear lines of accountability, and the fact that the tools of implicit social rationing had been statutorily eliminated, resulted in a responsible budgetary decision. The new appropriation funds all condition/treatment pairs through line 587 on the list of 709, resulting in a benefit package which covers virtually all current Medicaid mandates, including all preventive and screening services, plus coverage for such things as dental services, hospice care, prescription drugs, and mammograms not required by Medicaid. The waiver application was submitted in August 1991. Because the employer mandate is trigered by the waiver, a positive decision by HCFA or Congress will allow Oregon to provide this benfit package to 420,000 currently uncovered Oregonians, over 250,000 of whom are women and children.

8

Rationing: The Alameda County Experience

David J. Kears and Rodger G. Lum

Every poor family in America knows what it is like to ration products or services that most Americans take for granted—food, clothing, shelter, and the use of health care. For many, however, America is a country of plentiful resources, where access to those resources is taken for granted because it is rarely denied. Given the American social conscience, many argue that the United States should provide every resident, particularly the poor, access to basic human services, such as comprehensive health care (Bass et al. 1989).

However, few will argue that access should include whatever is medically necessary regardless of cost. The staggering price tag of certain medical procedures, along with rising health care premiums or copayments, have all heightened the public's awareness of cost (Janeway 1989). As Americans come to grips with the stark reality that health care is limited, perhaps by our own unwillingness to adequately finance it, there may then be greater pressures to debate who gets served, when they will get served, and what service they will get. What is already being discussed is rationing. However, for many Americans the idea of rationing, particularly on an explicit basis, is discomforting because of the moral issues raised.

Many Americans shy away from asserting that health care for the poor should be rationed—especially where policy or individual patient decisions will affect the quality of life or of life itself. Perhaps any definitive stance on explicit rationing is perceived as contrary to notions of American social ethics, in which certain human rights are considered inalienable, yet health care, interestingly, has never been declared such an inalienable constitutional right.

The most widely publicized and controversial effort to ration health care for a broad segment of the poor and uninsured is the state of Oregon's Medicaid priority-setting process begun in July 1987 (Kitzhaber 1988). Oregon's attempt to develop a value-based process for defining what medical services will be available for Medicaid recipients has generated national interest, as well as skepticism about its feasibility and criticism about its consequences. These concerns crystallized after seven-year old Adam ("Coby") Howard, in desperate need of a $100,000 bone marrow transplant, died of leukemia six weeks after the Oregon State Legislature decided it would no longer fund organ transplants for welfare recipients. The legislature was unwilling to fund such procedures at the expense of higher priorities such as prenatal care.

As in the state of Oregon, budgetary problems in California have worsened over the last ten to fifteen years. In 1978 and 1979, the passage of two measures in California to limit property taxes (Proposition 13) and government spending (the Gann Initiative) curbed the ability of counties to raise and utilize revenues. Consequently, counties experienced greater difficulty in subsidizing the difference between what the state mandates and what it will fund. Realizing that limits must be drawn on health care priorities, the county of Alameda, the fifth largest county in the state with a population of 1.3 million residents, embarked in the spring of 1989 on a process to examine its resources and the growing demands for health care, and to begin formulating explicit principles for rationing or allocating services.

This process was inspired by efforts in Oregon and drew heavily upon the expertise of prominent health care providers and advocates in the community. The county hired a bioethicist to frame the issues and facilitate the work. By reviewing and attempting to prioritize (and, in most cases, reprioritize) services and target populations, as well as those not provided or served, Alameda County had hoped to identify specific methods and policies to make the county system more equitable and responsive and to educate the public on the limitations of services available.

Background

Counties in the state of California function as providers of last resort, or as the "safety net," for the poor and the uninsured. They are the only governmental bodies that are responsible for the health care of all their people, and they rely heavily on public funding. The counties' mission includes the provision of comprehensive and accessible health care to those in need and unable to obtain care privately; health promotion and disease prevention; and environmental health protection. Over the last twenty-five years, scientific and technological advances have dramatically improved the quality and effectiveness of medical care, while standards and costs have risen accordingly. These advances have increased the public's expectation regarding access and quality of care and exceed the level of services made possible by funding. Initially, the state and federal governments promoted and financed this progress. Medicare/Medicaid set the groundwork for a public policy that promised equitable access to health care for all. As health care costs soared, however, state and federal government's willingness to sustain this funding commitment began to recede. In the last decade, counties have seen:

- Medicaid (or Medi-Cal, as it is known in California) reimbursement and negotiated contract rates frozen or increased at a rate lower than actual costs, which then discourages provider participation. Many physicians cite low Medi-Cal rates (currently about 58 percent of outpatient costs), cumbersome claims procedures, and high malpractice premiums as reasons for dropping out of Medi-Cal participation. Since 1988, 13 percent fewer physicians in northern California will accept Medi-Cal obstetric patients (*California Hospitals* 1990). In Oakland, the largest city in the county with its 360,000 residents, only two to three physicians in Oakland will do so.
- Direct state and federal subventions diminished or increased at subinflation levels (County Medically Indigent Services Program, Mental Health, Revenue Sharing, etc.).
- More state dollars categorically linked (tied to new mandates, programs, or targeted problems) and thus not available on a discretionary basis to address broad system deficits.
- Numbers of uninsured adult Californians under sixty-five years of age increasing steadily from 17 percent in 1979 to 22 percent in 1985 (Brown et al. 1987:4) and fast becoming a large percentage of the providers' uncompensated patient mix.
- State and federal mandates and regulations increased without corresponding allocation of funds, which then requires a growing commitment of county funding (Alameda County's net county cost has increased 76 percent, or $30 million, since fiscal year 1983–84).
- Local health resources drained by the epidemics of crack cocaine

and AIDS, the growing cost of trauma care for gunshot victims of drug wars, and the failure of the state-initiated deinstitutionalization of the mentally ill.

Private industry and insurance companies looking for ways to control exploding health care costs by shifting the cost of medical care from company to patient, or to counties.

The reality, then, is that health care for the poor and uninsured is rationed because of the widening gap between what the public needs and demands from its public health care system and what available resources will support. Clinics and programs operated or contracted by Alameda County all have extended waiting lists. The county's Highland General Hospital has experienced a 30 percent increase in outpatient and emergency room visits in just over two years, exacerbating already untenable waiting times. Patients needing an acute medical/surgical or ICU bed can wait up to sixteen hours and several days for a psychiatric bed to be available. Patients might wait up to eight hours in the emergency room for non-acute problems; six to thirty hours for an available acute-care bed; or seven to eight weeks for a clinic appointment. Approximately 176 patients per month leave the emergency room without being treated because they tired of the long waits. The disposition of these patients, including those with socially transmittable diseases, remains unknown.

Highland General Hospital's experience with restricted access is but one of many examples that pervade Alameda County's health care system and reflect a statewide problem. In effect, health care is rationed on the basis of increased inconvenience, delays in receiving care, and, in some cases, outright denial of care. Everywhere patients are turned away, and the care that is provided is often compromised by system overload. For instance, thirteen of fifty-five trauma centers in California have closed since 1980 because of heavy financial losses associated with a high volume of uncompensated care; this has exacerbated the access problem and has meant the difference between life and death for some patients diverted to trauma centers farther away.

Feeling that the county could no longer compromise care to the poor, particularly in light of the governor's proposal for massive reductions in health care for fiscal year 1989–90, the Alameda County Health Care Services Agency requested the County Board of Supervisors in April 1989 to establish a formal agency-wide process to examine available resources and to begin prioritizing services to benefit those most in need. The goal was to formulate a rational basis or policy for rationing health care, and to make explicit what was implicit.

Process

County health officials examined a variety of approaches, and eventually decided on a prioritization process similar to that utilized by the state of Oregon, but modified to reflect the manner in which the county health care system is organized. A Jesuit priest, Dr. John Golenski of the Bioethics Consultation Group who had assisted the state of Oregon, was hired to help frame the issues, organize and facilitate the process, and assist in preparing a report to the County Board of Supervisors.

However, the county's process was different from that used in Oregon in several key respects. First, the process used by the state of Oregon was far more involved, complicated, and extensive. Oregon's focus groups considered actuarial data and many more variables before developing a rank ordering of medical procedures that the Medicaid system would cover for welfare recipients. Second, the state of Oregon is a payer of health care services and does not directly provide services, as does a county. Each faces different demands and challenges.

Like Oregon's process, however, Alameda County utilized focus groups representing various service areas. Five such groups, each with ten members, were formed to represent alcohol and drugs, community health services (nonhospital-based primary care and public health), mental health, Fairmont Hospital (acute medical, rehabilitation, and skilled nursing care), and Highland General Hospital (emergency, trauma, and acute medical services). Department heads selected participants from a pool of prominent health care advocates, clinicians, and administrators in the community. Every effort was made to ensure balanced representation by sex, ethnicity, area of expertise, and geography.

The tasks of each group were to list the health care needs of people served by Alameda County; outline the services provided, as well as the needs not met; assess better ways to respond to the needs of target populations; and prioritize services and populations, where appropriate. The focus groups each met twice for all-day sessions, with a week between sessions.

Every group drafted individual reports and selected one representative from each group for an executive group that also included a representative of the Alameda-Contra Costa Medical Association, the agency director of the Health Care Services Agency, and three other members chosen by the agency director to provide technical and professional balance. The tasks of the executive group were to review the findings of the five focus groups, address issues not dealt with by the focus groups, and prepare an integrated report for submission to the Board of Supervisors, which is responsible for the final review, scheduling of public hearings, and adoption of any policy recommendations.

Objectives

The process had four key objectives:

1. Produce a document that describes and prioritizes target populations and services, and estimates costs associated with meeting these needs;
2. Publicize the links between levels of funding and services provided, and the gap between public expectations or needs and what funding will support;
3. Promote public dialogue regarding the crisis in health care and the need for major reform; and
4. Influence, however slightly, the state budget process so that further reductions in state funding to counties do not occur.

Findings

Common themes

Although a major objective was to prioritize existing services and client populations, none of the focus groups was able to reach consensus to do so. The failure to elicit the desired product from the review reflects both the difficulty of the task and the anguish participants felt over the county's existing health care system. Many participants believed that the current system of care for the poor was already overburdened, inadequate, and immoral, and that no amount of prioritizing could make it fairer or more rational. Furthermore, most focus group members were unwilling to ration care prior to an exhaustive review of cost-containment and revenue-enhancement strategies.

Many feared that a formal prioritization process would leave the system more vulnerable to further reductions in services. Many were fearful that opting for an explicit rationing process would play into the hands of fiscal and political conservatives who would want to maintain or reduce existing levels of government support for indigent care once local options to prioritize and reallocate services had been identified. Assurances that the prioritization would not be used to reduce care, but rather identify ways to make the system more responsive to those most in need, were not persuasive. The fact that the Health Care Services Agency and its departments prioritize now and would continue to do so in the face of increased demands and reduced revenue did not overcome participant concerns or fears. Others objected to the idea of prioritizing or rationing care for the poor only, and argued that this or any other health care reform process should occur statewide and address the health needs of the entire state. Panelists all felt that the state should debate the merits of major reforms that emphasize universal, not rationed, access to affordable, comprehensive health care.

All groups, however, were willing to identify and prioritize unmet needs in each departmental area, and to argue that new revenues should be directed to specific target populations or services. The executive group reviewed these suggestions and recommended the following five groups, ranked in order of priority:

- high-risk obstetric patients, especially substance-abusing pregnant women lacking access to prenatal care who were more likely to deliver low-birth weight and high-risk infants;
- minority populations whose access to care is limited by language and cultural barriers;
- high-risk youth and children, especially those from abusive and substance-abusing environments, or those from families with histories of mental illness;
- isolated and frail elderly people; and
- minority AIDS patients.

A number of criteria were considered in developing the list of priorities. First, the economic, social and quality-of-life consequences of denying or of not providing care had to be significant. Second, gaps in serving particular populations had to be large relative to need. The overriding concern, however, was to provide equal access for all, even to an inadequate system.

All five focus groups examined this general dilemma and the obstacles to obtaining health care access. Participants realized the difficulty of separating situational life problems from medical problems, and the futility of treating medical symptoms without addressing root causes. Beyond the immediate issues of long waiting lists and limited clinic hours, participants felt that access was further restricted by the lack of bilingual and bicultural services or the relative unavailability of telephones, child care, and transportation for the physically and developmentally disabled and the poor.

All participants called for a comprehensive approach to health care that (1) addresses the *root* causes of poor health—poverty, inadequate housing and educational opportunities, or alcohol and drug abuse; (2) balances emergency services and acute care with health promotion, disease prevention, and primary care; and, (3) emphasizes leadership, teamwork, and comprehensive planning. Two groups further recommended a comprehensive annual process of examining the health status of Alameda County and that such efforts document, monitor, and evaluate the impact of prior-year decisions or actions.

Although all participants articulated the need for a comprehensive approach, they also wanted to emphasize the needs of the individual. Unfortunately, categorical funding and reimbursements based on diagnosis-related groups (DRGs) tend to focus attention on symptoms, and not people, and provide little incentive for cooperation with other caregivers. Meanwhile, single-diagnosis patients are fast becoming the exception, making it difficult to distinguish the effects of drugs or the physical and social environments on mental and physical illnesses. A few mental health panelists suggested the use of "categorical" funding either from mental health or alcohol-and-drug services to help dual-diagnosis patients by developing creative, multidisciplinary programs. The community health group argued that care coordinators, by having been placed at the center of the delivery system, would help refocus attention on the needs of the person.

Focus group members believed that local health care providers could no longer bear primary responsibility for health care delivery, because doing so would be economically impossible and generally futile. Instead, they urged the county to emphasize health promotion, disease prevention, and early intervention, and to build stronger ongoing links between clients, communities, and providers. This broader focus would require a greater coordination and sharing of resources possible only with public and private sector involvement.

Program issues and concerns

In addition to common themes from all groups, each focus group identified issues and concerns specific to their department or service area.

Alcohol and drug programs. The alcohol and drug focus group felt that any comprehensive program must emphasize primary prevention and address social injustices, such as the lack of jobs or affordable housing, that result in alcohol and drug abuse. These programs would incorporate a social or public health model, emphasize intensive community interventions and citizen participation, and restructure social environments to reduce support for alcohol and drug use (e.g., by removing alcohol billboard advertisements in poor neighborhoods). To accomplish these goals, the group recommended that funding for prevention be increased 10 percent each year to achieve a fifty-fifty balance between treatment and prevention within five years.

The focus group recommended that more resources and greater attention must be given to the homeless, teens in the criminal justice system (including those on probation), women in their childbearing years, and people who are both HIV seropositive and intravenous drug users. However, the group stopped short of arguing that existing services or funding should be diverted to serve these priority populations.

Community health. The community health focus group argued that health promotion and disease prevention must be the cornerstone of any public health care system, without which at-risk populations would eventually require more expensive care. In addition, panelists felt that the lack of early primary care would overburden and destroy the health system's infrastructure by forcing people with preventable, nonacute needs to rely on expensive acute and emergency medical services later.

Participants advocated increased spending for community health services in proportion to the unmet needs, with 70 percent of any increase to go to primary care and the balance to health promotion and disease prevention. Consistent with this, members wanted to target schools, teenagers, and women of childbearing age. They advocated that school-based clinics be reinstated to provide early intervention and prevention and, in general, serve a significant population receiving inappropriate help through an acute care model. They believed that teenagers and women of childbearing age would benefit greatly from health-promotion efforts, particularly those enhancing self-esteem and increasing understanding of the negative effects of alcohol and drug use.

Mental health. Due to years of chronic statewide underfunding of the mental health system, Alameda County's Mental Health Services had gone much further than the rest of the health care areas in prioritizing services. As a result of a major prioritization process in 1982 (ACDMH 1982), and through more recent efforts, the department had already narrowed services to those with severe and persistent mental illnesses. The group also acknowledged that large numbers of nonpsychotic people needing treatment were excluded from care, largely due to stricter admission criteria. Acutely mentally ill patients who do not yet meet involuntary treatment criteria are often turned away from the psychiatric emergency service as "not yet sick enough" to require hospitalization. None felt that access to these high-risk populations could afford further compromise through funding reductions.

Despite these problems, the group acknowledged and struggled with the reality that other populations, in addition to those traditionally served by the system, were emerging with needs that were not even minimally addressed. These included:

- ethnic minorities, including immigrants and refugees, whose language and culture pose barriers to obtaining adequate care;
- dual-diagnosis clients, especially those with mental illness and substance abuse;
- children and adults whose mental health is severely impacted by substance abuse in the community; and
- AIDS patients, especially those with previously diagnosed mental illness and AIDS dementia.

Fairmont Hospital. The Fairmont Hospital focus group felt that the hospital was losing its identity as a skilled nursing facility (SNF) providing rehabilitation, and was instead becoming a multiservice center for the southern area of the county, with little planning or clear decisions to move in new directions. This expanded role, however, had taxed the capacities of the hospital. For instance, waiting times for the clinics and the inadequate hours for working people were sending people to the hospital's urgent-care facilities, and the SNF waiting list contained anywhere from twenty to fifty people, with the wait approaching a year in some instances. The group felt that the development of a comprehensive approach to health care in Alameda County would require the active involvement of providers in both the public and private sectors and ongoing evaluations of programs or services to maximize performance and effectiveness.

The group members argued that unless health promotion, early intervention, and postacute follow-up are addressed through local primary care centers, any coordinated approach to health care would be futile. In turn, unless some sort of managed care coordination were initiated (with case management for high-risk people), public hospitals in the county would be choked by patients who could be better served in less acute facilities.

Highland General Hospital. The Highland General Hospital focus group, representing the "choked" part of the system (or "the narrow end of the funnel," as they termed it), focused on the increasing number and acuteness of the patients they saw. They spoke of nonacute patients using an overloaded acute service and of problems created by high-risk patients with multiple diagnoses needing more attention than available resources permitted.

Patients turned away from overfilled primary-care services in public and private clinics utilize Highland General Hospital as the first—and last—resort. Not only does this mean that Highland becomes congested with primary-care patients who feel they have nowhere else to go, but they perceive Highland as the center—or the "shopping mall"— of the health delivery system. Not surprisingly, 25 to 33 percent of emergency room visits are essentially for primary-care services. To address this dilemma, panelists felt the system should be enhanced so that patients could obtain primary care from primary-care centers and their acute care and emergency services from Highland, as they had been intended.

The group further recommended that an urgent-care center be developed for the southern part of the county to ease the burden on the northern-based Highland General Hospital, that available facilities be purchased or leased for use in providing local primary-care services, and that the county support a bond measure for adequate physical facilities at Highland. In addition, the group members recommended that Highland General Hospital's perinatal program, in which physicians from the hospital worked in primary-care clinics for the purpose of prevention, early intervention, and enhanced communication, be studied for application to all other subspecialties, and that the teaching mission of Highland General Hospital be expanded to outpatient services. The group also recommended that services should not be reduced or staff forced to ration care at a time when Highland General Hospital was becoming more agressive in its fundraising efforts.

Definition of adequate care

All of the focus groups felt that any discussion of health care reform or rationing must first define what constitutes adequate care. Participants eventually agreed by consensus that for the purposes of this process the definition of "adequate care" would be based on *specific timelines by which patients ought to be seen or provided a bed*. The decision to define care in this way was primarily pragmatic. First, a detailed definition of care that specifies treatment interventions relative to diagnostic categories or symptomatology was beyond the scope of work and was best left for another process. Second, since one of the values of a definition is its utility as a measuring tool for the public to gauge the extent and responsiveness of care, it was felt that using timelines for broad categories could be more easily understood by the general public. Finally, this approach allowed the many departments within the Health Care Services

Agency to define standards of access and associated costs in a consistent fashion.

The definition proposed during the rationing debate was considered a preliminary one. Eventually, the costs of expanding services to meet standards must be more carefully formulated. Finally, a comprehensive, practical definition of adequate care that includes standards of access and an analysis of existing services in relation to those standards must be adopted and used by the state to develop budget and health care policies.

In developing this list, members considered (1) the principles of equity and equal access to care by underserved populations, however limited or inadequate that care may be; (2) the financial impact of not providing the services; (3) the human suffering and familial and societal disruption caused by neglect; and (4) the availability of adequate services or the presence of major service gaps. The following categories were formulated for each program area:

1. primary care,
2. emergency care,
3. acute care,
4. subacute care, and
5. long-term care.

For each category of service a more specific definition was developed and acceptable standards of access were established. The standards operating in the current system were then evaluated, and appropriate recommendations were made as to what and how much funding was needed to bring the current system up to standard. The outcome of this effort is reflected in tables 8.1 to 8.5.

In order to achieve an adequate level of health care, or an acceptable level of access to such care, Alameda County would have to spend at least $168.7 million more. Clearly, Alameda County with its already overburdened $300 million health care program has no such resource, nor could the county ever hope for funding from the state or federal governments to make the local system more equitable or accessible. Despite the finding that huge gaps exist which require priority setting, the focus groups argued that rationing such care to those already lacking adequate access was unthinkable and unconscionable. However, limited incremental increases in funding, particularly in light of the $168.7 million gap, simply will not suffice in making the system here in Alameda County, or in other overburdened counties, more fair or morally acceptable. At some point, we will all have to come to grips with the reality that Americans will not, or cannot, spend themselves out of a tough, excruciating moral quandary.

From the beginning, the process to ration care was both arduous and controversial. Few people deny that health care for the poor and uninsured is not now rationed, and almost all argue that our public health care system is in crisis and in need of major reform and augmentation. To advocate more funds is certainly a supportable and necessary position. To suggest that current health care expenditures may be better spent, or at least scrutinized to ensure that those most in need are those most served, provokes controversy, concern, and resistance.

It is understandable that a health care system under siege believes that it will be made more vulnerable through open review and prioritization of existing services and mandates. Nevertheless, the county, as the provider of last resort, must face the ethical issues associated with allocating limited resources. Alameda County tried to confront unpleasant realities and to propose solutions that include policy changes. Efforts were made to define adequate care and to educate the community on how far removed the system is from reasonable standards. This process was not initiated as a primer on how to best allocate limited health care dollars; it was intended as the first step toward a broader dialogue, and more importantly, as a commitment to an ongoing process.

In effect, rationing is a reality, whether publicized or not. Alameda County attempted to be open about this process and the ethical dilemmas it poses. Rationing health care is controversial, but it should not be imponderable. We need to define and debate what rationing is and is not, and face the fact that unless additional revenue is allocated or major reform implemented health care services will be stretched more thinly. We need to enter into a public dialogue about how much service we expect or want and are willing to pay for. At the very least, open forums on whether the public is willing to finance adequate health care for the poor are needed, and if the public is not willing, then broad ethical choices must be made about who among the disadvantaged and the disenfranchised will be served, about who shall live and who shall die. However difficult these moral choices are, they are everyday realities for those who help the poor. Aside from outright denial of health care to the poor, the most repugnant choice available is one where no action is taken, suggesting that the status quo is acceptable and morally defensible.

Those responsible for organizing the rationing process learned very quickly, however, that the outcome would not include a prioritized list of needs, services, or client populations. From the beginning, opposition

Table 8.1 Primary Care

Service components and definition	Standard of access	Current access	What needed to achieve standard	Cost of bringing to standard
A. Health promotion and prevention				
Various clinical, educational, nutritional, and consultation services designed to prevent disease and protect and promote public health	Early outreach training to prevent transmission of communicable diseases	County clinics: none Community clinics: none Hospitals: none	Staff and associated resources	$10,900,000
	Periodic public health nursing follow-up to high-risk infants during first year of life	County clinics: none Community clinics: none Hospitals: limited	Sufficient staff and resources for all services reflected below	Community health services: $950,000
	Outreach and assistance to high-risk groups in obtaining needed health and social services	County clinics: limited Community clinics: limited Hospitals: none		
	Availability of multilingual/cultural county-wide health promotion and prevention campaign for healthier life-style and reduction of risk of disability or death	County clinics: limited Community clinics: limited Hospitals: none		

Table 8.1 Primary Care (continued)

Service components and definition	Standard of access	Current access	What needed to achieve standard	Cost of bringing to standard
B. Mental health services				
A spectrum of services provided for prevention of hospitalization, stabilization, crisis or therapeutic intervention, and advocacy for clients. These services include acute day treatment for severely disordered, out-patient services for mentally disordered, case management for chronic mentally disordered at risk of re-hospitalization, community support services for those in need of living and vocational skills, mental health advocacy, and outreach services	1-month wait for outpatient acute day treatment Immediate access for severely disturbed patients and weekly or monthly outpatient visits for stabilized patients Case management, community support services, and advocacy services available when needed	Adults: up to 2 months Children/Adults: 4–6 months Adults: 1–7 week wait list Children: 1–3 month wait list	Staff and resources necessary to handle volumes, e.g. additional 150 slots for day treatment, additional 4,000 slots for visits, additional case managers and rehabilitation programs	$5,531,649

Table 8.2 Emergency Care

Service components and definition	Standard of access	Current access	What needed to achieve standard	Cost of bringing to standard
A. Medical				
Range of services provided for alleviation of severe pain or immediate diagnosis and treatment of unforeseen medical conditions that may result in disability or death if services are not provided immediately	Care provided immediately for life-threatening conditions, and within 2 hours for non–life-threatening emergencies	Highland: Wait up to 8 hours for non–life-threatening conditions	Sufficient staff and resources to expand capacity.	$12,198,000
B. Psychiatric				
Services designed to provide crisis intervention and immediate therapeutic response to clients exhibiting acute psychiatric symptoms	Immediate if life threatening. Available as needed if not life-threatening	1–3 hours for non–life-threatening	Meets standard	$1,129,284
	Immediate availability of 24-hour crisis intervention	8 hrs/day, 7 days/wk (including mobile unit)	24 hrs/day, 7 days/ week, (including mobile unit)	

Table 8.3 Acute Care

Service components and definition	Standard of access	Current access	What needed to achieve standard	Cost of bringing to standard
A. Inpatient				
A wide range of medical surgical, and ancillary services provided for treatment of illness or injuries requiring 24-hour intensive care	Availability of bed when admission is required	Waiting time ranges from 6–30 hours. Lack of staff may preclude admissions	Sufficient staff and capital resources to increase bed capacity and provide for required consultative and diagnostic services	$6,163,700
B. Psychiatric inpatient				
Intensive 24-hour psychiatric treatment services provided to severely mentally disordered experiencing acute symptoms	Availability of bed when admission is required	Nearly 100% occupancy in current unit results in inappropriate housing of patients in emergency room	Staff and resources to increase capacity by 70 beds	$12,296,850
C. Crisis residential care				
Alternative treatment to acute hospital care for treatment of those experiencing situational distress	Availability of bed when admission is required	100% occupancy	20 beds	$234,520
D. Inpatient rehabilitation services				
Restorative inpatient care including intensive therapeutic regimes for severely impaired in need of intensive 24-hour service to develop function beyond what would occur in the normal course of recovery	Availability of bed within 72 hours of referral	Bed is typically available; however, lack of staff may preclude admission	Adequate manpower	Fairmont: $283,000

Table 8.4 Subacute Care

A. Rehabilitation Services

Restorative inpatient care including less intensive therapeutic regimes than those provided in acute setting. Length of stay usually does not exceed 3 months	Availability of bed within 1 week of referral	Lack of staff resulting in diversion of patients to other facilities	Manpower to handle volume	Figure included in acute service

B. Mental health

Transitional inpatient care provided to severely mentally disordered and emotionally disturbed. It is usually used as an alternative or follow-up to hospitalization	24-hour transitional care within 1–3 days Sub-acute care within 1 week Bed available in state hospital within 1 week	Adult: 2 weeks–3 months Child: 1–4 months 2 days–3 months 2 months–2 years	Resources to increase capacity by 102 transitional, 66 subacute, and 36 specialty beds in lieu of state hospital	$8,461,560

Table 8.5 Long-Term Care

Service components and definition	Standard of access	Current access	What needed to achieve standard	Cost of bringing to standard
A. Medical				
Inpatient care requiring medical and therapeutic services exceeding 3 months. This includes services appropriate for chronically ill and severely disabled individuals	Availability of bed within 1 week of referral	Neurorespiratory: 3 months Skilled nursing: 2–12 months	Staff and resources to increase capacity by 36 SNF beds and 4 neurorespiratory	Fairmont: $4,981,000
B. Mental health				
Inpatient and out-of-home placements for severely and persistently mentally disordered and chronically disabled	1-week wait for available bed in Institutes of Mental Diseases within 1 week Supplemental rate program (SRP) board and care within 1 week	1–9 months for IMD 100 additional board and care residents have been identified as needing SRP program	Staff and resources to increase capacity by 50 IMD beds and 100 board & care beds	$2,043,019

to rationing was readily apparent. In fact, many of those invited to serve on the focus groups had labored for years to ensure a more equitable system of care. It was inconceivable for them to argue for anything less than expanded services. Rationing was unacceptable. However, these advocates were invited to serve on the focus groups because they represented a key component of our county health system, either as providers or as advocates. Any representative panel simply cannot exclude people just because of differing health policy views. For many of these people, the invitation to serve elicited conflict—would their participation imply acceptance of rationing? Would they be outvoted and then be counted as a member of a group that endorsed explicit rationing? However, the opportunity to participate and to influence other members was too irresistible.

Many people will ask whether the health care system be reformed in such a way as to render rationing academic or unnecessary. However, we need to acknowledge that even with the move toward national health insurance, no one, including advocates, has argued for unlimited access to comprehensive medical care with no regard for cost. All health insurance proposals presented to date involve limiting access, eligibility, and services. These limits are especially necessary, since compromises are necessary to achieve broad support from those asked to finance universal access, namely employers and taxpayers.

Although the attempt to develop explicit policies on rationing failed, the process did dramatize the crisis in county health services in terms of underfunding, the many unmet needs, the stretching of limited resources, or the unrealistic standards set by governmental agencies that expect local jurisdictions to do more with less. Alameda County captured the attention of many health care policymakers because it wanted to explore rationing on a rational, explicit, and public basis. The failure to adopt a plan does not signal the impracticality or foolhardiness of such attempts. Rather, it emphasizes how different it is to confront problems directly and to assume accountability for decisions all policymakers would just as soon not make.

Regrettably, the repugnancy or unnecessariness of health care rationing for the poor will not alone stem the tide. Health care access will be improved only when public funding parallels public expectations. Until then, tough decisions regarding what services are provided and to whom will continue to be made. The only real question is whether or not those decisions will be made openly, and whether or not anyone will assume responsibility for them.

References

Alameda County Department of Mental Health (ACDMH). 1982. *Management by Priorities.*

Bass, Carol, Judy Bramson, Kathy Glasmire, and Patricia Staton. 1989. *California Health Decisions: Involving the Public in Health Care Choices (Sacramento Area).* Final Report of a Two-Year Education Program and Study of Public Opinion on Ethical Issues in Health Care, May 23.

Brown, E. Richard, R. Burciaga, Hal Morgenstern, Tom Bradley, and Chris Hafner. 1987. *Californians Without Health Insurance: A Report to the California Legislature.* Berkeley: Regents of the University of California.

California Hospitals. 1990. 4(5):52–53.

Janeway, Richard. "The Costs of Medical Care in a Society with Changing Goals: A Longitudinal View." In Jack D. McCue, ed., *The Medical Cost-Containment Crisis: Fears, Opinions, and Facts,* pp. 15–40. Ann Arbor, Mich.: Health Administration Press Perspectives.

Kitzhaber, John. 1988. "Uncompensated Care—The Threat and the Challenge." *Western Journal of Medicine* 148(6):711–716.

9

Organizing a Health Care Vision

Daniel Callahan

The United States is notorious for lacking any formal national health care planning process. There are those who think that is a strength. They laud the plurality of health care possibilities and plans in the United States, at both the federal and the state level and for both government and private programs. The evidence is beginning to suggest, however, that the lack of a national planning process is one of the major impediments to a cost efficient and equitable health care system. Pluralism is a wonderful value for a cultural and political system. In the case of health care, however, it has led inexorably to a great confusion of goals, purposes, and strategies. The result is not only a lack of planning but an absence as a consequence of effective means of managing the present system even on a day-to-day basis. A thousand flowers have been allowed to bloom, and they have created a weed garden. This is a great deficit.

Yet there is something even more fundamental lacking in the American health care system; a vision of long-term goals and ends. To be sure, many statements and declarations appear to suggest some long-term goals. They include "equal access," the meeting of all "health needs," and, for some, the conquest of the great killer diseases. But these are not the kinds of goals the nation needs; first, because they are either inherently unattainable or illusory, and, second, because they really deal with means rather than ends. "Equal access" to what in the name of what?

Meeting the "need" to stay alive—forever? Conquering the great diseases—which will then be replaced by what other diseases? Questions of this kind are rarely addressed; doing so forces a contemplation of ultimate purposes, and they are in short supply.

Instead, Americans have a full-court pluralism, both about means and ends. We might well agree that pluralism in health care is a value that we should respect, recognizing different cultural, economic, and political values. But at the same time we might concede that there ought to be a general vision or sense of overall direction that would provide some shape and direction to the pluralism; something more is needed than a pluralism that represents a free-for-all, with everyone competing against everyone else.

The idea of pluralism is not incompatible with some shared vision. Indeed, the idea of a society that embodies an active and viable pluralism must share some underlying agreement about the common good in order to have gained acceptance of the tolerance and diversity—and continuous disagreement—that pluralism entails. At the same time, there must be some agreement on the boundaries of the pluralism; at the least, values destructive of pluralism itself cannot be tolerated. The notion of pluralism as total chaos is not only impractical, it means that there can be no agreement on the values to be shared even in pursuing pluralism. In the case of health care, we now have diversity—the facade of pluralism—but increasingly seem bereft of some guiding vision and direction to give it form and substance.

Americans need to begin this work of shaping a common vision of the future of the nation's health care system in a comprehensive fashion. Even if we cannot agree on practical plans at the moment, we might begin the work of trying to envision where we want to go, where we would like to see things ten or twenty or thirty years from now, and at least begin sketching a direction. Perhaps because our country has been affluent for a number of decades, perhaps also because the pursuit of health has had unlimited public support in many respects, a general direction or plan has seemed unnecessary. It was sufficient simply to deal with the illnesses and diseases before us, go after them on all fronts, and not ask any further questions.

But we are now coming to a critical juncture in the American health care system, indeed in the health care systems of all developed countries. Letting all flowers bloom, or all choices be made, will not be possible in the future. The escalating costs of health care in the face of aging populations and technological advances mean that some clear directions must be chosen. Yet doing so will be impossible unless there is at least some rough consensus on what, in general, a health care system ought to provide and how it should cope with the kinds of problems it is likely to meet in the future. This is pertinent not only because of pressing economic and social issues, but also because the American health care system is bound to change, indeed will be forced to change, over the next few decades. It is time we anticipated where things might possibly go and try to sketch a vision of the possibilities.

As a concrete matter, in any case, most of the practical proposals for reform now before us cannot work effectively unless they are set in the context of some agreement on the general direction of the health care system. The one direction that cannot work, the historical evidence suggests, is one that simply allows each individual social unit to set its own goals and pursue them with as much vigor as possible. That leads to chaos, and the marks of such chaos are all around us: a maldistribution of access, enormous variation in practice standards, and significant regional differences in quality. Beyond that, the reform methods that are now being urged will not work unless they have something to be measured against. The system has been urged for a number of years now to engage in effective cost containment. Yet it seems increasingly evident that cost containment cannot be achieved short of some agreement on what ought to be limited or regulated as a way of better managing costs, on where discipline should be applied, and on what ought to be sacrificed for what.

Let me give some examples. Cost-benefit analysis, widely promoted, cannot operate unless there is some agreement on what counts as a benefit and on what counts as a cost. We have left those decisions in the hands of individuals or local institutions, thus making it difficult to use cost-benefit analysis effectively as a national policy tool. The widespread belief in technology assessment is bound to be misplaced unless, with that form of analysis, we come to some agreement on the burdens and benefits of different technologies, and some agreement on the weight to be given to different outcomes. The idea that we can simply do technology assessment in a politically, socially, and ideologically neutral context makes no sense.

Finally, there have been numerous efforts in recent years to apply theories of justice to health care. Most of them have been unrewarding and unilluminating because they have not been complemented by some agreements on the goals of the health care system. Somehow it has been assumed that the goals for the system can be set independently of questions of justice, and that questions of justice really pertain only to distributional matters. In one sense that is true, of course. But lacking a clear notion of where a health care system is supposed to go, and thus a notion of how much should be allocated to health care in the first place and what its purpose should be, it is impossible to carry out an effective analysis based on any known theory of justice.

In sum, practical questions of cost containment and more general questions of equity require a background vision of where the health care system should be heading, and what kind of system it should be in terms of its overall goals and values. We have lacked such a vision in the United States; indeed, we have even lacked agreement on whether it is good to have such a vision or picture. But it is practical to argue that we need such a vision as a theoretical substrate in order to give us some way to shape conceptually the problems that face us. Lacking a vision, the most popular remedies for efficiency and for economic and technological assessments simply cannot be used effectively.

A number of steps are necessary in developing a general picture, or vision, of the health care system of the future: (1) determining the place of health in human life, (2) achieving a sufficient level of good health, (3) setting health care priorities, and (4) specifying moral obligations. By setting out a general framework, we might at least agree upon a vision that is sensible. If not, then this framework might serve to identify some important junctures from where we could choose different directions.

The Place of Health in Human Life

The first step in creating a vision for a health care system is to confront the question of the place of health in human life. This is the most basic question of all. Unless there can be some agreement on the relative value of health in relationship to other goods, it is difficult to see how, as a society, we can have any kind of coherent discussion—at least one set, as it must be politically, within a whole range of other social and political needs—of the health care system at all. We will have to find a way of thinking about health in relationship to other human needs, and about what different forms and degrees of health mean to human flourishing. A fair amount of information is available on the effects of education, housing, and income on general health, along with a great deal of knowledge on the educational, housing, welfare, and other needs of our society. Engendering a discussion of the relative place of health among all these needs ought to be possible.

The pursuit of good health should enhance individual flourishing and societal welfare. We need a focus on health that looks both to the individual and to society, not to one or the other alone. Yet health is a means to human well-being, not an end in itself. If we are in terrible health, it is probably nearly impossible to be happy as human beings. Yet to be in perfect health does not in itself guarantee that we will be happy. No obvious symmetry exists between health and human happiness, and in any event, we cannot create a society that makes health its overriding purpose, just as we would find it implausible to make health alone the purpose of a human life. If we make health an end in itself, then inevitably it will trump all other social needs and will admit no boundaries or limits at all.

In thinking about health, it is important also to recognize the obvious: that aging, sickness, decline, and death are an inherent part of the human condition. Good health is, in this respect, a necessarily temporary, not a permanent, human condition. At some point, our health will decline, we will sicken, and we will die. We cannot afford to ignore this primary reality, as our present health care ideology too often does. One of the great problems with this ideology is that it tacitly assumes we can pursue health in such a way as to do away, eventually, with aging, sickness, and death. No one says that, of course, but it seems very much implicit in many of the patterns and practices of contemporary medicine, and surely in contemporary medical research. To pursue a conquest of those conditions that make us mortal human beings as though such a conquest were the highest goal of human life and society would be a distortion of sensible human ends and purposes. In the nature of the case, we can never have perfect health. Even if we could achieve it momentarily, we would not sustain it indefinitely; bodies do not last forever.

Achieving a Sufficient Level of Good Health

The second step in devising a vision is to determine when some sufficient level of health has been achieved, both for the individual and for society. What would count as "enough good health"? This is a fundamental question because, given the finitude of the human body, there is now, and always will be, the possibility of something going wrong. If "enough health" is perfect and enduring health, we cannot have it. It seems to be a biological truth that no matter what diseases we cure, there will always be successor diseases. Hence, we cannot even define as "enough good health" the conquest of disease and illness, since they are going to be ever present, and since the possibility of meeting human needs in the context of inevitable biological decline is going to be open-ended.

Determining when a society has "enough good health" may be easier than deciding when an individual does. At least we might come to some agreement on the former more readily than on the latter. Let me address both problems, however. A society might be said to have enough good health when a majority of its citizens are able to manage their social obligations effectively and run the necessary institutions of society. Put another way, a society will have a sufficient level of health when its major social, political, and familial institutions are not impeded by the poor health of its citizens. When we recollect that one of the major consequences of plagues and epidemics in the past was the (at least temporary) wrecking of all the important social systems, one can understand the importance of health as a foundation for an economic, educational, and political system. If a population in general has enough health that its institutions flourish, and an absence of good health among some of its population cannot be advanced as a main reason for the failure in those institutions, then one might say that a society has "enough health."

At the same time, if various groups within the society—as is the case with the poor and minority groups in the United States—are themselves not functioning effectively in the general institutional systems because of poor health, then that would be inequitable, and also harmful to the society as a whole. A society would be deprived of their social contributions while simultaneously being forced to bear the cost and other burdens that the poor health of one group can bring to the society as a whole. One can, therefore, make a distinction between the good health of the society in general and the good health of particular groups within the society. At present, white, middle-class, reasonably affluent Americans have enough good health to do everything they as a group need to do in society, and society is already able to get from this group what it needs for its own purposes. There is no important societal need for an overall improvement in the health status of this group, however much an improvement might benefit individual members of our group. We are already the healthiest people in the history of the human race.

Matters are different at the individual level. The problem here is that there are no potential limits to individual desires to want more life and better health. In particular, the pursuit of the cure of illness is of necessity infinite in its possibilities: unless we achieve immortality, we can be sure that something will go wrong with our bodies, and that as one condition is cured, another eventually will appear to take its place. Therefore, it becomes very difficult for individuals to say when they have enough good health. Nonetheless, individuals could be said to have enough good health when they are able to take their place within the political and cultural institutions, carry out the normal expectations of society, and live long enough to become elderly. This does not require perfect health; people can be effective citizens and function well in a society even if they are to some extent disabled, suffer from a chronic illness, or are otherwise burdened with some degree of mental or physical illness. When those burdens become genuinely inhibiting is a matter of degree. But individual functioning does not require a total absence of all illness or disability.

Whatever its definition, it is important that we talk about the question of enough good health because unless we do so, the very plenitude of potential human needs, forever open to invention, manipulation, and escalation, will constantly overwhelm us. The fact that we can always want more, even reasonably want it, does not mean that it is impossible to say that we have enough good health. The question is whether we ourselves, and our society, can get by without that "more," and still at the same time have a decent society. In many cases we surely can.

Setting Health Care Priorities

The third step, once we have agreed on the general place of health in human life, and on what would count as a sufficient level of good health, is to determine which priorities should be the most important within the health care system. My own particular priority is that a society ought first of all to aim for the overall good health of its citizens and not for the individual good health of particular members of its society. The reason is rather simple: if we can pursue the overall health of society effectively, we can be sure that we will also in general be improving the health of most individuals. Our pursuit of a decent general level of health care should be measured by the overall ability of a majority of individuals in that society to function well. Our first standards about health should be societal and communal in nature, not focused on individual needs.

The important point with this third step is to begin to come to some agreement on what is comparatively more or less important in the health care system. We can do this in a variety of ways. We can ask what might be the least expensive way of achieving the most health for the most people, using a general, utilitarian standard for doing so, and some objective (e.g., functional) standard to measure good health. We could, alternatively, ask what would create a subjective sense of good health, and that in turn might be utilitarian, depending upon individual preferences. This approach, however, has potential drawbacks. Some health needs, for instance, are so imperative that even if meeting them would not pass a utilitarian standard, they should be pursued, perhaps on the grounds that a failure to meet such needs would be in itself a sign of an inhumane society. Some health needs—those involving great pain, or a radical shortening of life, or an enormous burden upon others—would likely qualify for special status. In any event, in trying to set health care priorities it would be important to determine whether certain individual and societal needs are so paramount and transcendent that they simply should not be measured against other potential needs in a priority system.

In trying to establish a general set of health priorities, it will be important to have a policy bias: not a rigid set of rules and hierarchies but a proclivity to move in one direction rather than another, admitting the possibility of many exceptions and stressing that variations and gerrymandering are not impossible. My own bias is to have a health care system organized in the direction of public health, the common good, and a sufficient level of health for the operation of the major institutions of society. This does not by any means preclude special arguments being made for individual needs, in particular some disease conditions so painful, so stressful, and so threatening to individuals that they ought on occasion to be able to transcend the group needs of the society. Indeed, even in trying to set priorities within the health care system, a countervailing set of individual biases to offset the more cruel possibilities of a strictly societal emphasis is a necessity.

How could this be achieved? At the very heart of the health care enterprise ought to be individual caring; that is, a dedication to relieving human suffering, to not abandoning individuals to their fate without human company, to doing everything possible to help people endure their disabilities and illnesses. Caring does not cure disease or extend life, but provides support and comfort for those who are afflicted. With caring as its first priority, the health care system could then move on to a public standard marked by immunization, public health, and the provision of primary and emergency medical services. Beyond these services, when the system moves into more expensive curative therapies, resource scarcity will call up the question of whether there is a sufficient societal level of good health; at some point, aggressive pursuit of those individual curative modes will diminish. However, if the system provided a decent level of caring, and taken care of the general public health needs of the population as a whole, it already would have established an adequate level of health care. The system should not have to try to meet all individual needs.

Specifying Moral Obligations

The fourth step in fashioning a health care vision is to come to some understanding of the obligations of individuals, families, and society in the provision of good health care. Regardless of political or ideological leanings, everyone these days seems to recognize that contemporary health care is enormously expensive, especially in the case of major illnesses, and beyond the resources of most individuals. This is why, quite apart from government support of health care for the poor, there is widespread agreement in our society that employers should provide health care coverage as part of their general fringe benefits. Society recognizes that not only is it important that individuals have that kind of protection, but that it is best provided in an organized way; that is why we turn to insurance systems.

Among those groups that should have major duties, the obligation of government should be to make certain that there is a decent general level of health care for all, whether this is achieved through specific entitlement programs that the government itself manages or finances or more indirectly through government encouragement and subsidy of individual employer programs. Since one major purpose of government is to ensure the overall welfare of society, government necessarily must be responsible for making sure that there is a sufficient level of good health to enable the major institutions of the society to function well. This role of government is consistent with a general bias toward public and communal health.

Government, however, cannot do everything. It cannot entirely replace the family, if only because the cost of providing government support for everything provided to the sick by family members would be prohibitive. More important, under many circumstances sick people need the help of loved ones, not strangers, however dedicated. It is reasonable for government to aim to provide a generally decent level of care for all, up to and including primary care, but at the same time to expect that family members will bear some significant degree of the care and function themselves.

What should be the limits here? My own answer is this: when family life itself is clearly being overburdened, or destroyed, because of the requirement that family members take care of each other. At this point, government has an interest in making sure that families are not overwhelmed. The consequences of this kind of burden are not only economic difficulties, but other forms of individual and social pathology that can extend beyond the immediate family into the surrounding community. If government leaves families to their own devices, any serious problems that emerge almost certainly will impinge upon the larger community. Hence, making a sharp distinction between what is going to benefit the family and benefit the larger community is very difficult.

Special Future Challenges

The four general steps discussed here have outlined the major problems our society must think about in envisioning a health care system for the future At the same time, it is important to recognize that there are going to be some special additional challenges in the future. Let me mention some of them, and suggest ways they might be built into the general scheme I have sketched above.

The first problem is the growing number and proportion of the elderly in our society. The great difficulty here is not simply that there will be a change in the ratio of old to young, with fewer young people available to provide financial support for the health and welfare needs of a larger population of elderly people. Rather, because of medical progress and the likely increase in morbidity associated with increased life spans, the needs of the elderly possibly will come to dominate, and distort, the needs of the health care system in general.

In trying to think about the health care needs of the future, then, it is imperative that we come to some agreement on relative age group priorities. We cannot afford (nor does it make good sense) to adopt an egalitarianism that treats each age group in absolutely the same way, and to accord equal health care standing to individuals regardless of age. A more sensible priority would be to say that, in general, the needs of the young ought to take precedence over the needs of the old; or put another way, every young person ought to have a basic right to the chance to become an old person. Once a person is old, that person has already achieved a major purpose of a health care system: that of avoiding premature death. To say this does not abandon the elderly but only suggests that in order for all age groups to have some equality of chances in life, we will have to make sure that the needs of one group do not inevitably—by virtue of increased need as a result of the success of becoming old—negate the possibility of meeting the needs of other groups.

The likelihood of open-ended progress in therapeutic interventions to save or improve the lives of the elderly means that some firm limits will have to be set for health care for the elderly; and this in turn requires that some priorities must be set (even if only a rough kind) between and among different age groups. This difficult task might best be thought of in terms of each of the four steps sketched earlier:

1. How should we think about the place of health in the lives of individuals at different stages of life?
2. What might count as a sufficient level of good health for a particular age group?

3. What are appropriate health care priorities for different age groups?
4. Who should have the primary obligation for the health care (and personal care) for each age group?

A second problem is that of expensive, virulent, and contagious diseases. AIDS provides the obvious contemporary example. How will it be possible to deal with the enormous human toll and economic impact of AIDS in the years ahead without thoroughly distorting the health care system? The emphasis should fall heavily on immunization research, prevention, and health education—a trio of methods that is likely to bring the broadest benefit in the long run. The most delicate and painful point will come as we increasingly develop expensive methods of prolonging—but not saving—the lives of people with AIDS. AZT, of course, is the obvious case in point, and the drug has made AIDS a very expensive chronic illness. In trying to deal with this problem, it is obvious that, by any standards, the threat of AIDS to the lives of individuals, and to whole groups, is so significant that it must be given a high priority. At the same time, the government would be justified in primarily emphasizing those features of the disease that have the most impact on public health, and leaving to the private sector, or to individuals, those aspects that bear most importance upon personal well-being.

This of course cannot be a hard-and-fast rule but only a priority. As a policy, it ought to be complemented by the primacy of caring: the major thing that we owe to all those who are suffering from AIDS is to make certain that they are not abandoned, that they receive comfort and palliation, and that they have health and social services that will make their lives as tolerable as possible.

A third problem is the growing likelihood of expensive individual cures for people of all age groups. We know it is now possible to save low birth weight babies at great expense, to provide organ transplantation for people in their adult years, and then to find very elaborate technological means of prolonging the lives of the elderly. It is at the borderline where individual needs become enormously expensive and begin to threaten the overall welfare of society that some of the most difficult moral problems of health care are to be encountered. No doubt the effort to meet individual curative needs often leads to more and more expensive solutions; and it is proper enough to note that we ought not morally reject the meeting of those needs simply on the grounds that they are expensive. But in setting overall priorities for a health care system, making certain that public health needs are reasonably well met before giving a high priority to the more expensive individual curative needs seems important.

A fairly plausible decision making procedure is possible here. We ought not to lavish money on expensive neonatal care unless we have made certain that we have supported prenatal care programs well. We ought not to lavish large amounts of money on organ transplantation until we have spent money devising less expensive ways of reducing risks for the kinds of illnesses that require organ transplantation. We ought not to spend large amounts of money in prolonging the lives of the elderly until we have made certain that we have also provided for quality, not simply extension, of life. In other words, we need to take the general bias of the health care system toward the common good and apply it rigorously in these cases as well. We will in fact often have enough money to go beyond simply meeting general health needs. But this is precisely how a bias functions: it points us in a certain direction, giving us a general framework within which to operate, but it also allows for exceptions and flexibility.

Hence, in giving priority to prenatal care in the case of pregnant women, to education and other modes of health promotion for other diseases, we should not abandon acute-care medicine, much less abandon efforts to improve it. Simply, such efforts should have a lower priority and should not be fully explored, elaborated upon, or developed unless we have made a powerful effort to put into place preventive measures. There can be no perfect formulas for any of this; hopefully the words *picture* and *vision* have conveyed the wish that our society will look for a broad orientation rather than a set of formulas.

Much future discussion of such a broad topic as the goals of the health care system will inevitably be vague and uncertain. As time goes on, it will be important to agree to some limits to pluralism in health care, and to some general biases and an overall direction on the part of government and society about the goals of health care. The great problem with our health care system is that we have not yet attempted to do any of these things, and we have paid a grievous price for that omission. If only we can begin talking about the ideal and long-term ends of the system, we might eventually be in a better position to plan a system that is more adequate, more efficient, and more equitable.

II

Emerging Issues in Genetic and Reproductive Technologies

Introduction: Emerging Issues in Genetic and Reproductive Technologies

Andrea L. Bonnicksen

The New Genetics

Nearly 100,000 genes, contained in the "microscopic macrame weaving" (Suzuki and Knudtson 1989:48–49) of DNA molecules, direct biological processes in virtually all of the 100 trillion cells in the human body. Those who study the "dance" of the genes are confounded by the wonder of gene-directed activities within the cell. Those who study the societal implications of the ability to splice and recombine genetic instructions are confounded by the uncertainty of what could lie ahead. Genetic manipulation, a field still in its infancy, has enraptured and frightened, intrigued and repelled observers in nearly equal measure. Agreement is growing, however, that the new genetics is unfolding at a rapid pace demanding attention, direction, and public choice.

Novelty is a notable feature of the new genetics. Cells taken from a person's body for genetic correction and reinsertion make the patient his or her own tissue donor. Genetic manipulation of animals produces new strains, but not new species, such as Oncomouse, a mouse genetically engineered to develop tumors rapidly for research purposes. People diagnosed as carrying a genetic disease with symptoms that will not appear for decades now fall into a new medical limbo in which they are classified as pre-ill, or presymptomatic ill. Emerging genetic techniques bring with them concepts that challenge the way we view illness, medicine, and health. New strains of animals, notions of tissue donation, and definitions of disease all propel genetics beyond the science laboratory to become part of the societal consciousness. The link between science and social thinking has rarely been so basic and intricate.

The new genetics, which is not universally praised or welcomed, has raised fundamental uncertainties about values and priorities. Is it appropriate, for example, to invest money and energy in the study of genetically linked diseases affecting a small number of people when basic health needs for a large number of people are not being met? Does the excitement about locating disease genes divert attention from seemingly intractable social health problems such as poverty, pollution, and substance abuse that depend upon will rather than technique for their resolution? Or will genetic discoveries have a ripple effect, eventually promoting health for the many citizens affected by a broad range of genetic diseases?

Will the infusion of genetic discoveries into society ultimately be liberating in its capacity to treat and perhaps end diseases? Or will it have an oppressive impact by creating new disease categories, reducing tolerance of genetic dysfunction, and opening the door to genetics-based discrimination? Will genetic discoveries place new, not necessarily wanted obligations on citizens as well as offer them expanded choices? What challenge do genetic technologies pose to our sense of responsibility to future generations? Is it our responsibility to prevent the passing of genetic disease, or to protect genetic variability, even if that means passing on harmful genetic predispositions?

From these and other uncertainties have come pressures for public action. At present, the new genetics is practiced among individuals. Scientists study genes in laboratories, genetics counselors set up clinics for prenatal screening, couples undergo amniocentesis or chorionic villi sampling during pregnancy, technicians develop delivery systems for gene therapy, and corporations genetically engineer organisms for the pharmaceutical market. Public acts by policymakers tend to be sparse and isolated. Debate is building, however, and we have entered a decade in which decisions about committing public money to the new genetics and/or imposing limits on the field cannot be avoided. Four categories of public choice stand out as the most compelling.

Affirmative Commitment to Basic Research in Genetics

Genes are biochemical units on DNA molecules codified with enough information to direct the assembly of amino acids into a polypeptide

(Suzuki and Knudtson 1989:52). Each human cell contains 46 chromosomes made up of long, spiraling DNA molecules in turn comprised of stretches of genes. The geneticist's dream is to locate, map, and sequence all of the 50,000 to 100,000 genes in the human cell. This will create "an encyclopedia of the human genome" (McKusick 1989:913) useful, among other things, for identifying the genes associated with diseases. Nearly 5000 diseases have been linked already to single genes; this number grows monthly, and many polygenic diseases are also being examined. Supporters of gene mapping predict that such work will yield an extremely useful "set of instruction books" (Watson 1991:44) and will have far-reaching implications for disease prevention and treatment.

The idea of mapping the human genome took shape in the mid-1980s, when scientists at the Department of Energy, looking for substitute research projects in anticipation of a declining need for weapons research, suggested examining mutations, if any, among children of the survivors of Hiroshima (Angier 1990:B8). Around the same time a scientist published an editorial in *Science* encouraging gene mapping as a way of making headway in the understanding and treatment of cancer (Dulbecco 1986). After several years, Congress allocated funds to map and sequence the entire human genome over a period of years. Oversight of the so-called genome project was placed in a specially created office in the National Institutes of Health (NIH) headed by James B. Watson (McKusick 1989:912).

The genome project as an affirmative, monetary commitment to basic research has met with controversy among scientists who fear that a centralized mapping scheme with an earmarked budget and big mapping centers will be less productive than the traditional decentralized system of small groups of scientists working together on selected problems. Robert A. Weinberg, in an essay reprinted in this volume, explains his belief that the genome project, with its goal of mapping and sequencing all human genes, is a misguided method for learning about genetics. Most of the DNA in the human genome is uninteresting, he says—"a vast sea of intronic babel." Moreover, he sees a danger of turning gene mapping into a project for meeting economic and political ends such as competition with the Japanese for ascendancy in biotechnology. In contrast, Daniel Koshland, Jr., the editor of *Science*, regards mapping of the entire genome as a worthwhile—and even obligatory—enterprise. Society is guilty of the "immorality of omission," he concludes in the essay published here, if genetic knowledge leading to disease prevention is not "boldly and confidently" sought.

Part of the issue, then, revolves around questions of management. Is centralized planning and coordinating appropriate? If so, who should do it? Should funding come out of the entire science allocation or should a specific amount be set aside for genetic mapping in particular? Another part of the issue relates to priorities and values. Under what conditions are public commitments to genetic research being made? Are costs and benefits stated clearly and carefully, with minimal hyperbole on both sides? Is sufficient attention being given to societal repercussions that will come when the genome has been mapped? How broad and diverse has been interest group participation in the goals and methods of the genome project?

Affirmative allocations for genetic screening

With genetic inquiry comes the ability to diagnose and screen for genetic disease. The gene associated with Tay-Sachs disease, a malady that leaves children with a short and largely vegetative life, is, for example, located on the long arm of chromosome 15. A gene related to cystic fibrosis, a disease that leaves children with a shortened but largely normal life, is located on the long arm of chromosome 7. A gene thought to be associated with one kind of alcoholism is located on the long arm of chromosome 11 ("The Human Genome" 1990; Blum 1990). If the ability to locate genes precisely and then test people for genetic status is known, is it desirable to use public money to organize screening, testing, information, and reimbursement programs?

If the idea is acceptable, how does one decide, with limited dollars available, which diseases will receive attention and money? Should attention and money be given primarily to diseases for which there is acceptable treatment? Should this be primarily for diseases affecting a fairly large number of people, such as cystic fibrosis? Or should attention and funding be primarily for diseases with the most devastating costs to society and family, even if relatively few people are afflicted, as with Tay-Sachs disease? Should screening be provided for predisposition to disease such as alcoholism or colon cancer?

Consensus also needs to be reached on whether screening should be done on all people or only on at-risk populations. and whether identification of at-risk populations based on race is appropriate. Screening programs have been both effective, for example, with Tay-Sachs, and ineffective, as with sickle cell anemia (Jasanoff 1987; Roberts 1990). The success of a program depends, among other things, on the involvement of community groups and on sensitive and informed communication between medical personnel and the people being screened.

Nancy Lamontagne, a scientist at the National Institutes of Health

(NIH), reviews in her essay the matter of screening for cystic fibrosis, a disease that occurs in one in 2,000 live births. In 1989, after at least five years of intensive study, a gene associated with cystic fibrosis was located. It is estimated that one in 25 white Americans carries the cystic fibrosis gene. If two carriers conceive a baby, the odds are one in four that the child will have cystic fibrosis. Locating the "CF gene" opened the possibility for accurate screening of adults to identify carriers. In response to media coverage of the 1989 finding, the NIH sponsored a workshop on the question of cystic fibrosis screening (Workshop on Population Screening 1990). Lamontagne's essay provides a reasoned overview of the questions asked when considering whether and how to screen populations. Among other things, she points out that the gene is thought to account for only 70 to 75 percent of all cases. The members of the workshop listed guidelines that encourage restraint in genetic screening. One could conclude from this that just as "instant crises" need to be seasoned before regulatory action is appropriate, so do "instant breakthroughs" require seasoning before affirmative policy is appropriate.

Limits and controls on genetic research

Medical geneticists have long predicted that the payoff for gene research will come in the ability to treat human disease. Important events that occurred in 1988 and 1989, when the NIH approved the first clinical protocols connected with somatic cell gene therapy, furthered this goal (Cournoyer and Casky 1990; Culliton 1990; Rosenberg et al. 1990). In somatic cell therapy, genetically engineered cells are inserted into a patient's body in order to take over the functions of cells that fail to work properly due to faulty genetic instruction. Somatic cell therapy poses few ethical problems inasmuch as the engineered cells are not passed from one generation to the next. Concerns about its safety for patients have led to intensive reviews by federal regulatory agencies, however ("Points to Consider" 1990:7443–7447).

Much more ethically troublesome are the prospects of (1) engineering cells in the human embryo that will be passed across generations (germline therapy) and (2) engineering cells to enhance traits deemed socially desirable rather than to correct medical deficiencies. W. French Anderson, a leader in somatic cell therapy and a scientist at the NIH, reviews in his paper both prospects and concludes that lines should be drawn limiting research and application. For reasons discussed in his essay, he argues that enhancement genetic engineering should not be pursued and that gene therapy is appropriate only to treat serious disease.

That germ-line therapy is a near possibility is evident from the article on transgenic animals by Janice A. Sharp, a biochemist and lawyer. The genes of these animals, such as mice engineered to grow tumors for research purposes, are manipulated at the embryonic stage to include sequences of DNA from another organism. Their traits are then passed on to the next generation (Church 1990). Although Sharp does not belabor this point, successful germ-line manipulation in animals brings the day closer when manipulations for medical ends will be technically possible in human embryos. Once being the topic of science fiction, germ-line manipulation is now a prospect for humans (Ferguson, 1990:12).

Concerns about genetic manipulation at the germ-line level for both humans and animals and the use of enhancement engineering command discussion about whether public choice limiting genetic research and development is appropriate. The NIH currently will not review research proposals involving germ-line manipulations in humans (NIH 1986). It has also developed containment guidelines to prevent the accidental release of engineered organisms (Watson and Tooze, 1981). These guidelines do not apply to private researchers, however, nor do they contain enforcement power other than withdrawal of federal money from institutions that do not comply with the guidelines. Are substantive controls on genetic engineering appropriate? If so, what form should they take? When Anderson suggests drawing lines, who does he believe should draw them: individual researchers or government agencies?

Sharp's essay suggests that patent law may be either affirmative or regulatory in impact. Patents are an integral part of applied biotechnology. Can engineered animals, such as Oncomouse, be patented? In 1980, the U.S. Supreme Court held that engineered microorganisms, as living matter, are patentable. At least 120 animal patent applications are pending at the Patent and Trademark Office, according to Sharp, and congressional hearings have been held on the impact of patent law on genetic technology (U.S. Congress 1987). Patent procedures, along with the NIH guidelines, are examples of indirect ways of limiting and affirming genetic techniques. Public policy includes significantly more than legislation by Congress.

Prevention of genetics-based discrimination

Assume an employer at a metallurgy research institute is ready to hire a certain Ph.D. in chemical engineering until it becomes known that the applicant has a genetic trait that gives her a slightly increased risk of developing a red blood cell disease if she comes into contact with certain chemicals in the laboratory. The employer, unwilling to take the risk, hires another applicant (Weiss 1989). Is this a case of unwarranted discrimination? Observers have long been concerned about the use of genetic information to discriminate against individuals (Jasanoff 1987). In 1990, in response to documented cases of discrimination, a bill, the Human Genome Privacy Act, to forbid discrimination on the basis of genetic status was introduced in Congress (Miller 1990; U.S. Congress 1990). Dorothy Nelkin, a sociologist and author with Laurence Tancredi of *Dangerous Diagnostics*, draws attention in her essay to the political repercussions of the new genetics. She argues that not only will individuals face discrimination in employment, education, and insurance because of their genetic status, but they will bear the brunt of a power realignment. Those who carry certain genes will bear a new label and will, consequently, deviate from the norm. Being termed a "carrier," "deviate," or "presymptomatically ill" leaves an individual open to manipulation. Moreover, genetic diagnosis can prolong the experience of being ill, when the infirm have minimal power in society. Nelkin bids us to look beyond the applications of the day to the long-range implications of genetic technologies as a whole. According to her, genetics-based discrimination is only the visible manifestation of a more insidious development—the rise of what might be called a "biological underclass."

The New Reproductive Technologies

Thirteen years ago the new reproductive technologies were, as the new genetics is today, on the eve of expansion and integration into society. Uncertainty and excitement greeted the news of the birth of the world's first baby fertilized externally in 1978. Ironically, however, in the midst of the debate about the effects of in vitro fertilization (IVF) on society, federal policymakers left the scene. The government disbanded the Ethics Advisory Board (EAB), the structure that would have provided a forum for discussion of the dilemmas and management of in vitro fertilization. In so doing, it removed the possibility of federally funded (and watched) research on human embryos. The government provided no affirmative or regulatory guidance, leaving it to the private sector and the states to decide what steps to take. This set the stage for trial-and-error, laissez-faire decision making. The government's withdrawal from this issue contrasts with its symbolic and financial support of genetics through the genome project.

The new reproductive techniques include a core of methods for circumventing infertility: in vitro fertilization; donated eggs and embryos;

frozen eggs and embryos; artificial insemination; and surrogate gestational motherhood, in which a surrogate carries a couple's genetic embryo. Added to this core are specialized and still developing techniques for manipulating eggs, sperm, and embryos. These include circumventing male infertility by microinjecting sperm into oocytes (eggs) (Fishel 1991); separating embryos by sex to prevent the passage of sex-linked disease (Griffin et al. 1991); and analyzing for chromosomal and genetic abnormalities human eggs (Coutelle et al. 1989), spermatozoa (Braekeleer and Dao 1991) and embryos (Hardy et al. 1990). The challenges likely to arise with the confluence of reproductive and genetic technologies in laboratory conception point to the need to build a creative yet stable policy model now, before the challenges become cumulative and unwieldy. Efforts have already been made to develop private sector policies as one type of response.

The alternative of private policy

As mentioned above, the federal government provides little policy guidance in the area of assisted reproduction. To ask about federal affirmative policy is valid but rather unproductive, given the government's disbanding of the EAB and subsequent inability and unwillingness to fund research involving human embryos. In 1985 Congress opened the door for discussion by allocating $3 million to set up a bipartisan Biomedical Ethics Board, but the prospect wavered when members of Congress, caught up in the abortion controversy, failed to agree on the board's members. Regulatory policy is also at an impasse due to the government's skittishness over issues it regards as too hot to handle; the presumed unconstitutionality of interference with procreation, the value placed on reproductive privacy, and the absence of deep-seated crises (Bonnicksen 1989).

Still, recurring concerns have been voiced. Are consumers being exploited by practices in clinics such as inflated estimates of success rates and inadequate safety precautions? Are societal sensibilities harmed if money changes hands in tissue donation? Should couples be told the identity of egg or embryo donors? How does tissue donation fit into adoption and divorce law? Under what conditions should couples be able to conceive for the purpose of donating their child's tissue?

Clearly misunderstandings, exploitative practices, and varied ethical and legal problems are possible partners in the future unfolding of novel reproductive choices. Who, then, ought to bear primary responsibility for the development of guidelines for fairness and norms for restraint? Is it preferable to incline toward voluntary self-control or to opt for government oversight? The first approximates a model of autonomy, in which practitioners and couples are seen as rational actors capable of drawing lines in their own best interest. The other more closely approximates a paternalistic model in which officeholders are seen as benevolent actors capable of drawing lines in what they perceive to be the public interest.

If government control seems preferable, it is fruitful to look abroad, where national governments have played a more active role in policy experimentation in matters of IVF and embryo research. Jacques Cohen, a leader in the field of IVF research, and Robert Lee Hotz, a science editor and writer, provide a timely review of some of the bills and laws—both successful and unsuccessful—extant in Europe and Australia. They also discuss the promises and challenges of microsurgery on embryos as an emerging field in reproduction.

If private policy is preferable, a number of models exist in this country that have arisen in response to reproductive technologies in the 1980s. Physicians and researchers in the private sector have powerful incentives for self-regulation: the need for satisfied clients, fear of lawsuits, a wish to preempt governmental control, and a tradition of autonomous decision making. By practitioners' choice, by governmental inaction, and by the societal value placed on procreative privacy, models of private policy are a growing feature of the new reproductive technologies.

Some private policy develops in clinics with well-known practitioners and/or innovative techniques. Martin Quigley, a pioneer in the practice of egg freezing and donation, describes in his essay a clinic's evolving policy about sperm, egg, and embryo donation. Among other things, the clinic switched from fresh to frozen sperm use and set up a payment plan for the services of egg donors. The essay contains data about patient use of services and success rates of different techniques.

It is not unusual for practices in one center to be adopted by other centers to provide a more or less standard set of expectations. Professional associations such as the American Fertility Society (AFS) periodically issue statements that encourage more continuity in the clinic-by-clinic evolution of practices. A particularly well-developed system of private sector monitoring is described in the essay by Stuart C. Hartz, Jane B. Porter, and Alan H. DeCherney. A subgroup of AFS members, the Society for Assisted Reproductive Technology, contracted with Medical Research International to collect and publish data about IVF from member clinics across the country. Reports on data from 1985 onward have been published yearly in *Fertility and Sterility*, as reviewed in the Hartz-Porter-DeCherney paper. This method has become standardized and may, the authors suggest, be expanded for the collection of data on genetic manipulation of embryos. Thus it will provide a data-gathering base while broader issues of ethics and public policy are debated by the society at large.

Voluntary policy in the private sector has several advantages: policy is developed by those closest to the practice who are able to analyze medical and legal problems; policies can be adapted readily in response to changing conditions and situations; private policies protect reproductive privacy; and self-monitoring conforms to the tradition of medical autonomy. On the other hand, enforcement power is only indirect, and policy is developed with a minimum of publicity. For private policy to meet public ends, the interests of different groups need to be taken into account to maintain a broad and equitable perspective. Thus the use of private policy in the absence of public policy itself generates questions about the preferred role of private policy. Are private sector policies to be interim arrangements while public policy options are weighed? A model for later policy? A long-term substitute for public choice? The articles by Quigley; Cohen and Hotz; and Hartz, Porter, and DeCherney suggest that private and public policy can interact to encourage the sharing of responsibilities by both practitioners and policy makers. Such models are examples of creative action needed in a time of government silence, public uncertainty, and continuing technological change.

Reproductive issues beyond infertility

The new reproductive technologies traditionally are associated with infertility. It is possible that the public will look back on this era as a relatively halcyon time, however, as newly quixotic activities, choices, and obligations emerge in which the participants are fully fertile. Early in 1990, for example, Mary and Abe Ayala made it known that they had conceived a baby in the hope that it would be a compatible bone marrow donor for their daughter who had leukemia. When making their plan public, they had little idea that their action would spark controversy. To the Ayalas their choice was a truism: of course they would do whatever it took to try to save the life of their daughter. The news prompted a blast of negative publicity, however, about the morality of conceiving a child at least in part for the motive of using its tissues for its sister's medical care.

Warren Kearney and Arthur L. Caplan of the Center for Biomedical Ethics carefully explicate the ethical ramifications of what they call parity (birth) for the purpose of bone marrow donation. They point out in their essay that the Ayala case may have been the first publicized birth for tissue donation, but it was not the first time that this had been attempted. It is clear from their essay that the Ayala case offers only a glimpse of what might become an increasingly frequent practice. Using as a starting point a survey of physicians and coordinators at fifteen bone marrow transplant centers, they offer guidelines to practitioners who assist in parity for tissue donation.

Another emerging issue that is likely to break into as-yet-unimagined avenues is that of enforced controls on pregnant women. In a timely and thorough essay about this, Martha A. Field, a law professor and author of *Surrogate Motherhood*, describes how the controversy is evolving, particularly around enforced cesarean sections on pregnant women and attempts to punish as criminals women who drink alcohol or take drugs during pregnancy. Apart from the implications for individual rights inherent in these two areas, the essay points to important potential directions for the future: efforts by legal authorities to obligate women, under pain of prosecution or civil suit, to use high-technology methods to detect abnormalities in embryos and fetuses and to undergo treatment for these abnormalities, either by microsurgery on embryos before transfer to the uterus, or in utero surgery on fetuses during gestation.

Field, like Nelkin in her essay on a genetic underclass, compels us to examine the power implications of biomedical technologies. When a technique is available, who uses it? Who benefits from its use? Who gains choice? Who, in the appearance of choice, actually loses it? Who gains authority to manage techniques? Do biomedical techniques magnify inequities in society?

Leonard S. Cottrell has observed that "there is nothing new in the scientist's upsetting the societal applecart," but that today's rate and scope of change challenge "as never before . . . the search for ordered change" (1966:115). The issues of embryo manipulation, controls over pregnant women, gene mapping, genetic enhancement, genetic discrimination, genetic screening, transgenic animal creation, egg donation, and procreation for tissue donation all testify to a steeply diagonal line of change. Biomedical ethics and policies clarify issues and point to principles and options. In the wake of unfolding dilemmas in biomedicine, we should guard against becoming distraught if public policies are not enacted immediately. Public choice must be ordered, not reflexively prompted by topical crises and discoveries. Concern *is* warranted, however, if we do not place a high priority on the weighing of private and public policy choices.

It is also essential periodically to take stock of the choices already made, the areas of consensus reached, and the values clarified since the first gene splicing experiments and since the birth of the world's first IVF baby. Each essay in part II of this book points to a unique set of applied technologies that will unfold, ripple-style, as expansive emerging issues in reproduction and genetics. Acknowledging the areas in which ordered change has already taken place, however, is as important as anticipating the multiple challenges to ordered change that will occur in this decade. The essays demonstrate that such a thoughtful cross-disciplinary effort to inform, clarify, and propose, is ongoing.

References

Angier, Natalie. 1990. "Vast, 15-Year Effort to Decipher Genes Stirs Opposition." *New York Times,* June 5:B5.

Bonnicksen, Andrea L. 1989. *In Vitro Fertilization: Building Policy From Laboratories to Legislatures.* New York: Columbia University Press.

Blum, Kenneth, Ernest P. Noble, Peter J. Sheridan, Anne Montgomery et al. 1990. "Allelic Association of Human Dopamine D2 Receptor Gene in Alcoholism." *Journal of the American Medical Association* (April 18) 263(15):2055–2066.

Braekeleer, M. De, and T.-N. Dao. 1991. "Cytogenetic Studies in Male Infertility: A Review." *Human Reproduction* (February) 6(2):245–250.

Church, Robert B., ed. 1990. *Transgenic Models in Medicine and Agriculture.* Proceedings of a UCLA Symposium Held at Taos, New Mexico, Jan. 28–Feb. 3, 1989. New York: Wiley-Liss.

Cottrell, Leonard S., Jr. 1966. "The Interrelationships of Law and Social Science." In Harry W. Jones, ed., *Law and the Social Role of Science,* pp. 106–119. New York: Rockefeller University Press.

Cournoyer, Denis, and C. Thomas Caskey. 1990. "Gene Transfer into Humans." *New England Journal of Medicine* (August 30) 323(9):601–602.

Coutelle, Charles, Carolyn Williams, Alan Handyside, Kate Hardy, et al. 1989. "Genetic Analysis of DNA From Single Human Oocytes: A Model for Preimplantation Diagnosis of Cystic Fibrosis." *British Medical Journal* (July 1) 299(6690):21–24.

Culliton, Barbara J. 1990. "Gene Therapy: Into the Home Stretch." *Science* (August 31) 249:974–976.

Dulbecco, Renato. 1986. "A Turning Point in Cancer Research: Sequencing the Human Genome." *Science* (March 7) 231:1055–1056.

Jasanoff, Sheila. 1987. "Biology and the Bill of Rights: Can Science Reframe the Constitution?" *American Journal of Law & Medicine* 13(2–3):249–289.

Ferguson, Mark W. J. 1990. "Contemporary and Future Possibilities for Human Embryonic Manipulation." In Anthony Dyson and John Harris, eds., *Experiments on Embryos,* pp. 6–26. London: Routledge.

Fishel, Simon, Severino Antinori, Peter Jackson, Joanne Johnson, and Leonardo Rinaldi. 1991. "Presentation of Six Pregnancies Established by Sub-Zonal Insemination (SUZI)." *Human Reproduction* (January) 6(1):124–130.

Griffin, D. K., A. H. Handyside, R. J. A. Penketh, R. M. L. Winston, and J. D. A. Delhanty. 1991. "Fluorescent In-Situ Hybridization to Interphase Nuclei of Human Preimplantation Embryos with X and Y Chromosome Specific Probes." *Human Reproduction* (January) 6(1):101–105.

Hardy, Kate, Karen L. Martin, Henry J. Leese, Robert M. L. Winston, and Alan H. Handyside. 1990. "Human Implantation Development in Vitro Is Not Adversely Affected by Biopsy at the 8–Cell Stage." *Human Reproduction* 5(6):708–714.

"The Human Genome." 1990. *Journal of NIH Research* (August) 2:133–160.

McKusick, Victor A. 1989. "Mapping and Sequencing the Human Genome." *New England Journal of Medicine* (April 6) 320(14):910–915.

Miller, Susan Katz. 1990. "Genetic Privacy Makes Strange Bedfellows." *Science* (September 21) 249:1368.

National Institutes of Health (NIH). 1986. "Points to Consider in the Design and Submission of Human Somatic-Cell Gene Therapy Protocols." In Eve K. Nichols, *Human Gene Therapy*, pp. 195–208. Cambridge, Mass.: Harvard University Press, 1988.

"Points to Consider for Protocols for the Transfer of Recombinant DNA into the Genome of Human Subjects." 1990. 55 *Federal Register* 7443 (March 1).

Roberts, Leslie. 1990. "To Test or Not to Test?" *Science* (January 5) 247:17–19.

Rosenberg, Steven A., Paul Aebersold, Kenneth Cornetta, Attan Kasid, et al. 1990. "Gene Transfer Into Humans—Immunotherapy of Patients with Advanced Melanoma, Using Tumor-Infiltrating Lymphocytes Modified by Retroviral Gene Transduction." *New England Journal of Medicine*, (August 30) 323(9):570–578.

Suzuki, David, and Peter Knudtson. 1989. *Genethics: The Clash Between the New Genetics and Human Values.* Cambridge, Mass.: Harvard University Press.

U.S. Congress, House of Representatives, Committee on the Judiciary, Subcommittee on Courts, Civil Liberties, and the Administration of Justice. 1987. *Patents and the Constitution: Transgenic Animals.* 100th Congress, 1st session.

U.S. Congress, House of Representatives. 1990. H.R. 5612. "Human Genome Privacy Act." 101st Congress, 2d session (September 13).

Watson, James D. 1990. "The Human Genome Project: Past, Present, and Future." *Science* (April 6) 248:44–49.

Watson, James D., and John Tooze. 1981. *The DNA Story: A Documentary History of Gene Cloning.* San Francisco: W. H. Freeman.

Weiss, Rick. 1989. "Predisposition and Prejudice." *Science News* (January 21) 135(3):40–42.

Workshop on Population Screening for the Cystic Fibrosis Gene. 1990. "Special Report: Statement from the National Institutes of Health Workshop on Population Screening for the Cystic Fibrosis Gene." *New England Journal of Medicine* (July 5) 323(1):70–71.

10

The Human Genome Sequence: What Will It Do For Us?

Robert A. Weinberg

The debate over sequencing the human genome seems to have been resolved now in the United States, not through a widely established consensus in the community of biologists but rather through the report of a panel commissioned by the National Academy of Sciences. Given this decision to go ahead, what form will this effort take, and how much will it cost? The last question will ultimately be the most contentious. Cost estimates beginning in the hundreds of millions of dollars and reaching into the billions have been justified in terms of the priceless anticipated returns for biologists.

What will this work yield for the biological community, and will the returns indeed be priceless beyond calculation? An initial, clear return will be the development of an entirely new set of tools for rapidly sequencing large amounts of DNA, analyzing the data, and integrating it in a usable way. Here, there seems to be little debate. Moreover, a consensus prevails that order-of-magnitude improvements in current sequencing technologies must precede the bulk of the genomic sequencing effort, and this will undoubtedly provide great impetus to improvements in technique over the next several years.

A second fallout of this large-scale project will stem from the extensive chromosomal mapping that will also precede direct sequencing. This effort to map and order a large array of single-copy probes is already well under way. The fallout of this will also prove invaluable in the long run, even if its results are only used as aids in the cloning of interesting genes that have already been identified through biological and genetic techniques.

But what of the results of the large-scale sequencing itself? The complete sequence of the human genome has been widely touted as a Holy Grail of modern biology. The proponents of this megaproject argue that this information will be of limitless value in resolving many of the problems that biologists presently confront. These statements seem to have been accepted at face value by many, but it is less than obvious that this information will have utility beyond measure.

Idiosyncrasies in the organization of the mammalian genome would seem to dictate that only a small proportion of the future sequence data base will ever be of much interest to anyone. Over the last decade it has become increasingly clear that only 3 to 5 percent of the human genome carries genetic information that is critical for organismic development and homeostasis. Much of the remainder would appear to encompass introns and the vast intergenic segments carrying pseudogenes, repeated sequences, and sequences whose connection to biological function will forever remain obscure. This arrangement seems to run counter to an intuition that suggests that our genome is lean and well designed, having been continually pared back by the optimizing forces of evolution.

There are those who dismiss this view as myopic; they live with the hope that this 95 percent of the genome's sequences represents a vast storehouse of undiscovered, potentially fascinating biological lessons. But the evidence for this is unconvincing. The more scientists have learned about genes over the last decade, the less persuasive is the case for an important role for most of these sequences, including the introns that make up the bulk of most genes. The extensive sequencing and functional tests of cloned DNA have not uncovered many unexpected treasures in introns and intergenic regions. The genome as a whole is best characterized as groups of small information islands swimming in a vast sea of genetic gibberish.

My own laboratory has been working on a human gene of about 200 kilobase pairs, termed Rb, whose inactivation provokes retinoblastoma. I cannot imagine what I would want with 195 kbp of its intronic sequence that will be presented to me on a platter some years hence. In this Rb-gene model, as in most others, all utility has come from the cDNA and the control sequences around the promoter; the rest appears as useless detritus and I wager will forever remain so.

Granted the possibly limited utility of the great majority of primary sequence data, will other benefits accrue? Will all this sequence rapidly lead to the identification and cloning of long-sought genes? Here there is also room for serious doubt. To begin with, the genomic sequence banks will not in most cases provide indications allowing precise definition of the starting and end points of genes. Even within the apparent confines of a gene, the genomic sequence will not readily indicate where the small and interesting exon islands merge with the vast sea of intronic babel. Reference to cognate cDNAs will be essential to determine essential coding, as is the case at present. Even then, the biological significance of one or another of the genes encountered in a sequence bank will be obscure and in most cases not indicated by attributes of sequence.

In the end, the rate-limiting steps in the progress of research will remain as they are now: defining a protein or genetically encoded trait, cloning a portion of the encoding gene through one or another trick often involving protein isolation or complex genetics, and spending decades figuring out how the encoded protein affects phenotype. Having reference to a genomic sequence bank will ameliorate these problems only to a minor extent.

A more useful alternative to genomic sequencing would be the sequencing of a complete or almost complete human cDNA library, each of whose clones carries a precise chromosomal assignment. Such a data bank would have much more utility in the end. Creating truly representative and complete cDNA libraries is not within our technical reach at present, but might well be after several years of concentrated effort. Such improvements in cDNA technology might be achieved for a fraction of the cost that would be spent on genomic sequencing. However, the most important decisions may have already been made and soon, the great sequencing juggernaut will begin its inexorable forward motion, flooding our desks with oceans of data whose scope defies conception and our ability to interpret meaningfully. The United States and Japan may soon make completion of the sequence a matter of national pride. Imagine two national teams may soon be racing neck-and-neck to finish almost 3 billion bases of sequence. We can only hope that the costs of these sequencing efforts will not impoverish efforts to solve the real problems in biology!

11

Sequences and Consequences of the Human Genome

Daniel E. Koshland, Jr.

The sequencing of the human genome involves big money, big consequences, and big controversies. Within the scientific community there is the question of money because of the "big science" image. The cost of the genome project ($3 billion in fifteen years) is much smaller than the cost of a supercollider or of a space station, and it is more of a mom-and-pop enterprise than the mass production assembly line of really big science. The Cystic Fibrosis Foundation has spent $120 million in the past four years on one illness, to say nothing of the other foundation and federal money spent on the same project. In this context, a price of $200 million per year, the figure for the human genome project, for work that applies to many diseases and untold discoveries in biology sounds cost-effective.

The benefits to science of the genome project are clear. Illnesses such as manic depression, Alzheimer's, schizophrenia, and heart disease are probably all multigenic and even more difficult to unravel than cystic fibrosis. Yet these diseases are at the root of many current societal problems. The costs of mental illness, the difficult civil liberties problems it causes, the pain to the individual all cry out for an early solution that involves prevention, not caretaking. To continue the current warehousing or neglect of sufferers of these and other diseases, many of whom are in the ranks of the homeless, is the equivalent of providing iron lungs to polio victims at the expense of working on a vaccine.

Other medical applications of a genome sequence include an early warning system that may help individuals predisposed to diseases such as alcoholism, colon cancer, and depression. The early warning may allow them to avoid problems by behavior adjustment or diet modification or frequent medical checkups. Family planning also will be made more accurate. No individual should be forced to obtain genetic information, but none should be denied information either.

The "sky is falling" group who denounce the genome project, sound like they are paraphrasing a Woody Allen admonition by saying, "We stand at the crossroads. One road leads to hopelessness, the other to utter despair. We must have the courage to make the right decision." The potential risks from the new knowledge gained by sequencing the human genome appear, on close examination, to be old problems revisited. Genetic counseling already exists for Down syndrome, Tay-Sachs, and sickle-cell anemia. Personal insurance policies already ask for lung x-rays, heart condition tests, and information on such behaviors as smoking. Group insurance is available without tests. Fingerprints are not required of the general population but are kept on file for those who commit a crime. The information in the genome adds accuracy and scope to many of these applications but no new or threatening principles. If the higher visibility of the genome project causes a qualitative change, then, of course, new procedures may be needed.

A genome sequence should not be a precondition of employment, and legislation might be needed if that problem were to arise. However, less accurate data of the same type would be available today from family histories, and that does not seem to be part of current employment forms. If more accurate information provides temptation for abuse, action will be needed.

The argument that dictators would alter genes to convert their enemies is farfetched. The idea that a Hitler or a Stalin would prefer the engineering of Jews into Aryans or capitalists into communists as cheaper or more satisfying than killing them (as they did) is absurd. We must be vigilant about ethical concerns but not paralyzed by outlandish scenarios.

The belief of biologists that studying simple organisms such as *Escherichia coli*, flies, and rats is relevant to human physiology and behavior has been brilliantly confirmed. But there are differences. One cannot extrapolate carcinogenic potency from the mouse to the rat with precision, and even less from the mouse to the human. Some diseases involve speech and mental states unique to humankind. Sequencing the human genome puts us on the threshold of great new benefits and some real but avoidable risks. There are immoralities of commission that we must avoid. But there is also the immorality of omission—the failure to apply a great new technology to aid the poor, the infirm, and the underprivileged. We must step boldly and confidently across the threshold.

12

Cystic Fibrosis: Identification of the Gene

Nancy Lamontagne

Cystic fibrosis (CF) is the most common life-threatening inherited disease in the Caucasian population, with an approximate incidence of one out of two thousand live births (Talamo, Rosenstein, and Berninger 1983). The disease is manifest only when a child inherits one copy of the mutant gene from both parents, who each also have a normal copy of the gene and are therefore designated as carriers (heterozygotes). This pattern of inheritance is termed *autosomal recessive*. The carrier frequency for cystic fibrosis approaches one in twenty in Caucasians of European ancestry, but is much lower in Native Americans, Africans, and Asians (Thompson 1980; Nadler and Ben-Yoseph 1984). If both parents are carriers, a child has a one in four risk of having CF.

In patients with CF the exocrine glands fail to function properly, so the disease is characterized by elevated sweat chloride levels, intestinal obstruction, pancreatic insufficiency, sterility in males, and chronic lung disease leading to respiratory failure and death (Mangos 1987). CF usually presents in childhood as failure to thrive in combination with recurrent lung infections and/or maldigestion, but a subset of patients have a milder phenotype and may not be identified until later in life (Talamo, Rosenstein, and Berninger 1983; Wood, Boat, and Doershuk 1976). The median survival age of patients has increased dramatically over the last two decades from approximately ten years in the 1960s to approximately twenty-five years today. The improvements in mortality and morbidity have been accomplished by aggressive symptomatic treatment of the chronic obstructive lung disease and pancreatic insufficiency.

For fifty years, CF has been the subject of a frustrating search for an underlying cause. Dorothy Anderson first identified CF as a distinct syndrome in 1938, and she coined the term "cystic fibrosis of the pancreas" (1938:344). In the 1940s, CF was characterized by a failure of the exocrine glands to clear their mucous secretions, which led to the term mucoviscidosis found in the medical literature of that time (Farber 1945). Also in the 1940s, antibiotics were used for the first time to treat the chronic lung infections of CF patients, and a hypothesis of the autosomal recessive pattern of the disease was formulated (Anderson and Hodges 1946). A major breakthrough in the understanding of CF came in 1953 when Paul di Sant'Agnese and colleagues demonstrated that the salt (sodium chloride) level is elevated in virtually all individuals with CF (di Sant'Agnese 1953). This discovery led to the pilocarpine iontophoresis method for sweat testing, which remains a diagnostic standard (Gibson and Cooke 1959) and also provided a clue to the underlying pathophysiology. Although the next thirty years saw a more comprehensive approach to the care of CF patients and a more refined description of the CF syndrome, there was little progress in the basic research on this disease.

In the early 1980s, Michael Knowles and colleagues associated the abnormal sodium and chloride transport with altered electrical properties of CF respiratory epithelium (Knowles, Gatzy, and Boucher 1981) and Quinton and Birman reported reduced chloride permeability of sweat gland ducts (1983). These observations provided for the first time a pathogenic role for salt and water movement in both sweat gland and lung dysfunction. Scientists now have evidence of abnormal electrolyte transport in the epithelia of all three organs classically involved in CF, i.e., the sweat glands, airways, and pancreas (Boat, Welsh, and Beaudet 1989). Therefore, although the basic biochemical defect is still unknown, there is a unifying hypothesis of a transport defect that relates the research observations to the pathophysiology. Because CF has a clear and consistent pattern of recessive inheritance, in the mid-1980s scientists also began to look for the CF gene that, when located, could reveal a protein product that presumably affected electrolyte transport.

The technique that allowed the search for the CF gene to begin is called *restriction fragment length polymorphism (RFLP) analysis*. In RFLP analysis, scientists seek variations among individuals in the chain of genetic material (DNA) that are closely linked to a gene and thus mark its location. The closer a marker is to a specific gene, the more frequently the marker and the gene will be inherited together. In order to visualize such markers, think of the individual's DNA as cleaved into pieces by special enzymes called restriction enzymes, because they each can cut the DNA only at places identified by a certain pattern in the sequence of chemical bases that make up the steps in the ladderlike DNA structure. Variations (RFLPs) in the lengths of the DNA fragments produced by restriction enzymes are determined by their differential migration in a size-dependent separation gel. The so-called bands on the gel are detected by using radioactively labeled, cloned human DNA sequences (probes) that bind to the markers (Donis-Keller et al. 1986). RFLP loci behave as codominant Mendelian alleles; that is, they are always fully expressed and thus can be used in family studies to trace the inheritance of a trait such as CF, even if almost nothing else may be known about the trait. This approach, identifying a gene responsible for an inherited disorder without reference to a known protein product of the gene, has been termed *reverse genetics* (Orkin 1986). The logic of reverse genetics is first to establish the location of the gene on one of the twenty-three human chromosomes—i.e., the "map position" on the human genome. The next step is to narrow the region on the chromosome in which the specific gene is located by correlating RFLP gel patterns with the presence of the CF trait.

The possibility of obtaining RFLP lineage data for CF became a major focus in many laboratories in 1985. At that time Hans Eiberg et al. demonstrated linkage between CF and a genetic variation in serum level activity of the enzyme paraoxonase (PON) (1985). This provided reassurance that CF represented a single gene locus, but PON was not mapped to a particular chromosome. Shortly thereafter, Lap-Chee Tsui and coworkers reported another CF-linked marker, which they designated DOCRI-917 and rapidly assigned to the long arm of chromosome 7 (Tsui et al. 1985; Knowlton et al. 1985). Two other polymorphic DNA markers also were located on the long arm of chromosome 7, the oncogene *met* (White et al. 1985:382) and the anonymous probe J3.11 (Wainwright 1985). A large collaborative study of more than two hundred families with two or more affected children showed that *met*, J3.11, and CF were closely linked (Beaudet 1986) but the precise order was not yet proven. Chromosome 7 is estimated to contain 150 million base pairs of DNA and therefore accounts for approximately 5 percent of the human genome (Tsui 1988). Now the search for the CF gene had become a reasonable quest. In 1986 and 1987 other markers for the CF gene were located on chromosome 7 (Boat, Welsh, and Beaudet 1989) and in 1988 the CF gene was definitely placed between *met* and J3.11 (Fulton 1989). Researchers estimated that the distance between *met* and J3.11 was 2 million base pairs.

Rather than continue to screen for new markers more or less at random, it was more systematic at this point to close in on the CF gene using a technique called "walking" the chromosome, in which the "steps" are overlapping segments of DNA (Rommens 1988). The steps in gene walking, however, are only 20,000 or so base pairs in length, making walking too arduous a process to cover the distance involved between the markers *met* and J3.11. Francis Collins and colleagues at the University of Michigan were using an important new technique analogous to gene walking, called "gene jumping" because it allowed a skip over 100,000 base pairs at a time (Collins et al. 1987:1046; Ianuzzi et al. 1989). So in 1987 Dr. Tsui and colleagues at the Hospital for Sick Children in Toronto, who were conducting the walking searches for the CF gene, began a collaboration with Dr. Collins and his team who performed the gene jumping experiments. In January of 1989 their collaborative effort succeeded in finding a 300,000-base-pair stretch of DNA from the long arm of chromosome 7 that matched the occurrence of the CF trait (Rommens et al. 1989).

This candidate DNA was verified to contain the CF gene by several techniques. One involved cutting the candidate DNA into fragments and determining if any of the fragments were active, that is, copied to make an RNA message that instructs a cell to make a protein. By a process of elimination, one such active fragment was designated to be the CF gene (Riorden et al. 1989). The Tsui and Collins research teams then "accessed" this candidate gene by verifying that it occurred in other animal species. This "zoo blot" technique is based on the theory that important genes are conserved throughout the animal kingdom. The final proof for the CF gene was the determination that it made a protein relevant to cystic fibrosis. Using a "library" of DNA copies from human sweat gland cells known to express the CF trait, one of the genes was demonstrated to make a membrane protein in sweat glands. The DNA sequence of the confirmed CF gene from people without cystic fibrosis was then compared with the CF gene from cystic fibrosis patients. In approximately 70 percent of the CF-patient genes analyzed, there was a deletion of three specific base pairs of DNA; thus the gene produced the identified membrane protein, but with the loss of one amino acid (Kerem et al. 1989). The detection of this major mutation had immediate important implications for genetic diagnosis.

A diagnosis of cystic fibrosis based on pathological and clinical features is difficult because CF presents in many different ways and mimics a number of other clinical entities. Before the advent of RFLP analysis for CF in 1985, the diagnosis of this disease was based on analysis of sweat chloride levels coupled with the following clinical criteria: (1) typical pulmonary manifestations, and/or (2) typical gastrointestinal manifestations, and/or (3) a history of CF in the immediate family (Boat, Welsh, and Beaudet 1989). Although there are a number of other clinical entities that can be accompanied by elevated sweat chloride concentrations, none of these disorders is easily confused with CF. Of individuals with CF, however, 1 to 3 percent have sweat chloride values in an intermediate or normal range. Evaluation of these atypical patients involved other diagnostic tests for pancreatic function, azoospermia (lack of spermatozoa) in sexually mature males, and, after 1985, the measurement of bioelectrical potential across respiratory epithelia (Knowles, Gatzy, and Boucher 1981). The sweat test, which became the diagnostic standard in 1953 and remained so for more than thirty years, was a procedure that required meticulous administration to avoid errors. Misdiagnosis because of false positive or false negative sweat test results occurred in as many as 40 percent of patients referred to CF centers (Boat, Welsh, and Beaudet 1989). Newborn screening by the sweat test was confounded by a difficulty in obtaining sufficient amounts of sweat and a normal elevation of sweat electrolyte levels in infants during the first few days of life (Boat, Welsh, and Beaudet 1989).

Other early attempts at newborn (Crossley, Elliott, and Smith 1979; King et al. 1975) and prenatal (Brock, Bedgood, and Hayward 1984) screening for CF were based on the alterations of certain intestinal enzymes in amniotic fluid or blood samples caused by the gastrointestinal abnormalities frequently associated with this disease. The discovery that newborns with CF had elevated levels of the enzyme immunoreactive trypsin, which could be detected in the dried blood samples already being collected from newborns, led to sophisticated enzyme immunoassays using radioactivity or antibodies as detectors (Crossley, Elliott, and Smith 1979; King et al. 1979). High-volume newborn screening using these methods began in the 1980s in New South Wales, Australia; Colorado, United States; New Zealand; and Veneto, Italy, with a detection rate of approximately 95 percent (Hammond, Naylor, and Wilcken 1987). A continuing program in Wisconsin is screening one-half of the population by random selection in order to evaluate the potential benefits of newborn screening (Farrell et al. 1988). The potential benefits and risks of newborn screening for CF, including the sensitivity and specificity of the test, the impact on reproductive decisions, psychosocial outcomes, and the effectiveness of presymptomatic treatment have been major issues since its inception.

The availability of RFLP markers for CF in 1985 quickly led to reliable prenatal and neonatal diagnosis that was fully informative in families with a DNA sample from an affected child (Beaudet et al. 1988). Identification of the cystic fibrosis gene in 1989 now opens the possibility of genetic testing for CF to the general population. The identification of the three-base-pair deletion (designated DF508) that removes the amino acid phenylalanine 508 from the gene protein product as the mutation that causes cystic fibrosis in the majority of cases allows screening for the mutation which is present in 70 percent of CF genes. In addition, mutation analysis is applicable to difficult clinical circumstances such as questionable CF in a deceased newborn, suggestive gastrointestinal obstruction on prenatal ultrasound, or diagnosis of a patient with borderline sweat test results.

The advent of mutation analysis has had an immediate and major effect on programs offering genetic counseling, heterozygote detection, and prenatal diagnosis for families with a history of cystic fibrosis (Lemna et al. 1990). This is particularly true for families in which no DNA sample is available from an affected child. A recent study (Lemna et al. 1990) of more than two hundred families who underwent DNA analysis for cystic fibrosis reported that a majority of families were either fully informative (58.2 percent) or partially informative (33.7 percent), providing a predictive tool for assessing occurrence of CF in the offspring of the majority of these families. Before the availability of mutation analysis, carrier testing in the relatives of patients with CF was not offered because carrier detection and definitive prenatal diagnosis of CF was virtually impossible except in siblings of a child with CF. Now if a parent has a close relative with CF and is found to be a carrier, the mutation analysis of the spouse can be offered. If the spouse tests positive, there is a one-in-four risk of an affected child, and prenatal diagnosis is possible. When the spouse has a normal result on mutation analysis, further analyses are problematic due to the 70 to 75 percent mutation-detection currently available. That is, if the spouse of a known carrier tests negative, he or she still has one chance in a hundred of having one of the rarer CF mutations (the one in twenty-five carrier risk reduced due to 25 percent occurrence of other mutations), giving a risk of approximately one in four hundred that the child of such a couple will have CF. This risk can be modified further by the use of other techniques such as DNA linkage data and intestinal enzyme analysis. Thus carrier testing in families with CF is informative, and researchers have recommended that such testing be offered to all individuals and/or couples with a family history of CF (Beaudet et al. 1990). For this purpose, the importance of medical care providers obtaining family history information, particularly for patients of reproductive age, is emphasized.

In September 1989, when the major CF mutation was reported, scientists hoped that the mutations accounting for the remaining 25 to 30 percent of CF genes would be few in number and quickly identified. Although to date more than twenty additional mutations have been identified, these all are rare mutations which together account for less than a few percent of CF genes. Thus carrier detection is still in the 70 to 75 percent range, making carrier testing in the general population a complex issue at this time (Beaudet et al. 1990:70).

Several recent reviews (Lemna et al. 1990; Beaudet et al. 1990; Wilfond and Fost 1990; ASHG 1990) and editorials (Roberts 1990; "Cystic Fibrosis" 1990; Brock 1990; Brody 1990) on the question of population screening for CF have been published. The authors of these articles generally agree in that a carrier detection rate of greater than 90 percent would substantially reduce the difficulties associated with CF genetic screening. The 70 to 75 percent detection rate possible at the present time means that only a little more than half of the couples at risk can be detected, whereas 90 percent of such couples would be detected if mutation analysis were 95 percent effective. These recent reviews have generally concluded that at present population screening should not be recommended for individuals or couples with no family history of CF. The reasons that routine carrier testing is not now recommended to be the standard of care in medical practice, in addition to the relatively low current detection rate of couples at risk, are: (1) the differences in the frequency of the disease and frequency of the major mutation in individuals of different racial and ethnic backgrounds, which will require significant modifications in testing and counseling among different populations; (2) substantial limitations foreseen in the ability to educate the population regarding the potential complexity of test results; and (3) the anxiety created in the approximately one out of fifteen couples in which one partner tests positive and the other negative, thus informing them of their increased risk of bearing a child with CF, without the availability of a more definitive test. In addition to the technical difficulties with carrier detection, procedures for informed consent, education, quality control of laboratories, and counseling need to be in place before population screening could be considered (Wilfond and Fost 1990).

Despite these reservations, a recent survey of the attitudes of geneticists from eighteen nations indicates that widespread screening for CF carriers is being discussed as a future probability in some countries (Wertz and Fletcher 1989) There is already a consensus on a number of screening guidelines that will be required if population screening becomes widespread. As listed in the statement from the NIH workshop on population screening for the CF gene (Beaudet et al. 1990), these suggested guidelines are: (1) screening should be voluntary and confidentiality must be assured; (2) screening requires informed consent; pretest educational material should explain the hazards (e.g., potential loss of insurability and psychosocial effects) and benefits of choosing to be tested or choosing not to be tested; (3) providers of screening services have the obligation to assure that adequate education and counseling are included in the program; (4) quality control of all aspects of the laboratory testing including systematic proficiency testing is required and should be implemented as soon as possible; and (5) there should be equal access to testing.

Pilot programs to work out the logistical and technical aspects of population screening for CF carriers have been suggested by many experts in the field. These pilot programs should address clearly the defined questions including effectiveness of educational materials, level of utilization of screening, laboratory aspects, counseling issues, cost, and beneficial and deleterious effects of screening (Beaudet et al. 1990).

The debate over carrier screening of the population for CF should not detract from the benefits already available due to identification of the CF gene. These include improved prenatal and neonatal diagnosis of CF and the ability to correlate the different CF gene mutations with variable disease presentation, for example, pancreatic insufficiency versus sufficiency. It is now apparent that the wide range in severity and clinical presentation of CF is at least partially due to the genetic heterogeneity of the CF gene locus.

Identification of the CF gene might address the unsolved problems regarding the population genetics of this disease. One question is why the CF gene has been maintained at such a high frequency in the Caucasian PG population; the possible answers being a high mutation rate, heterozygote advantage, meiotic drive, or simply random genetic drift. Other questions are, how long ago did the CF mutation(s) arise (3,000 to 6,000 years?), and what has been the rate of variant introduction of the original mutation? Identification of the CF gene protein product has now opened many additional lines of research in the quest for defining the basic biochemical defect(s). Additional knowledge on the molecular mechanisms of the defect will ultimately lead to improved methods of treatment.

References

American Society of Human Genetics (ASHG). 1990. "Statement on CF Screening." *American Journal of Human Genetics* 46:393.

Anderson, D. H. 1938. "Cystic Fibrosis of the Pancreas and Its Relation to Celiac

Disease: A Clinical and Pathological Study." *American Journal of the Disabled Child* 56:344–399.

Anderson, D. H., and R. G. Hodges. 1946. "Celiac Syndrome v. Genetics of Cystic Fibrosis of the Pancreas with a Consideration of Etiology." *American Journal of the Disabled Child* 72:62–80.

Beaudet, A., A. Bowcock, M. Buchwald, L. Cavalli-Sforza et al. 1986. "Linkage of Cystic Fibrosis to Two Tightly Linked DNA Markers: Joint Report from a Collaborative Study." *American Journal of Human Genetics* 39:681–693.

Beaudet, A., H. H. Kazazian, Jr. et al. 1990. "Statement from the NIH Workshop on Population Screening for the Cystic Fibrosis Gene." *New England Journal of Medicine* 323:70–71.

Beaudet, A., J. R. Spence, M. Montes, W. E. O'Brien et al. 1988. "Experience with New DNA Markers for the Diagnosis of Cystic Fibrosis." *New England Journal of Medicine* 318:50–51.

Boat, T. F., M. J. Walsh, and A. L. Beaudet. 1989. "Cystic Fibrosis." In Charles R. Scriver, ed., *The Metabolic Basis of Inherited Disease*, pp. 2649–2679. New York: McGraw-Hill.

Brock, D. 1990. "Population Screening for Cystic Fibrosis." *American Journal of Human Genetics* 47:164–165.

Brock, D., D. Bedgood, and C. Hayward. 1984. "Prenatal Diagnosis of Cystic Fibrosis by Assay of Amniotic Fluid Microvillar Enzymes." *Human Genetics* 65:248–251.

Brody, J. S. 1990. "Discovery of the Cystic Fibrosis Gene: The Interface of Basic Science and Clinical Medicine." *American Journal of Respiratory Cell and Molecular Biology* 1:347.

Collins, F. S., L. M. L. Drumm, J. L. Cole, W. K. Lockwood et al. 1987. "Construction of a General Human Chromosome Jumping Library, with Application to Cystic Fibrosis." *Science* 235:1046–1049.

Crossley, J. R. B. Elliott, and P. A. Smith. 1979. "Dried-Blood Spot Screening for Cystic Fibrosis in the Newborn." *Lancet* (March 3) 1:472–474.

"Cystic Fibrosis: Prospects for Screening and Therapy, 1990." 1990. *Lancet* (January 13) 1:79–80.

di Sant'Agnese, P. A., R. A. Darling, G. S. Perera, and E. Shea. 1953. "Abnormal Electrolytic Composition of Sweat in Cystic Fibrosis of the Pancreas: Clinical Significance and Relationship of the Disease." *Pediatrics* 12:549–563.

Donis-Keller, H., D. F. Barker, R. G. Knowlton, J. W. Schumm, J. C. Braman, and P. Green. 1986. "Highly Polymorphic RFLP Probes and Diagnostic Tools." Paper read at Symposia on Quantitative Biology, Cold Spring Harbor, N.Y.

Eiberg, H. K. Schmiegelow, L.-C. Tsui, M. Buchwald et al. 1985. "Cystic Fibrosis: Linkage with Paraoxonase." *Cytogenetics Cell Genetics* 40:623.

Farber, S. 1945. "Some Organic Digestive Disturbances in Early Life." *Journal of the Michigan Medical Society* 44:587–594.

Farrell, P., et al. 1988. "Infant Screening Test for Cystic Fibrosis." *Pediatric Research* 23:563A (supplement).

Fulton, T. R., A. M. Bowcock, D. R. Smith, L. Daneshvar et al. 1989. "A 12

Megabase Restriction Map at the Cystic Fibrosis Locus." *Nucleic Acids Research* 17:271–284.

Gibson, L. E., and R. E. Cooke. 1959. "A Test for Concentration of Electrolytes in Sweat in Cystic Fibrosis of the Pancreas Utilizing Pilcarpine by Iontophoresis." *Pediatrics* 23:545–549.

Hammond, K., E. Naylor, and B. Wilcken. 1987. "Screening for Cystic Fibrosis." In B. L. Therrell, ed., *Advances in Neonatal Screening*, pp. 377–382. New York: Excerpta Medica.

Ianuzzi, M. C., M. Dean, M. L. Drumm, N. Hidaka et al. 1989. "Isolation of Additional Polymorphic Clones from the Cystic Fibrosis Region, Using Chromosome Jumping from D758." *American Journal of Human Genetics* 44:695–703.

Kerem, B., J. M. Rommens, J. Buchanan, D. Markiewicz et al. 1989. "Identification of the Cystic Fibrosis Gene: Genetic Analysis." *Science* 245:1073–1080.

King, D. N., A. F. Heeley, M. P. Walsh, and J. A. Kuzemko. 1979. "Sensitive Trypsin Assay for Dried Blood Specimens as a Screening Procedure for Early Detection of Cystic Fibrosis." *Lancet* (December 8) 2:1217–1219.

Knowles, M., J. Gatzy, and R. Boucher. 1981. "Increased Bioelectric Potential Difference Across Respiratory Epithelia in Cystic Fibrosis." *New England Journal of Medicine* 305:1489.

Knowlton, R. G,, O. Cohen-Iaguenauer, V. C. Nguyen, J. Frezal et al. 1985. "A Polymorphic DNA Marker Linked to Cystic Fibrosis is Located on Chromosome 7." *Nature* 318:380–382.

Lemna, W. K., et al. 1990. "Mutation Analysis for Heterozygote Detection and the Prenatal Diagnosis of Cystic Fibrosis." *New England Journal of Medicine* 322:291–296.

Mangos, J. A. 1987. "Clinical Progress in Cystic Fibrosis." In G. Mastella and P. M. Quinton, eds., *Cellular and Molecular Basis of Cystic Fibrosis*, pp. 1–7. San Francisco: San Francisco Press.

Nadler, H. L., and Y. Ben-Yoseph. 1984. "Genetics." In L. M. Taussig, ed., *Cystic Fibrosis*, pp. 10–24. New York: Thieme-Stratton.

Orkin, Stuart H. 1986. "Reverse Genetics and Human Disease." *Cell* 47:845–850.

Quinton, P. M., and J. Birman. 1983. "Higher Bioelectric Potentials Due to Decreased Chloride Absorption in the Sweat Glands of Patients with Cystic Fibrosis." *New England Journal of Medicine* 308:1185.

Riorden, J. R., J. M. Rommens, B. Kerem, N. Alon et al. 1989. "Identification of the Cystic Fibrosis Gene: Cloning and Characterization of Complementary DNA." *Science* 245:1066–1073.

Roberts, L. 1990. "To Test or Not to Test?" *Science* 247:17–19.

Rommens, J. M., M. C. Iannuzzi, B. Kerem, M. L. Drumm et al. 1989. "Identification of the Cystic Fibrosis Gene: Chromosome Walking and Jumping." *Science* 245:1059–1065.

Rommens, J. M., S. Zengerling, J. Burns, G. Melner et al. 1988. "Identification and Regional Localization of DNA Markers on Chromosome 7 for the Cloning of the Cystic Fibrosis Gene." *American Journal of Human Genetics* 43:645–666.

Talamo, R. C., B. J. Rosenstein, and R. W. Berninger. 1983. "Cystic Fibrosis." In

J. B. Stanbury et al., eds., *The Metabolic Basis of Inherited Disease*, pp. 1889–1971. New York: McGraw-Hill.

Thompson, M. W. 1980. "Genetics of Cystic Fibrosis." In J. M. Sturgess, ed., *Perspectives in Cystic Fibrosis*, pp. 281–291. Toronto: Canadian Cystic Fibrosis Foundation.

Tsui, L. C. 1988. "Genetic Markers on Chromosome 7." *American Journal of Medical Genetics* 25:294.

Tsui, L. C., M. Buchwald, D. Barker, J. C. Braham et al. 1985. "Cystic Fibrosis Locus Defined by a Genetically Linked Polymorphic DNA Marker." *Science* 230:1054–1057.

Wainwright, B. J., J. Scamler, J. Schmidtke, E. A. Watson et al. 1985. "Localization of Cystic Fibrosis Locus to Human Chromosome 7 cen-q22." *Nature* 318:384–385.

Wertz, D. C., and J. C. Fletcher. 1989. "An International Survey of Attitudes of Medical Geneticists towards Mass Screening and Access to Results." *Public Health Reports* 104:35–44.

White, R., S. Woodward, M. Leppert, P. O'Connell et al. 1985. "A Closely Linked Genetic Marker for Cystic Fibrosis." *Nature* 318:382–384.

Wilford, B. S., and N. Fost. 1990. "The Cystic Fibrosis Gene: Medical and Social Implications for Heterozygote Detection." *Journal of the American Medical Association* 263:2777–2783.

Wood, R. E., T. F. Boat, and C. F. Doershuk. 1975. "State of the Art: Cystic Fibrosis." *American Review of Respiratory Disease* 113:833–878.

13

Genetics and Human Malleability

W. French Anderson

Just how much can (and should) our society change human nature . . . by genetic engineering? A response to this question hinges on the answers to three further questions: (1) What *can* we do now? Or, more precisely, what *are* we doing now in the area of human genetic engineering? (2) What *will* we be able to do? In other words, what technical advances are we likely to achieve over the next five to ten years? (3) What *should* we do? An examination of these questions supports the argument that a line can be drawn, and should be drawn, to use gene transfer only for the treatment of serious disease, and not for any other purpose. Gene transfer should never be undertaken in an attempt to enhance or "improve" human beings.

What Can We Do?

A 1980 paper published in the *New England Journal of Medicine* delineated what would be necessary before it would be ethical to carry out human gene therapy (Anderson and Fletcher 1980). As with any other new therapeutic procedure, the fundamental principle is that the probable benefits should be determined in advance to outweigh the probable risks. For somatic cell gene therapy, three risk/benefit questions need to be answered from prior animal experimentation before such therapy is carried out on humans: Can the new gene be inserted stably into the correct target cells? Will the new gene be expressed (that is, function) in the cells at an appropriate level? Will the new gene harm the cell or the animal? These criteria are very similar to those required before use of any new therapeutic procedure, surgical operation, or drug. They simply require that the new treatment should get to the area of disease, correct it, and do more good than harm.

A great deal of scientific progress has occurred in the years since that paper was published. The technology now exists for inserting genes into some types of target cells (Anderson 1984; Friedman 1989). The procedure being used is called "retroviral-mediated gene transfer." In brief, a disabled murine retrovirus serves as a delivery vehicle for transporting a gene into a population of cells that have been removed from a patient. The gene-engineered cells are then returned to the patient.

The first clinical application of this procedure was approved by the National Institutes of Health and the Food and Drug Administration on January 19, 1989 (Wyngaarden 1989). The protocol for this procedure received the most thorough prior review of any clinical protocol in history: it was approved only after being reviewed fifteen times by seven different regulatory bodies. In the end it received unanimous approval from every one of those committees. But the simple fact that the NIH and the FDA, as well as the public, felt that the protocol needed such extensive review demonstrates that the concept of gene therapy raises serious concerns.

The initial question, "What can we do now in the area of human genetic engineering?," can be answered by examining this approved clinical protocol. Gene transfer is used to mark cancer-fighting cells in the body as a way of better understanding a new form of cancer therapy. The cancer-fighting cells, called TIL (tumor-infiltrating-lymphocytes), are isolated from a patient's own tumor, grown to a large number, and then given back to the patient along with one of the body's immune growth factors, a molecule called interleukin 2 (IL-2). The procedure, developed by Steven Rosenberg of NIH, is known to help about half the patients treated (Rosenberg et al. 1988).

The difficulty is that there is at present no way to study the TIL once they are returned to the patient to determine why they work (that is, killer cancer cells) when they do work, and why they do not work when they do not work. The goal of the gene-transfer protocol was to put a label on the infused TIL: to mark these cells so that they could be studied in blood and tumor specimens from the patient over time.

The TIL were marked with a vector called N2 containing a bacterial gene that could be easily identified through recombinant DNA techniques. The protocol was called, therefore, the N2–TIL Human Gene Transfer Clinical Protocol. The first patient received gene-marked TIL on May 22, 1989. Five patients have now received marked cells. No side effects or problems have thus far arisen from the gene transfer portion of the therapy. Useful data on the fate of the gene-marked TIL are being obtained.

But what was done that was new? Simply, a single gene was inserted into a population of cells that had been obtained from a patient's body. There are an estimated 100,000 genes in every human cell. Therefore the actual addition of material was extremely minute, nothing to correspond to the fears expressed by some that human beings would be "reengineered." Nonetheless, a functioning piece of genetic material was successfully inserted into human cells, and the gene-engineered cells did survive in human patients.

What Will We Be Able to Do?

Although only one clinical protocol is presently being conducted, it is clear that several applications for gene transfer probably will be carried out over the next five to ten years. Many genetic diseases that are caused by a defect in a single gene should be treatable, such as ADA deficiency (a severe immune deficiency disease of children), sickle cell anemia, hemophilia, and Gaucher disease. Some types of cancer, viral diseases such as AIDS, and some forms of cardiovascular disease are targets for treatment by gene therapy. In addition, germ-line gene therapy, that is, the insertion of a gene into the reproductive cells of a patient, probably will be technically possible in the foreseeable future. (The author's position on the ethics of germ-line gene therapy is published elsewhere [Anderson 1985].)

But successful somatic cell gene therapy also opens the door for enhancement genetic engineering, that is, genetic engineering for supplying a specific characteristic that individuals might want for themselves (somatic cell engineering) or their children (germ-line engineering), which would not involve the treatment of a disease. The most obvious example at the moment would be the insertion of a growth hormone gene into a normal child in the hope that this would make the child grow larger. Should parents be allowed to choose (if science should ever make it possible) whatever useful characteristics they wish for their children?

What Should We Do?

A line can and should be drawn between somatic cell gene therapy and enhancement genetic engineering (Anderson 1989). Our society has repeatedly demonstrated that it can draw a line in biomedical research when necessary. The Belmont Report illustrates how guidelines were formulated to delineate ethical from unethical clinical research and to distinguish clinical research from clinical practice. Our responsibility is to determine how and where to draw lines with respect to genetic engineering.

Somatic cell gene therapy for the treatment of severe disease is considered ethical because it can be supported by the fundamental moral principle of beneficence: it would relieve human suffering. Gene therapy would be, therefore, a moral good. Under what circumstances would human genetic engineering not be a moral good? In the broadest sense, when it detracts from, rather than contributes to, the dignity of humankind. Whether viewed from a theological perspective or a secular humanist one, the justification for drawing a line is founded on the argument that, beyond the line, human values that our society considers important for the dignity of humanity would be significantly threatened.

Somatic cell enhancement engineering would threaten important human values in two ways: it could be medically hazardous, in that the risks could exceed the potential benefits and the procedure therefore would cause harm. It would be morally precarious in that it would require moral decisions our society is not now prepared to make. And it could lead to an increase in inequality and discriminatory practices.

Medicine is a very inexact science. We understand roughly how a simple gene works and that there are many thousands of housekeeping genes, or genes that do the job of running a cell. Scientists predict that there are genes which make regulatory messages that are involved in the overall control and regulation of the many housekeeping genes. Yet we have only limited understanding of how a body organ develops into the size and shape it does. We know many things about how the central nervous system works—for example, we are beginning to comprehend how molecules are involved in electric circuits, in memory storage, in transmission of signals. But we are a long way from understanding thought and consciousness. And we are even further from understanding the spiritual side of our existence.

Even though we do not understand how a thinking, loving, interacting organism can be derived from its molecules, we are approaching the time when we can change some of those molecules. Might there be genes that influence the brain's organization or structure or metabolism or circuitry in some way so as to allow abstract thinking, contemplation of good and evil, fear of death, awe of a "God"? What if, in our innocent attempts to improve our genetic makeup, we alter one or more of those genes? Could we test for the alteration? Certainly not at present. If we caused a problem that would affect the individual or his or her offspring, could we repair the damage? Certainly not at present. Every parent who has several children knows that some babies accept and give more affection than others in the same environment. Do genes control this? What if these genes were accidentally altered? How would we even know if such a gene were altered?

At this point in the development of our culture's scientific expertise, we might be like the young boy who loves to take things apart. He is bright enough to disassemble a watch, and maybe even bright enough to get it back together again so that it works. But what if he tries to "improve" it, maybe put on bigger hands so that the time can be read more easily? But if the hands are too heavy for the mechanism, the watch will run slowly, erratically, or not at all. The boy can understand what is visible, but he cannot comprehend the precise engineering calculations that determined exactly how strong each spring should be, why the gears interact in the ways that they do, and so forth. Attempts on his part to improve the watch will probably only harm it.

We are now able to provide a new gene so that a property involved in a human life would be changed—for example, a growth hormone gene. If we were to do so simply because we could, we would be like that young boy who changed the watch's hands. We, too, do not really understand what makes the object we are tinkering with tick.

In summary, it could be harmful to insert a gene into humans. In somatic cell gene therapy for an already existing disease the potential benefits could outweigh the risks. In enhancement engineering, however, the risks would be greater while the benefits would be considerably less clear.

Yet even aside from the medical risks, somatic cell enhancement engineering should not be performed because it would be morally precarious. Assuming that there were no medical risks at all from somatic cell enhancement engineering, there would still be reasons for objecting to this procedure. To illustrate, consider some examples: What if a human gene were cloned that could produce a brain chemical resulting in markedly increased memory capacity in monkeys after gene transfer? Should a person be allowed to receive such a gene on request? Should a pubescent adolescent whose parents are both five feet tall be provided with a growth hormone gene on request? Should a worker who is continually exposed to an industrial toxin receive a gene to give him resistance upon his, or his employer's, request?

These scenarios suggest three problems that would be difficult to resolve: Which genes should be provided? Who should receive a gene? And how do we prevent discrimination against individuals who do or do not receive a gene?

Using somatic cell gene therapy for treatment of serious disease would be ethically appropriate. But what distinguishes a serious disease from a "minor" disease from cultural "discomfort"? What is suffering? What is significant suffering? Does the absence of growth hormone that results in limitation of growth to two feet in height represent a genetic disease? What about a limitation to a height of four feet, or five feet? Each observer might draw the lines between serious disease, minor disease, and genetic variation differently. But all can agree that there are extreme cases that produce significant suffering and premature death. Here, then, is where an initial line should be drawn for determining which genes should be provided: treatment of serious disease.

If society establishes the position that only patients suffering from serious diseases are candidates for gene insertion, then the issues of patient selection are no different than in other medical situations: the determination is based on medical need within a supply-and-demand framework. But if we extend the use of gene transfer to allow a normal individual to acquire, for example, a memory-enhancing gene, profound problems would result. On what basis should the decision be made to allow one individual to receive the gene but not another? Should it go to those best able to benefit society (the smartest already)? To those most in need (those with low intelligence; but how low? Will enhancing memory help a mentally retarded child?)? To those chosen by a lottery? To those who can afford to pay? As long as our society lacks a significant consensus about these answers, the best way to make equitable decisions in this case should be to base them on the seriousness of the objective medical need, rather than on the personal wishes or resources of an individual.

Discrimination can occur in many forms. If individuals are carriers of a disease (for example, sickle cell anemia), would they be pressured to be treated? Would they have difficulty in obtaining health insurance unless they agreed to be treated? These are ethical issues raised also by genetic screening and by the human genome project. But the concerns would become even more troublesome if there were the possibility for "correction" by the use of human genetic engineering.

Finally, we must face the issue of eugenics, the attempt to make hereditary "improvements." The abuse of power that societies have historically demonstrated in the pursuit of eugenic goals is well documented (Ludmerer 1972; Kevles 1985). Might we slide into a new age of eugenic thinking by starting with small "improvements"? It would be difficult, if not impossible, to determine where to draw a line once enhancement engineering had begun. Therefore, gene transfer should be used only for the treatment of serious disease and not for putative improvements.

Our society is comfortable with the use of genetic engineering to treat individuals with serious disease. On medical and ethical grounds we should draw a line excluding any form of enhancement engineering, and we should not step over that line that delineates treatment from enhancement.

References

Anderson, W. French. 1985. "Human Gene Therapy: Scientific and Ethical Considerations." *Journal of Medicine and Philosophy* 10(3):275–291.

Anderson, W. French. 1989. "Human Gene Therapy: Why Draw a Line?" *Journal of Medicine and Philosophy* 14(6):681–693.

Anderson, W. French. 1984. "Prospects for Human Gene Therapy." *Science* 226:401–409.

Anderson, W. French, and John C. Fletcher. 1980. "Gene Therapy in Human Beings: When is it Ethical to Begin?" *New England Journal of Medicine* 303(22):1293–1297.

Friedman, Theodore. 1989. "Progress Towards Human Gene Therapy." *Science* 244:1275–1281.

Kevles, Daniel J. 1985. *In the Name of Eugenics.* New York: Knopf.

Ludmerer, Kenneth M. 1972. *Genetics and American Society.* Baltimore: Johns Hopkins University Press.

Rosenberg, Steven A., Beverly S. Packard, Paul Aebersold, Diane Solomon et al. 1988. "Use of Tumor-Infiltrating Lymphocytes and Interleukin-2 in the Immunotherapy of Patients with Metastatic Melanoma." *New England Journal of Medicine* 319(25):1676–1680.

Wyngaarden, J. 1989. "Human Gene Transfer Protocol." *Federal Register* 54 (47):10508–10510.

14

The Patenting of Transgenic Animals

Janice A. Sharp*

In the latter half of the twentieth century, humankind has witnessed an explosion of scientific discoveries, particularly in the field of molecular biology, popularly known as biotechnology. The advancements in this field will have an enormous impact on society. Yet the extraordinary harvest to be reaped from these new technological abilities must be balanced against the moral and legal issues created by "human-made" life forms. The possible dangers associated with the use of these new and revolutionary, but as yet unfamiliar, technological advances must be weighed against the almost certain benefits they will engender.

On April 12, 1988, the U.S. Patent and Trademark Office issued the first patent on a vertebrate animal (May 1988). The patent's subject matter is a mouse that has been genetically engineered so that it, and all of its offspring, will be highly susceptible to the development of cancer. The patent, granted to Harvard, gives the university exclusive control over the use of the mouse strain during the seventeen-year patent term. Issuance of this patent refueled the ongoing debate about the 1980 Supreme Court decision that living organisms, in that case bacteria, were patentable (*Diamond v. Chakrabarty* 1980).

After the April 12 announcement of the Patent and Trademark Office

*The author wishes to thank Kirk Hoiberg for his valuable assistance in the research for this article.

decision, numerous interest groups have voiced their opinions about the mouse patent. Religious groups have expressed concern about the ethics of changing nature; environmentalists about the unknown threat of altered animals released into the wild; ranchers and farmers about the possibility of added cost resulting from royalties for the progeny of patented animals; and animal rights activists about the potential for inhumane treatment of patented animals (Booth 1988; "Activists, Farmers," *Los Angeles Times* 1988).

Background

Biotechnology

Biotechnology relates to the use of biological processes in an industrial setting. Over the last twenty years humankind's ability to manipulate the genetic material of organisms has steadily grown, leading to a rapid development of new products and production processes in many industries. While extraordinary advances are being made in biotechnology, it should be noted that the use of living organisms in biological manufacturing processes are as old as the history of humanity. Humanity has used biological entities for eons in the preparation of beer, wine, and bread. In these processes, a living organism, yeast, converts sugar to alcohol and carbon dioxide. Bacteria and fungi, as well, have long been used commercially in the production of such commodities as yogurt and cheese.

Often, naturally occurring organisms have undesirable traits or produce less than the manufacturer would like, and, as a result, new strains with the preferred properties are sought. New strains are found by screening large numbers of naturally occurring organisms until one with the desired characteristics is found. Alternatively, naturally occurring organisms can be mutated and selected for their expression of the required characteristics.

Microorganisms such as bacteria and yeast are not the only organisms bred and selected to display characteristics which please and profit humanity. The manipulation of animal species has been extensive. New breeds of dogs, all of which at one time were derived from the wolf, or farm animals that are commercially superior to naturally occurring animals as a result of their resistance to disease or their superior ability to produce meat, wool, or other products, are examples of humankind's extensive manipulation of the natural "starting material." Modern, domesticated cows, pigs, and sheep bear little resemblance to the wild animals from which they originally were derived.

The plant world has also been a target of humanity's manipulations for economic gain. Most commercial strains of plants have been selected and crossed to obtain plants with resistance to disease and pests, a more pleasing appearance for their fruit, improved yields, and more economical production.

Until recently, all improved species resulted from mutations which had been artificially induced in the organism or which had arisen spontaneously. The individual organisms with the desired characteristics were then selected and purified from the organism's "brothers and sisters" which did not carry these traits. Using mutations as the means of generating new strains of organisms is a random and time-consuming process that frequently takes many years to finally produce an improved organism.

The ability of an organism to produce a particular chemical or protein, or to exhibit a particular trait, is conferred by the genes the organism carries. Genes are segments of DNA that contain the instructions required by an organism to produce proteins. A protein is produced when its corresponding gene is in an "active" form. When the protein is produced, the trait that it confers on the organism is expressed. If the gene is in an "inactive" form, the protein is not produced, and the trait is not exhibited by the organism. If an organism does not possess a particular gene, the trait that the gene confers can never be expressed by the organism.

One method of obtaining new traits, or genes, is by crossing animals or plants (i.e., breeding different but compatible organisms). When two organisms each have desirable characteristics, they are crossed to produce a new organism with both characteristics in a single offspring. This method of producing a new strain of animal or plant can take many years and is limited by the gene pools from which the desired traits can be selected. For example, a bacteria or a cow will never be able to develop the ability to express human genes, since breeding between genetically unrelated species is impossible. Some exceptions to this rule exist. For example, mules result from cross-breeding between a horse and a donkey. However, the progeny of such a match is sterile and unable to reproduce its own kind.

Chemicals or pharmaceuticals produced by a yeast or bacteria have tremendous commercial potential, since microorganisms grow very quickly. A new generation of bacteria occurs about every twenty minutes and of yeast every few hours, as compared to twenty years or so for humans. A further advantage to microbial production of chemicals is that microorganisms can be grown cheaply and in large quantities. Until recently, the products that these organisms were able to produce was limited by their natural gene pool. A yeast can never naturally acquire the ability to produce insulin, since yeast do not have a gene for this protein. However, the ability to produce insulin, particularly insulin that is identical to human insulin, in an organism such as yeast or bacteria would represent a tremendous boon not only to the pharmaceutical industry but also to diabetics who rely on injections of this protein for their survival. No longer would diabetics be dependent on the animal sources of insulin, such as pigs and horses, that are currently used. With human insulin available from microorganisms, diabetics would no longer face the possibility of allergic reactions from continued injections of animal proteins that the human body recognizes as foreign. The ability to produce a product such as insulin in a microorganism would result in an unlimited, relatively cheap, and safe supply of the drug. Also, the ability to produce other compounds, such as Factor VIII, the antihemophilic factor, in microorganisms would overcome the need to extract this or other important factors from blood that could potentially be contaminated with viruses such as the AIDS virus.

Advances in biotechnology in fact have resulted in the ability to take the step beyond the limitations of the gene pool of naturally compatible organisms and allow the transfer of genes from one species to another. This transfer is performed not in a random way, as occurs with mutations, but in a planned and controlled manner. The gene of interest, such as the insulin or Factor VIII gene of humans, can be taken from one species, any species, and transferred to a microbial host, where it can be expressed to produce the desired protein, for example, insulin or Factor VIII. Now technology has advanced to the point where human insulin is produced in microorganisms and is commercially available.

An extension of this technology is not only to transfer genes into microorganisms, but to transfer them into higher organisms such as mice, cows, sheep, pigs, or even humans. The genes of interest are injected into the fertilized egg of an animal, where they are incorporated into the embryo's chromosomes. The offspring that results from this procedure is called a transgenic animal; it expresses all of the genes that it would normally express, plus the gene that was injected. In such cases, it is possible for a dairy cow to produce not only milk, but milk that contains insulin, interferon, growth hormone, or other compounds that are of pharmaceutical and commercial importance.

Even though the technique for creating a transgenic animal is more directed than the methods that have been used in the past, the time, effort, and cost involved in the development and production of these organisms are great. Unless manufacturers of such organisms can be guaranteed protection for their inventions so that they can recoup their costs and profit from their investment, the motivation for future research and development may be lost. Traditionally, the business world has employed patents or trade secrets as a means of securing protection for technological advances.

Patent Protection

The concept of patents has existed since the time of ancient Greece. The present form developed from British common law. In the United States, intellectual property rights are granted by the Constitution (Article I, Section 8). Congress enacted the first patent and copyright laws in 1790.

Patents are a government grant giving the patent owner the right to exclude others from making, selling, or using the patented invention for a period of seventeen years, within the United States. Patents may be granted to a person or entity who invents or discovers any new, useful, and nonobvious process, machine, manufacture, composition of matter, or improvement of existing inventions.

Patents are an essential means of protecting vital commercial interests. This form of protection has been as important to the development of the biotechnology industry as it has been for other industries. Without patent protection, inventions could be easily copied and economic advantages lost. Large, prosperous entities would be able to market new innovations at the expense of smaller, less competitive businesses. Patent protection gives small businesses competitive advantages against large organizations and creates vitality in all businesses.

Until 1980, the Patent and Trademark Office had refused to grant patents on any living organisms with the exception of plants, because, as living entities, they were considered to be "products of nature" and, therefore, unpatentable. This exception to the patentability of living organisms was carved out in the Plant Patent Act of 1930. However, the Plant Patent Act did not include microorganisms explicitly. Later, the 1970 Plant Variety Protection Act specifically excluded bacteria. Thus until 1980, the courts interpreted the patent statutes as excluding bacteria from patentability The Supreme Court, in its landmark decision on the patentability of life forms in the case of *Diamond v. Chakrabarty*, in which a strain of bacteria was held to be patentable, eliminated this long-standing exclusion.

The next step toward the patenting of higher organisms was taken in

Ex parte Allen (2 U.S.P.Q. 2d 1425 [BNA] [1987]). *Allen* concerned a method that had been developed for the production of sterile, polyploid (containing more than the normal number of chromosomal copies) oysters. Polyploid oysters offer a significant advantage over naturally occurring oysters because they do not devote a significant amount of their body weight to the seasonal development of inedible reproductive organs and are thus edible year round. "In the wake of Allen the Patent and Trademark Office announced that it would consider 'non-naturally occurring non-human multicellular living organisms, including animals, to be patentable subject matter within the scope of 35 U.S.C. 101'" (Chisum 1988).

After the decision in *Allen,* and at the request of Representative Robert W. Kastenmeier (D-Wis.), the Patent and Trademark Office agreed to a voluntary eight-month moratorium on further animal patents, to give Congress time to debate the various issues involved. The moratorium expired on April 12, 1988, and on the same day, the Patent and Trademark Office announced its decision to grant the mouse patent to Harvard. The patent, which was filed on June 22, 1984, covers "[a] transgenic non-human eukaryotic animal whose germ cells and somatic cells contain an activated oncogene sequence introduced into the animal, or an ancestor of the animal, at an embryonic stage" (Leder and Stewart 1988). An activated oncogene, a cancer-producing gene (in this case the mouse *c-myc* gene sequence), was introduced into a fertilized mouse oocyte (egg). This gene, when incorporated into the mouse genome, the chromosomal DNA of the mouse, results in an animal that exhibits an increased probability of developing malignant tumors. Since the activated oncogene sequence is incorporated into the animal's germ cells, all the progeny of the animal will also exhibit increased susceptibility to cancer. The importance of these animals is that they can be used as a test system for screening suspected carcinogens or for selecting materials that protect against cancer.

The important advantage of these transgenic mice, in the words of Philip Leder, is that they "have taken the first step toward cancer. . . . With them you can learn some rather powerful and telling lessons about the genesis of cancer *in vivo*" (Booth 1988:718). The patent is not limited to mouse genes nor to transgenic mice, but lists thirty-three oncogenes from seven different animal sources. The patent further suggests that, in some circumstances, it may be advantageous to use a species that is more closely related to humans than mice, such as rhesus monkeys, as the transgenic host for the oncogenes. The mouse patent began a wave of new applications in this field—about 120 other animal patent applications are now pending at the Patent and Trademark Office (Manbeck 1990).

The legislative response to the issuance of the patent

Many groups seized on the controversy initiated by the issuing of the mouse patent as a means of forcing Congress to address the broader moral and economic questions related to genetic engineering. These groups contend that the issue of genetic engineering was not adequately addressed when the Supreme Court, in 1980, deemed microorganisms to be patentable subject matter. In sum, the main concerns that arose over the Chakrabarty decision were twofold: (1) humans had no ethical or moral right to create new life forms; and (2) the new life forms created could be hazardous, resulting in human-made plagues or agents dangerous to the world's environment.

The patenting of transgenic mice has given these groups a new forum in which to express their continuing fear of the new genetic engineering technology. Therefore, some have characterized the patent as an "arrogant abuse of power," as president of the Foundation on Economic Trends Jeremy Rifkin does, and have claimed that "a handful of bureaucrats at the patent office have set themselves above Congress . . . in establishing a public policy that will have profound economic, environmental and ethical consequences for the U.S. and world community" (Hart 1988). However, as pointed out by Commissioner of Patents Donald J. Quigg, "issuance of the patent does not preclude regulation of the subject matter by Congress or other governmental agencies" (Quigg 1988). Commissioner Quigg further stated, "The patent office would welcome guidance on where to draw the line between patentable and unpatentable life forms as well as the moral questions raised by the decision to patent genetically altered animals" ("U.S. Grants Patent" 1988).

On August 5, 1987, in response to the decision in *Ex parte Allen*, Representative Charles Rose (D-N.C.) introduced a bill to amend Title 35 of the United States Code to prohibit the patenting of genetically altered or modified animals. This bill did not survive subcommittee vote, and the House-Senate conference committee rejected the proposed moratorium in June 1988. On June 30, 1988 Representative Kastenmeier introduced legislation, the Transgenic Animal Patent Reform Act, designed to govern the use of animal patents and to create an exemption for research organizations and family farmers.

Kastenmeier's bill introduced "limitations similar to those applicable to patented plants in the Plant Variety Protection Act." The bill was intended to amend Section 271 of Title 35 to state that it would not be an infringement to use patented animals for research or experimentation. This exemption was designed to encourage "parties to invent around the patent" and was limited to persons who are not involved in commercial endeavors (*Congressional Record* 1988:16602).

A second proposed exemption provided for reproduction of genetically engineered animals on the farm. Under the exemption on-farm reproduction would not be a patent infringement. According to Kastenmeier, "Under the current patent law, a farmer who obtains a patented animal would likely also obtain the right to use the animal for the intended use, such as milking and slaughter. It is uncertain, however, whether the farmer would be liable for an act of patent infringement if the farmer reproduced the animal." The bill provided exemptions for small family farmers to reproduce through breeding and to use or sell a patented animal. It also would grant regulatory authority to the Environmental Protection Agency to monitor the "release of genetically altered animals into the wild" (*Congressional Record* 1988:16602).

Other bills relating to animal patenting have been introduced, including a bill by Senator Mark Hatfield (R-Ore.) on February 26, 1990, to amend Title 35 of the United States Code to impose a five-year moratorium on the granting of patents on genetically altered or modified animals. The intention is first to establish a federal regulatory and review process to deal with the ethical and environmental issues raised by the patenting of animals.

Is the Patenting of Animals in the Public Interest?

As expected, different interest groups have aligned on opposite sides of the controversy surrounding the issue of patenting animals. Each side has expressed its concerns about the future of animal patents and of the application of the transgenic technology. Advocates of patent protection argue that patenting provides a necessary incentive to conduct research on transgenic animals; is necessary to protect American business from foreign competition; and will reduce animal suffering, enhance medical research, and improve human health by, for example, creating leaner meat and new drugs to treat human diseases. Opponents of patent protection argue that animal suffering in research and production will increase; that patent protection produces economic concentration; that farmers will be disadvantaged by paying higher prices for animals; and that the federal regulatory framework is inadequate to protect human health and the environment from the effects of such patents (*Congressional Record* 1988:16602).

Potential disadvantages

One of the concerns raised by those opposed to animal patenting is the fear that transgenic technology will be used to create animal-human hybrids. In answer to such claims, Commissioner Quigg stated that "[a] claim directed to or including within its scope a human being will not be considered to be patentable subject matter under 35 U.S.C. Section 101. The grant of a limited but exclusive property right in a human being is prohibited by the Constitution" ("Animals—Patentability" 1988:328).

The constitutional prohibition would be on the grounds that patents grant a personal property interest in the patented subject matter, and the holding of a proprietary interest in a human being would be prohibited under the Thirteenth Amendment of the U.S. Constitution. However, while the patenting of a human being would be prohibited under the Constitution, it is possible that Congress may eventually be required to address the problem of defining what constitutes a human being. At what stage does a transgenic animal cease to be an animal and become a human being? This problem would be significant if primates, in particular higher apes that are evolutionarily, and therefore genetically, closely related to human beings, were used as the starting animal in transgenic experiments and if human DNA were used as the source of the transferred genes.

A further consideration, one that first arose with the original patent on a living organism, is whether humans, by creating transgenic animals, are meddling in the realm of deities in an interference that should not be encouraged by the Patent and Trademark Office. Religious leaders such as Arie R. Brouer, general secretary of the National Council of Churches, argue that "the gift of life is from God, in all forms, and species, [and] should not be regarded solely as if it were a chemical product, subject to genetic alteration and patentable for economic benefit. . . . Moral, social, and spiritual issues deserve far more serious consideration before binding decisions [patent awards] are made in this area" (Crawford 1987:480).

To counter such arguments, the biotechnology industry contends, at least as represented by patent attorney William H. Duffey in congressional hearings, that "the act of issuing a patent is morally neutral and ought to be kept that way. . . . [It is] wrong . . . to consider limiting protection for biotech inventions in response to those groups who play upon the emotional components of a burgeoning science" (Crawford 1987:480).

Other issues relate to humanity's control over and responsibility toward nature. From the point of view of animal rights activists, "what the patent office has done—apparently without authority—is to open a Pandora's box that can unleash extraordinary consequences. The inhuman effect is to equate animals with other patentable human inventions such as the pocket-size fishing rod or the cordless microphone" ("Activists, Farmers" 1988). Such arguments focus on the potential of developing grotesque monsters, often citing as an example the "Beltsville pig" engineered by USDA researchers (Hart 1990:27). These pigs were developed by the transfer of the gene for bovine-growth hormone into pigs, in an attempt to produce low-fat pork. The pigs that resulted were bow-legged, arthritic, cross-eyed, and lethargic.

Another concern is species integrity. John A. Hoyt, president of the Humane Society, says that "the patenting of animals reflect[s] a human arrogance toward other living creatures that is contrary to the concept of the inherent sanctity of every unique being. . . . It also reflects a dehumanistic and materialistic attitude towards living beings and precludes a proper regard for their intrinsic nature" (Hanson and Nelkin 1989:78). In addition, Jeremy Rifkin has argued that "animals have an intrinsic value independent of people, and they have the right to experience their own nature" (Hart 1990:22). Others contend, however, that such arguments overlook the history of humans and their relationship with animals. The concept of animal ownership was not created by the new developments in biotechnology, nor was the concept of creating new animals that do not exist in nature. Farmers and pet lovers have been the stimulus in the development of many new and unnatural strains of animals. Farmers and pet owners would certainly consider that they have a right to own, sell, and use the animals in their possession as they wish, with few restrictions being placed on them by society.

Others in the debate say that patenting animals undervalues nonhuman life, asking, "Is there no dignity in separate species, or is it permissible to blend these species into creatures never imagined by nature? Are animals biological machines that can be engineered and cloned?" (Gorner and Kotulak 1990). Similarly, theologians remind us of the responsibility humans have toward animals. Wesley Granberg-Michaelson of the

National Council of Churches asserts, "The Judeo-Christian view says that the Creation is, in essence, held in trust. . . . We have the responsibility to see that its integrity is preserved" (Hanson and Nelkin 1989:78). Critics of this view contend, however, that such arguments overlook the reality of the long historical dominion humans have had over domestic animals. The modern cow is certainly not a product of nature.

Opponents of patenting animals state that other countries do not allow animal patents and that no advantage is gained by issuing such patents in the United States. In fact, the patent laws of other countries do, in theory, allow patenting of animals. These countries include Argentina, Australia, Brazil, Hungary, Japan, Turkey, and the USSR, which allows an inventor's certificate (Bent et al. 1987). Most other countries have statutory prohibitions against the patenting of animals. However, this is likely to change as the commercial potential of these animals becomes apparent. Also, attempts to harmonize the patent laws of different countries may contribute toward making animal patents universally acceptable.

Some opponents point out that patenting could have an adverse impact on third world countries, since this new technology may be too expensive to adopt and because these countries lack the resources to develop the technology for themselves. Such arguments express the legitimate concerns of advanced societies for their less fortunate counterparts. However, the inability of the third world to afford technology has not yet stopped development of new products that our society can afford. Some third world countries currently cannot afford the technical developments that are thought of as commonplace in the U.S., including vaccines to prevent death from childhood diseases such as measles and polio. However, should those who can pay be denied access to such technology? Such an attitude does not appear to be consistent with the capitalistic values of Western society. While these attitudes may be less than admirable, they will not be cured by preventing the development of new technologies.

Another concern is the adverse effect transgenic animals might have on the environment if they were released or escaped. "In a recent experiment, a gene for growth hormone was implanted in fish to increase their size. Environmentalists question how the release of these fish will affect the existing ecosystem" (Hart 1990:22). They fear that such animals might take over the natural ecosystems and displace native animals. The proponents of such arguments point to the monumental problems that have resulted when exogenous wild animals have been introduced into a number of ecosystems throughout the world and proceeded to establish themselves so completely in the new environment that they became uncontrollable pests.

Many genetically altered animals, such as the Beltsville pigs, would be poor candidates for competing against natural populations of wild animals. In most cases, the transgenic animals probably would be less fit for survival than their wild counterparts. The genetic makeup of wild animals is the product of many eons of evolution that has steadily adapted the animals to become efficient survivors in their own environment. Genetic alterations such as those introduced by the transgenic technology would not be expected to give the animals a selective advantage to survive in the wild. In fact, the genetic alterations would be expected to be burdensome to such an extent that the animals would survive very poorly. However, such arguments are only probable results, and sufficient experimentation with transgenic animals should be conducted to ensure that they will not survive in the wild before they are allowed to be released. Or, alternatively, transgenic technology could be used to introduce genes into the animal that would ensure its death in a natural environment.

Still other arguments are the expected higher costs to consumers of food produced by transgenic animals. Critics worry that consumers will have little or no control over the technology, and that the technology will be controlled by a small segment of the community which will derive a profit from the new life forms at the expense of consumers (Sugarman 1989). Again, this appears to be capitalism at its best, and consumers have already demonstrated that they are more than ready to pay a higher price for new products that they find attractive. Cholesterol and calorie watchers will predictably be eager to pay for such products as low-fat meat and low-cholesterol eggs.

Seven years ago, animal rights activists and farmers took action by filing suit in U.S. District Court in San Francisco to halt patenting of genetically altered animals, claiming that the government had no authority to issue patents for higher orders of life ("Activists, Farmers" 1988). Commenting on the filing of the suit, one of the plaintiffs, Steven Wise, stated that "this is not an attack on the merits of genetic engineering, . . . it is simply an allegation that the patent office, by attempting to shoehorn all animals into the category of a 'new and useful . . . composition of matter,' has exceeded the authorization Congress has given" ("Activists, Farmers" 1988). The district court determined that this action should have been brought before the Court of Appeals for the Federal Circuit and dismissed the action. The decision of the district court was upheld by the Court of Appeals for the Ninth Circuit.

Undoubtedly, new patents will spawn further lawsuits, as did the

Supreme Court decision in *Diamond v. Chakrabarty*. According to Senior Circuit Judge MacKinnon, concurring in *Foundation on Economic Trends v. Heckler*, "the use of delaying tactics by those who fear and oppose scientific progress is nothing new. It would, however, be a national catastrophe if the development of this promising new science of genetic engineering were crippled by the unconscionable delays that have been brought by litigants" (756 F. 2d 143, at 161).

Potential advantages

While interest groups on one side of the controversy have raised concerns over the patenting of animals, the "biotechnology industry cheered the April 12 decision . . . calling the move a logical extension of the patenting process" (Booth 1988:718). What is seen as possibly the greatest potential of the new technology is its promise in helping understand and treat cancer and other diseases.

Among other potential benefits of this new technology, some of which have already been realized, is the availability of new drugs. Currently, pharmaceutically important drugs such as insulin, growth hormone, Factor VIII, and interferon are being synthesized by organisms that have been genetically altered by incorporating foreign genes. These products are being produced either in bacteria or in higher transgenic animals. Another benefit, of course, is the potential to improve the quality of food to suit the needs of our society. Such improved products would include low-fat meats and milk and low-cholesterol eggs.

Transgenic technology undoubtedly will produce animal models for the investigation and development of cures for diseases in addition to cancer. A prime candidate for such investigation at the moment is AIDS. This disease has remained difficult to investigate since humans are the only animals who are afflicted. The development of animal models will allow researchers to investigate the course of the disease, to develop effective drug treatments, or, hopefully, to effect a cure.

As stated earlier, a few countries do theoretically permit patenting of animals. The most notable of these is Japan. With patent protection of animals, the United States will be in a competitive position in what promises to be a lucrative and ever-growing international market. Without patent protection, United States businesses will be in a poor position to remain competitive with other countries that offer protection for human-made animals. Additionally, even if other countries do not permit animal patents, the granting of patents in this area by the United States will still protect the nation's businesses from importation of animals that have been patented in the United States. Even if foreign countries do not permit patent protection for animals, this is not a prohibition on the use of the technology. Other countries will still be active in the development of transgenic animals, and importing these animals into the United States will compete with American industrial innovations.

An alternative to patenting new technology is to maintain new inventions as trade secrets. The option of trade secrets is not, in general, an attractive alternative for biotechnology, since many of the inventions easily could be "back-engineered" if a competitor should determine the exact nature of the invention and copy it. Alternatively, if the inventions actually can be maintained as secrets, the result is not an ideal solution for society. In this case, the inventions would remain in the hands of a small group of people or one company and would not be available to the community as a whole. In general, employment of this option would deprive the public of the advances, or at least slow the progress, that is to be made or could be made by science, through fostering a free exchange of ideas and technological advances. Patenting also ensures that technological advances will be available for public scrutiny and comment. Such public scrutiny would be impossible under the trade-secret approach.

Another benefit to the field of biotechnology is the potential for increased funding from a source previously untapped for basic research in the biological sciences. Such funding would be in the form of royalties and grants from pharmaceutical companies and other industries for the right of first refusal on potentially patentable experimental results, or under licensing agreements for the use of patented inventions. Harvard University has granted exclusive rights to the mouse patent to DuPont, "which has donated about $6 million in open-ended grants to Leder's group at Harvard in exchange for the right of first refusal to license" (Booth 1988:718). This form of funding basic research may become more attractive in the future as traditional sources of funding become scarcer.

The National Institutes of Health currently is the major source of funds for basic research in the biological sciences. This funding is in the form of research grants to academic researchers. Federal grants to basic research have been dropping since 1987, even though the number of applications has grown dramatically (Lindgreen 1990). The potential to gain funding from private, industrial sources through grants will stimulate the formation of academic and industrial alliances that will foster a transfer of technology from the academic world to that of private industry. Patenting will promote this transfer of technology.

The insight of the Supreme Court in *Diamond v. Chakrabarty* is still applicable to the latest biological patenting decision of the U.S. Patent and Trademark Office:

> The grant or denial of patents on a micro-organism is not likely to put an end to genetic research or to its attendant risks. The large amount of research that has already occurred when no researcher had sure knowledge that patent protection would be available suggests that legislative or judicial fiat as to patentability will not deter the scientific mind from probing into the unknown any more than Canute could command the tides. Whether respondent's claims are patentable may determine whether research efforts are accelerated by the hope of reward or slowed by want of incentives, but that is all.
>
> What is more important is that we are without competence to entertain these arguments—either to brush them aside as fantasies generated by fear of the unknown, or to act on them. The choice we are urged to make is a matter of high policy for resolution within the legislative process after the kind of investigation, examination, and study that legislative bodies can provide and courts cannot. (447 U.S. 303, at 317)

Granting of a patent will not prevent the continuation of research. However, patenting will ensure the general availability of the advances made by biotechnology to the public at large and ensure that the public will be able to receive the benefits of that research.

Inevitably, there will still be continuing political and legal battles before a compromise is reached by all the parties who have conflicting interests in the outcome, as the benefits to be gained from the use of the new technology are weighed against its perceived disadvantages and dangers. The questions inevitably will be resolved by the involvement of the legal, scientific, and industrial communities, and the public. However, we also have to ensure that "we . . . increase the scientific literacy so the questions involved can be resolved with full public debate" ("How to Cope with the Genetic Genie" 1990).

References

"Activists, Farmers File Suit to Halt Genetically Bred Animal Patents." 1988. *Los Angeles Times*, (July 30):II12.

"Animals—Patentability." 1988. *Journal of the Patent and Trademark Office Society* 69:328.

Bent, Stephen A., Richard L. Schwab, David G. Conlin, and Donald D. Jeffery. 1987. *Intellectual Property Rights in Biotechnology Worldwide*. United Kingdom: Stockton Press.

Booth, William. 1988. "Animals of Invention." *Science* 240:718.

Chisum, Donald S. 1988. *Patents*. Section 1.02(7):*n*24.6.

Congressional Record. 1988. House of Representatives. 2d Session. 134, Pt. 12 (June 30, 1988):16602.

Crawford, Mark. 1987. "Religious Groups Join Animal Patent Battle." *Science* 237:480–481.

Diamond v. Chakrabarty. 1980. 447 U.S. 303.

Ex parte Allen. 1987. 2 U.S.P.Q.2d (BNA) 1425.

Foundation on Economic Trends v. Heckler. 1985. 756 F2d 143.

Gorner, Peter, and Ronald Kotulak. 1990. "Cattle-Cloning Labs Transform the Barnyard." *Chicago Tribune* (April 10):1.

Hanson, Betsy, and Dorothy Nelkin. 1989. "Public Responses to Genetic Engineering." *Society* 27(1):76–80.

Hart, Kathleen. 1990. "Making Mythical Monsters." *The Progressive* 54:22.

"How to Cope with the Genetic Genie." 1990. *Chicago Tribune* (April 15):C2.

Leder, Philip, and T. Stewart. 1988. "Transgenic Non-Human Mammals." U.S. Patent No. 4736866 (abstract).

Lindgreen, Kristina. 1990. "Research, Talent Win UCI Record Amount of Grants." *Los Angeles Times* (August 13):A1.

Manbeck, Harry F. 1990. "Entering Our Third Century." Keynote address before the American Bar Association, Section of Patent, Trademark and Copyright Law.

May, A. 1988. "Role as 'Cancer Detectives' Seen for Patented Mouse." *Los Angeles Times* (April 13):I1.

Quigg, Donald J. 1988. *Patent, Trademark and Copyright Journal* 35:508.

Sugarman, Carole. 1989. "Biological Wizardry: Genetic Engineers Set the Table with New Products." *Washington Post* (April 19):E1.

"U.S. Grants Patent to Genetically Altered Mouse." 1988. *Reuter's Business Report*, April 12.

15

Diagnosis: The Social Implications of Emerging Biological Tests*

Dorothy Nelkin

Metaphorical constructs are commonly used to conceptualize the body and mind. The particular metaphors that have shaped our understanding of the body have changed over time, following scientific and medical developments, but even as they evolved, they have continually reinforced the view of the body as a mechanical system. Advances in organ transplantation, for example, projected an image of the body as a set of replaceable parts. The development of antibiotics created the image of the body as a chemical system, and discoveries elucidating the chemical basis of cellular activity pushed this metaphor to the forefront. Similarly, research on neuronal activity and electrical impulses shaped a perception of the brain as a complex system of electric wires. The growing role of computers evoked the metaphor of the mind as a computerized system, but later biochemical research has suggested that the brain, more than a computer, is also a producer of neurochemicals.

Today, research in genetics and the neurosciences is shaping the popular discourse on body and mind. Centered on the importance of biology in predicting future behavior and health, this research presents an image of the body and mind as machine-like "systems" that can be visualized on a computer screen and understood simply by deciphering a code. Objectifying the person as a set of mechanical parts or processes

*This essay was drawn from Dorothy Nelkin and Lawrence Tancredi, *Dangerous Diagnostics: The Social Power of Biological Information* (New York: Basic Books, 1989).

to be calibrated and defined, this metaphor underlies the development of new diagnostic tests that are able to detect more and more subtle biological differences among individuals and predict diseases prior to the manifestation of symptoms. The expectations derived from this metaphor are shaping how these predictive tests are interpreted and their results employed.

What are these diagnostic tests? Briefly, they include improved imaging technologies such as computer electroencephalogram (CEEG), positron emission tomography (PET), and technologies with acronyms such as BEAM, SPECT, and SQUID. In experiments with these devices, researchers study the relationship between brain functioning and particular behaviors. Such devices will one day be used to diagnose behavioral disorders and psychiatric diseases before their symptoms are expressed. According to the National Institute of Mental Health, "presymptomatic detection of psychiatric disease will be routine" (NIMH 1988:20).

Other predictive tests are emerging from scientific advances in genetics. For many years, we have been able to identify chromosomal and biochemical abnormalities in utero through amniocentesis. Current research is yielding methods of scanning the sequences of DNA that form the basis of our biological inheritance. These methods involve the location of RFLPs (restricted fragment length polymorphisms), sections of DNA on specific chromosomes that are considered to be genetic markers. When a variation, detected by a radio-labeled probe, cosegregates with illness in members of a family in which a hereditary disease occurs, this variation is assumed to be linked to the presence of a defective gene. In this way, hundreds of genetic markers indicating predisposition to a growing number of hereditary diseases have been identified to date. Presymptomatic tests are becoming commercially available for a number of single gene disorders. They now exist for about thirty disorders, including Huntington disease, cystic fibrosis, and hemophilia. As more genes are identified, tests will be able to indicate predisposition not only to purely genetic diseases, but also to very complex disorders suspected of having a genetic component: mental illness (including bipolar diseases, schizophrenia, and anxiety disorders), hyperactivity, early-onset Alzheimer disease, heart disease, certain forms of cancer, and predispositions to alcoholism or addition (Holtzman 1989).

Many of the more sophisticated genetic and neurological tests are still limited to experimental investigation. Moreover, as has usually been the case in the history of medical invention, diagnostic techniques are far ahead of therapeutic possibilities. The most important social consequence of these new diagnostic tests in the short term is their bearing on the definition of disease. They are providing theoretical models to explain complex human behavior in simple biological terms. Genetics, says the president of the American Society of Human Genetics, has "made inroads into the medical mind" (Scriver 1987).

What do such tests tell us? All diagnostic tests function by establishing a statistical measure of the "normal" against which to measure individual differences. In addition, these recent technologies share several related characteristics:

1. They pierce the external frame of the body to reveal the biological substrata from which physical or psychological characteristics emerge. Able to detect very early biological changes, they enhance diagnostic predictability, allowing anticipation of future problems that may not be visibly expressed in manifest symptoms for years. They are, in effect, creating a new category of people called the "asymptomatic ill."

2. They can detect ever-more-minute individual differences with increased precision. Just as the testing of food products has allowed greater sensitivity in the detection of carcinogens, so improved diagnostics have refined our capacity to identify deviations from the norm. In both cases, the number of products or persons defined as problematic has greatly expanded.

3. These new diagnostic technologies are useful not only for clinical diagnosis, that is for providing an explanation of an individual's health status, but also for screening, where the purpose is to identify from a large population those individuals who deviate from the norm.

These characteristics enhance the appeal of biological diagnosis not only in medical contexts but in nonclinical settings, as employers, insurers, schools, and the courts are seeking ways to conform their constituents to institutional needs. This is a time when many organizations are facing difficult economic, legal, and administrative pressures. They are seeking strategies that will increase economic efficiency and predictability, and allow them to minimize future risks. Biology-based tests that tap into biological understanding of how the body functions and predict how an individual body can be expected to function in the course of a person's life can serve these organizational needs.

Physicians look at biological diagnosis in terms of its contribution to defining therapeutic modalities. While genetic therapies are far in the future, knowledge of genetic defects can be clinically useful, allowing control, in some cases, through dietary measures, in others through reproductive choice. But diagnosis is more than a medical procedure; it is also a way to create social categories, to preserve existing social arrangements, and to enhance the control of certain groups over others (Brown 1987). Michel Foucault, for example, wrote about the medical examination as a strategy of political domination, a means of "normalization." He described the examination as "a normalizing gaze," that "introduces the constraints of conformity . . . [that] compares, differentiates, hierarchizes, homogenizes, excludes" (1979:183–184). Anthropologists have observed the institutional tendency to conform individuals to institutional values. As Mary Douglas put it, "Institutions bestow sameness. . . . They turn the body's shape to their conventions" (1986:63, 92). In the context of these sociological perspectives on diagnosis, certain cultural and social conditions legitimate the growing use of tests in nonclinical settings. These tests, in turn, contribute to institutional goals.

The Appeal of Testing

The increased preoccupation with testing in American culture reflects our prevailing approach to problems—an approach that rests on what may be called an "actuarial mind-set." Actuarial thinking requires calculating the cost of future contingencies, taking into account expected losses, and selecting good risks while excluding bad risks. To do so it is necessary to understand the individual—the body—with reference to a statistical aggregate. In this context the information derived from tests becomes a valuable resource.

Reflecting the actuarial mind-set, the gathering of personal information by government agencies, employers, and schools has greatly increased in the last twenty years. Testing is part of this trend. The screening of prospective employees for drug use, for example, continues despite concerns about the accuracy and legitimacy of tests. The pressure to test for AIDS is relentless, despite well-documented discriminatory implications. And the use of standardized tests in schools is growing, despite questions about their validity as a measure of intelligence and predictor of performance. Indeed, the faith in "facts," in the numbers derived from testing, has obscured the uncertainties intrinsic to most tests, and such tests are widely accepted as neutral, necessary, and benign.

Just as the value of facts is part of the actuarial mentality, so too is the tendency to reduce social problems to measurable biological dimensions; that is, to dimensions that can be revealed through a test. Since World War II, geneticists have been reluctant to extend their ideas into the realm of social values (Kevles 1985). However, scientific advances in the

1980s have inspired more frequent references to the application of genetic understanding to social policy. Geneticist Marjorie Shaw, for example, has recently asserted that "the law must control the spread of genes causing severe deleterious effects, just as disabling pathogenic bacteria and viruses are controlled" (1984:63). The editor of *Science*, Daniel Koshland, Jr., has asserted that in the warfare between nature and nurture, nature has clearly won—with all that this implies for the idea of genetic determinism and the immutability of inherited traits (1987:1445). The psychiatric profession, inclined in any case toward deterministic explanations, is largely committed to the notion of behavioral genetics.

Social policies are mediated through institutions. Schools, courts, and insurers increasingly are using biological concepts and diagnostic tests to serve their organizational goals. Conceptually, biological tests are but an extension of earlier pedagogical and psychiatric tests. Like these tests, they can serve as gatekeepers, controlling access, for example, to employment or insurance. They allow organizations to shape their clients as a projection of their economic and administrative needs.

Tests can be used to redefine a socially derived syndrome as a problem of the individual, placing blame in ways that reduce public accountability and protect routine institutional practices. The availability of biological tests gives an organization a scientific means of dealing with failures or unusual problems without threatening its basic values or disrupting its existing programs. For example, at a time when public schools face pressures for accountability, it is convenient to explain learning difficulties or behavior problems in terms of individual disabilities. Once explained in terms of cultural deprivation or nutritional deficiencies, educational failures have been redefined over the past decade as "learning difficulties"—that is, problems located in the student's brain. Hyperactivity, once defined as a problem in classroom dynamics, has been redefined as attention deficit disorder—a problem intrinsic to the child. Of course, the behavioral or learning difficulties of many children are very real. But diagnostic labels are also an institutional convenience, removing blame from the schools and other social influences and satisfying demands for accountability. Meanwhile, they can stigmatize slow learners as inherently, and therefore permanently, disabled, and they can draw attention away from the social interactions that influence learning (Coles 1988:14).

Testing in the workplace can also be used to justify routine institutional practices. Biological tests are used to identify the susceptibility of particular workers to toxic exposure. Justified in the first instance as a way of protecting workers' health, testing and then excluding vulnerable individuals can be used to avoid costly changes in the work environment. Through testing, the employee assumes responsibility and can be made to conform (U.S. Congress 1990).

The predictive capacity of biological diagnosis is also useful to organizations as a means of facilitating efficient long-term planning. Companies, as insurers, increasingly are reluctant to employ those whose lifestyle or genetics may predispose them to future illness. In the context of growing economic competition, screening techniques that will identify those predisposed to genetic disease can become a cost-effective way to control absenteeism, reduce compensation claims, and avoid future medical costs for workers and their families.

In the medical sector, efficient planning is urgent in the context of prepaid medical plans, the financial dilemmas of insurance companies, and government policies linking reimbursement decisions to diagnostic categories. These pressures, as well as the threat of malpractice suits, create powerful incentives to back up health care decisions with objective and predictive information. They encourage competition for the "profitable" patient, the person who carries no dangerous genetic characteristics and who has predictable and reimbursable illnesses. Diagnostic technologies help to categorize patients; they provide the technical evidence to support controversial decisions and patient profiles to control access to health care facilities (U.S. Congress 1988).

The need for efficiency also has implications for the use of fetal tests. A number of studies have documented the cost of genetic disorders, believing them to occur in about 5 percent of all live births, and to account for nearly 30 percent of all pediatric hospital admissions and 12 percent of all adult admissions in the United States. While the presumed beneficiary of fetal testing is the prospective parent, health care providers and insurers also benefit from genetic information that may have consequences for future medical obligations.

This brings us to the third use of biological tests—to justify difficult decisions about the exclusion of high-risk individuals from situations in which their future health status may be costly. The use of testing as a means of exclusion from work is well established. About half of American employers require preemployment medical exams (Rothstein 1984:10). But the biological status of a person's body, indicated by tests, may also be grounds for exclusion from insurance. Today, about 37 million people in the United States have no public or private health insurance. About 15 percent of those who are insured are individually covered and must meet underwriting standards by providing their health history, information on their family illnesses, and evidence of their current state of health. Sometimes tests are required. In 1987, 20 percent of individual applicants were issued policies that excluded preexisting conditions, or else they paid a higher premium in the presence of such conditions; 8 percent were denied coverage for diseases including obesity, alcoholism, cancer, schizophrenia, and AIDS. Similarly, HMOs in 1987 denied membership to 24 percent of individual applicants. As genetic tests become available, the medical directors of insurance companies expect to have access to the diagnostic information to make judgments about coverage and to calculate rates (U.S. Congress 1988).

Finally, tests may facilitate controversial decisions about the disposition of those who will not or cannot conform to institutional norms. Consulting psychiatrists are brought into hospitals to test, for example, the competency of patients who fail to comply with controversial decisions about recommended treatment or placement in a nursing home. The courts increasingly are predisposed to admit "hard" evidence to sort out conflicting psychiatric opinion in decisions about the responsibility, culpability, and disposition of defendants. In a remarkable response to such demands, a neurologist in California has introduced the use of PET scans in the courts as a scientific basis for sentencing decisions that require consideration of the responsibility and rehabilitation potential of convicted criminals. Legal scholars writing on biological psychiatry anticipate that the courts will increasingly use information from brain scans to evaluate responsibility and predict the likelihood of future dangerousness (Jeffrey 1985:82).

Diagnostic technologies, grounded in science, are compelling. Images on a screen have an appearance of precision. Statistical findings processed by computers appear to be objective, neutral, beyond refutation, equivalent to truth. However, the use of such tests is subject to many interpretive fallacies. The evidence produced by most diagnostic tests is only inferential, and interpretation rests on statistical definitions of the normal. Moreover, interpretation often assumes causation when there is only correlation. And in the present state-of-the-art biological testing, the error rate—the false positives and false negatives—remains high for many conditions. Even if tests are totally reliable predictors of disease, they tell us little about the character of its actual expression. For in most diseases, the manifestation of symptoms, their severity, and when they will appear, rests on random events, or on intervening factors such as diet, lifestyle, or the influence of environmental or social interactions (Nelkin and Tancredi 1989).

The interpretive assumptions underlying the use of biological tests become especially critical when they are used to screen large populations—as, for example, when workers are screened for genetic susceptibility to toxic substances. Unlike clinical tests, the point with biological tests is not to discover the cause of particular symptoms but to deduce statistical levels of a disease in a population. Actual behavior of symptoms in such circumstances can be ignored or, worse, interpreted to support the biological indicator.

The Social Implications of New Diagnostic Tests

As advances in genetics and the neurosciences provide powerful instruments for predicting disabilities and behavioral abnormalities, tests that are efficient, inexpensive, accurate, and nonobtrusive can be developed. Testing every newborn child will become simple. Establishing national DNA data banks to store information about a person's parentage and predisposition to disease also will be feasible. Every person could have a genetic map on file. The medical benefits of anticipating genetic disease, the social benefits of records that would facilitate control of "criminal elements," and the economic benefits of having data for rational planning could serve as powerful justification for the development of such records. Thus despite the technical limits of predictive tests, their potential uses are generating a large and competitive industry.

Data banks today already contain considerable personal information about a large number of people. In some states, information on hospitalized mental patients is stored in state files. State genetic registries record birth defects, often including identifying information such as Social Security numbers. The FBI has begun a DNA data bank containing the DNA fingerprints of suspected criminals and paroled ex-convicts as a means of crime control.

Diagnosis can be viewed in terms of its psychological implications for the individual or the family. What does it do to an individual to find out he or she is sure to get a devastating illness like Huntington disease or early-onset Alzheimer disease. Beyond the psychological effect of knowing one is "presymptomatic," however, such knowledge has social and economic implications. The possibilities for discrimination are evident. Many cases of "genetic discrimination" have been documented, cases in which genetic predisposition to a disease has been reified as the disease itself, even when no obvious manifestations of illness exist. The asymptomatic ill, people who have no symptoms but are known to have a genetic disease, have been barred from insurance and employment because of their genetic labels (Rowley 1988:105–106).

The significance of biological profiles rests, of course, on how they will be used. Schools, employers, insurers, and law enforcement agencies can and do use the information from tests. But other groups also have an intrinsic interest in the genetic or neurobiological condition of the people in their domains. The Department of Motor Vehicles, immigration authorities, creditors, adoption agencies, organ transplant registries, professional sports teams, sexual partners, and the military all may have reasons for wanting access to diagnostic information about the present and future health status of individuals. Families might demand information about their genetic roots; adoption brokers could probe the genetic history of children in order to find appropriate matches; or commercial firms could store genetic profiles and sell them to interested agencies. Considering such possibilities for exclusion, stigmatization, and discrimination, there has been little discussion about the use and abuse of testing, or about questions of access to biological information.

References

Brown, Phil. 1987. "Diagnostic Conflict and Contradiction in Psychiatry." *Journal of Health and Social Behavior* 28:37–50.
Coles, Gerald S. 1988. *The Learning Mystique.* New York: Pantheon.
Douglas, Mary. 1986. *How Institutions Think.* Syracuse, N.Y.: Syracuse University Press.
Foucault, Michel. 1979. *Discipline and Punish.* New York: Vintage.
Holtzman, Neil. 1989. *Proceed with Caution: The Use of Recombinant DNA Technology for Genetic Testing.* Baltimore: Johns Hopkins University Press.
Jeffrey, C.R., R. V. Del Carmen, and J. D. White. 1985. *Attacks on the Insanity Defense: Biological Psychiatry and New Perspectives on Criminal Behavior.* Springfield, Ill.: Charles C. Thomas.
Kevles, Daniel. 1985. *In the Name of Eugenics.* New York: Knopf.
Koshland, Daniel, Jr. 1987. Editorial. *Science* 235:1445.
National Institute of Mental Health (NIMH). 1988. *Approaching the 21st Century: Opportunities for NIMH Neurosciences Research.* Report to Congress on the Decade of the Brain. Washington, D.C.: U.S. Department of Health and Human Services.
Nelkin, Dorothy, and Lawrence Tancredi. 1989. *Dangerous Diagnostics: The Social Power of Biological Information.* New York: Basic.
Rothstein, Mark. 1984. *Medical Screening of Workers.* Washington, D.C.: Bureau of National Affairs.
Rowley, Peter. 1988. "Genetic Discrimination." *American Journal of Human Genetics* 43:105–106.
Scriver, Charles R. 1987. "Presidential Address." *American Journal of Human Genetics* 40:199–211.
Shaw, Marjorie. 1984. "Conditional Prospective Rights of the Fetus." *Journal of Legal Medicine* 63:63–116.

U.S. Congress, Office of Technology Assessment. 1990. *Genetic Monitoring and Screening in the Workplace.* OTA-BA-455. Washington, D.C.: U.S. Government Printing Office.

U.S. Congress, Office of Technology Assessment. 1988. *Medical Testing and Health Insurance.* OTA-H-384. Washington, D.C.: U.S. Government Printing Office.

16

Toward Policies Regarding Assisted Reproductive Technologies

Jacques Cohen and Robert Lee Hotz

Some important enigmas of early human conception—the union of one female egg and one male sperm—have now been solved. The basic scientific discipline of biology and the practice of medicine have joined, perhaps for the first time, in the clinical application of assisted reproductive technology. Some specialists, seeking a novel acronym to define this new field, call it ART. These new technologies usually are aimed at women who cannot carry their own child and at those numerous couples—an estimated 2.4 million married couples in the United States (U.S. Congress 1988:3)—who are infertile and cannot conceive unaided. More recently, ART specialists have developed the biopsy techniques necessary to investigate the gender and genetic health of an embryo in the first several days of its life without jeopardizing its ability to develop into a normal fetus. As a result, early embryos can now be clinically selected on the basis of their genetic health to avoid the birth of a genetically disabled child, i.e., one who would develop muscular dystrophy, cystic fibrosis, or some other potentially lethal condition. Several normal births resulting from this technique have been reported in England (Handyside 1990). This newest reproductive technology raises questions regarding the possibility that in future decades abnormal human embryos could be repaired by altering their genetic structure. Instead of discarding a genetically diseased embryo, it might be repaired by inserting new genes or by deleting the abnormal gene. Such germ-line gene therapy would require several molecular biology techniques yet to be developed. However, the technology, once it is available, will raise ethical, social, and legal issues far more complicated than anything reproductive scientists, physicians, and lawmakers have previously encountered. Other potentially controversial techniques such as embryo gender selection, embryo transplants or cloning—commonly used in the cattle industry today—may one day find clinical application among human beings. Earlier controversies concerning donor insemination, in vitro fertilization, gestational surrogacy, and embryo freezing will have served as a prelude to these larger controversies.

The moment for state and federal lawmakers to join with philosophers and ethicists to address such reproductive technologies systematically is long overdue. The overriding characteristic of the field in the United States is the absence of state or federal regulation and the refusal of the National Institutes of Health—the world's largest biomedical research establishment—to fund or monitor human embryo research. Clinical embryo laboratories have been exempt from basic medical licensing procedures. In litigation concerning human embryos, two lower courts in the United States have explicitly rejected policy positions developed by the relevant medical societies (*Davis v. Davis* 1989; *York v. Jones* 1989). State and federal insurance plans have not extended their coverage to include such procedures, and many private insurers routinely reject claims for the most high-tech infertility procedures, raising troubling questions of equal access to these emerging technologies.

A number of other industrialized nations including England, Australia, Germany, and Spain recently have enacted comprehensive legislation to regulate the emerging technologies. The Council of Europe has drawn up extensive recommendations for its member countries (Gunning 1990). At least eighty-five national bioethical committees and law reform commissions representing twenty-five countries have reviewed some or all of the reproductive technologies. More than 110 additional formal governmental assessments of the new reproductive techniques have been prepared but never formally published (Walters 1987). The laws and commission reports reveal an absence of any international agreement even on such fundamental questions as whether human embryos should be created specifically for research purposes. There is little national or international consensus on research into the beginnings of human life or on the appropriate application of the resulting clinical technologies.*

---

*Information on the international policies concerning reproductive policies and embryo experiments cited here and elsewhere in the text is the product of Robert Hotz's ongoing research on advanced reproductive technology. The results of his research will appear in his book, *Designs on Life: Exploring the New Frontiers of Human*

Research into the first days and weeks of embryonic development—into the genetic framework dictating an embryo's growth and its differentiation from its earliest single cell into fetal organs, tissue, and placenta—yielded the techniques embryologists needed to fertilize a human egg outside the body and cultivate the resulting embryo in the laboratory. From such research, embryologists also learned how to perform microsurgery on a human egg or early embryo to improve the chances that an embryo will successfully implant in the womb when it is transferred several days after fertilization. Several births have been reported in the United States in 1990 and 1991 from this technique.* As embryologists absorb the lessons of molecular biology, in vitro fertilization will find broader medical applications.

Many of these scientific developments challenge traditional notions of family and social customs. Recent developments allow for the union of sperm and egg, even if a couple is separated by great distance or by death. They create the possibility that one generation may donate sperm and eggs to another generation. A daughter, for example, may donate her eggs to her infertile mother. A grandmother may donate her frozen embryos to her infertile grandchild or carry her daughter's embryos to term. Such arrangements cross sensitive barriers of social and sexual custom. Spurred by the social innovations such reproductive technologies make possible, courts already are reassessing traditional notions of parentage on a case-by-case basis.

There is no single place in the legal code where such issues are addressed. Troubling legal dilemmas are scattered through adoption law, divorce codes, inheritance statutes, product liability ordinances, negligence standards, and patent law. Lord Meston, during a 1990 debate in the British House of Lords over legislation to license human embryo research, said, "If an embryo is to be treated by the law as a thing, it could obviously be owned. If, however, an embryo is treated as a person, it cannot be owned. If it is to be treated as a person how are such disputes to be resolved?" He went on to observe, "I do not envy the court which has to decide what is or may be in the best interest of an embryo, particularly if the choice is between being implanted or not being implanted" (*Hansard* 1990). In light of further advances, a systematic political, philosophical, and legal appraisal of assisted reproductive technologies is necessary.

Fertility, to be published in 1991 by Pocket Books. The author conducted more than 300 interviews with embryologists, patients, and policymakers in the United States, Europe, and Australia in the course of extended site visits in those nations.

*According to unpublished data from Jacques Cohen, the Center for Reproductive Medicine and Infertility, the New York Hospital-Cornell University Medical Center, New York, and Reproductive Biology Associates, Atlanta, Georgia.

The Onset of New Human Life

When does an embryo become a fetus? When does a fetus become a child? The answers to these questions will in all likelihood never cease to be controversial. The answers involve not only scientific findings, but social and religious beliefs. The world's 920 million Roman Catholics believe, as a matter of theological doctrine, that human life begins at conception, in the precise moment when sperm and egg combine. The world's 860 million followers of Islam, in contrast, believe as a matter of religious faith that human life begins forty days after conception. Protestant Christian groups do not even agree among themselves.

In a pluralistic society, unanimity on such issues may be beyond the ability of any secular authority. Whether governments should actually have to address issues concerning the embryo and the fetus in order to regulate further research and emerging medical technologies is, for some people, an open question. However, policy makers and legislators need some consensus on which to base rule-making decisions. This can only be accomplished if they are given some clear guidance in determining fact from reproductive fiction. Unfortunately, scientists and medical professionals who deal with these questions on a daily basis disagree sharply. Hence, confusion begins where it might least be expected—with embryologists, endocrinologists, physicians, and reproductive technicians. Some of them define the onset of new human life as the time when the neural system has reached a stage in development in which it can receive and interpret signals—in other words, when the fetus can "feel." This stage is reached many weeks after the embryo comes into being. In his dissent from the court's ruling in *Webster v. Reproductive Services*, Supreme Court Justice John Paul Stevens, commenting on the State's right to protect the life of a fetus, noted, "As a secular matter, there is an obvious difference between the state interest in protecting the freshly fertilized egg and the state interest in protecting a nine-month-gestated, fully sentient fetus on the eve of birth. There can be no interest in protecting the newly fertilized egg from physical pain or mental anguish because the capacity for such suffering does not yet exist. . . . A State has no greater secular interest in protecting the potential life of an embryo that is still 'seed' than in protecting the life of a sperm or an unfertilized ovum" (*Webster v. Reproductive Services* 1989).

Some scientists pinpoint the development of an individual's life at about the fifteenth day of the embryo's primitive streak—the precursor of the spinal cord (Ford 1988:164–177). Until that point, it is possible that the embryo could develop into twins or triplets. Other specialists define the onset of life earlier, at the time of implantation, when the free-floating embryo emerges from its protective membrane, called the zona pellucida, and adheres to the uterine wall—about seven days after fertilization. Shortly after this time, the woman's body receives chemical messages from the implanted embryo that signal the onset of a pregnancy. Still other scientists believe that new life is created when the sperm cell and the egg cell fuse, a moment that is now routinely observed in laboratories handling reproductive cells from hundreds of couples seeking treatment for infertility. The technique that makes direct observation of the human embryo possible, in vitro fertilization (IVF), is the best known of all the assisted reproductive technologies. IVF has been applied clinically worldwide on such a scale that by the year 2010 as many as one million people will owe their conception to this technique.

What is the moral status of these human embryos? Do they require legal status? Should their status differ from that of any other human cell or from that of the unfertilized egg? Such questions have put embryo research in the center of a national debate over abortion. Antiabortion activists and many religious groups offer a single, principled view on this issue: egg plus sperm equals human life; an absolutist position that focuses on fertilization. The Duke of Norfolk, during the 1990 House of Lords debate, said, "The answer is simple. I believe that an embryo is the start of life and must be given the same status in life as a child, a grown-up person or a Member of your Lordships' Chamber. I can see no distinction between that and the life of an embryo (*Hansard* 1990)." In the Missouri abortion law at issue in the case of *Webster v. Reproductive Services*, reviewed by the U.S. Supreme Court in 1989, that state's legislators embedded such a view in the preamble they had adopted—"The life of each human being begins at conception"—and they defined conception as "the fertilization of the ovum of a female by the sperm of a male." Such a view places severe constraints on embryo research, infertility treatments, fetal tissue research, and research into new forms of contraception. However, no Biblical guidance to sustain such a notion of human life exists. Many passages in the Bible and the Talmud refer to human life in the womb without asserting precisely when the individual human comes into being. Aristotle believed that it took forty days to form a male and ninety days to form a female. Saint Thomas Aquinas believed that a developing fetus acquired a soul only after its first forty days (Ford 1988:21–57).

Specialists again add to the confusion by adopting new language to describe the fertilized egg in order to distinguish its status from that of the more developed, hundred-cell embryo that eventually attaches to the wall of the uterus. In 1986, the American Fertility Society, following the lead of a British parliamentary committee inquiry into in vitro fertilization and embryology, adopted the term "pre-embryo." The

British committee adopted the term as a matter of legislative convenience to describe the first fourteen days of an embryo's development (United Kingdom 1984). But in the United States, some medical policy makers have sought to elevate the term to a formal, biological distinction in an effort to circumvent a political debate with antiabortion activists.

Such concerns also shape the clinical application of reproductive technologies. For example, the early human embryo can be frozen safely at any stage between the moment of fertilization until about five days later, when it has become a hollow ball of fifty cells called a blastocyst. Several clinical IVF programs, however, will freeze the fertilized egg only at the moment when the sperm has traversed the layers surrounding the egg and formed a nucleus within it but before the actual process of fertilization is complete. The textbook view of fertilization is that the process culminates hours after the initial union of sperm and egg, when the genetic material from the two individual nuclei have fused and the cell has divided into two daughter cells. Clinics that freeze the "prefertilized egg" do so largely to avoid the ethical debate over the status of the human embryo. By appearing to comply with the absolutist view of conception, they may avoid interference with their clinical affairs, but they confuse matters for policymakers by suggesting that the two-cell embryo has a more significant ethical status than an egg which has been penetrated by a sperm.

All of the embryo's early stages—the two-cell embryo, the egg in the process of fertilization, even the unfertilized egg and the single sperm cell—represent crucial moments in the creation of a new human life. Each stage is deserving of respect. No one phase can be circumvented or replaced by another. It is a stately progression that must proceed in its own order and in its entirety to reach its goal. During each cell division in the first days of embryonic development, dramatic molecular and physical changes occur. Although the process can be described scientifically only by defining each moment of development separately, no single stage is any more or less important than any other. New life does not appear suddenly; it is created gradually, with each new phase differing from that which preceded it. Life, death, and the creation of new life can be regarded as a continuum. "We are constantly trying to apply distinctions which pertain in ordinary life but which do not actually apply in a particular respect. For example, lawyers try to put everything in one of two baskets; it is either a person or a thing," said the Archbishop of York before the House of Lords. "However, there are entities which are neither persons or things. What we are referring to in the case of a conceptus is an organism of human origin which given the right conditions has the potential to develop and may become a full human person" (*Hansard* 1990).

Some policymakers have proposed that the unique genetic structure embodied in the embryo endows it with special status. Lawmakers in the Australian state of Victoria, who were the first in the world to regulate embryo research and in vitro fertilization, attached great significance to the moment of syngamy (the moment the male and female pronuclei fuse) (Australia 1989). As noted, many clinics will freeze only embryos that have not yet reached this stage. Each of the two daughter cells resulting from the initial union of sperms and egg contains two sets of chromosomes that consist of genes made up of the twisted strands of DNA. The DNA molecules code for each essential protein that make every cell unique and functional. Scientifically speaking, the two-cell embryo is not as genetically mature as later stages of the embryo. Cells of the two-cell embryo are genetically similar to those of the implanting blastocyst, fetus, and subsequent child, but the embryo's genes are inactive. The inactive DNA of the newly formed two-cell embryo is not able yet to produce its own proteins. Its two cells are completely dependent on the presence of proteins produced by certain maternal molecules already present in the unfertilized egg. The embryonic genes only become active—switched on—two days later, when the embryo has reached the eight-cell stage. That stage usually is not studied in the laboratory because IVF embryos created in the course of clinical infertility treatment are transferred to their mother at the four-cell stage. Genetically, therefore, one could define the completion of fertilization and the moment of conception as the formation of the eight-cell stage of the embryo three days after the sperm has penetrated the egg.

Fertilization may be redefined, perhaps, as a series of events which is completed three days after a sperm enters the egg, when the resulting embryo has grown into eight cells. The moment when the embryo becomes a fetus, however, resists definition. Only one of that embryo's eight cells will differentiate into "precursor cells" that later develop into the actual fetus. The other seven cells form the placenta, which is almost entirely embryonic in origin. No one considers the placenta, which comprises the majority of embryonic material, to be of any special moral or ethical significance.

Assisted Reproductive Technologies and Embryonic Research

There are basically four modes by which to establish conception artificially and to handle eggs and sperm under laboratory conditions. The first variation, artificial insemination technologies, involves obtaining human spermatozoa and eggs and using them for an otherwise natural conception inside a woman's body. The second set of methods, in vitro fertilization technologies, requires that the creation of the embryo take place outside the human body in the laboratory. The third group, embryo transfer technologies, involves the removal of a naturally conceived embryo or egg from a woman's uterus and the placement of the embryo or egg in a second woman's uterus. The fourth, surrogate mother technologies, involves transferring an embryo conceived in a petri dish by any of the artificial laboratory methods into a host mother for the duration of the pregnancy.

Each of these modes has numerous variations. Insemination techniques, for example, have been practiced clinically for decades. The most common, known as AID, is insemination with donor semen, is utilized by couples in which the male partner is infertile or has a hereditary disease that could be transmitted to his children. The American Fertility Society (AFS) and the American Association of Tissue Banks (AATB) urge that all donor semen be frozen for at least six months to exclude any donor who might later test positive for the AIDS virus. The second most commonly used method is artificial insemination with the husband's semen (AIH), which is used in cases of unexplained fertility and in some instances of male infertility. Deposit of semen directly into the uterus is called intra-uterine insemination (IUI). Some clinicians deposit spermatozoa in the cervical canal between the vagina and the uterus; others place it in the fallopian tube or the pelvic cavity. Yet another approach, called gamete intrafallopian transfer (GIFT), requires a surgical procedure and the use of a laparoscope, which is inserted through an incision in the woman's abdomen. Eggs retrieved from the ovaries are combined with sperm, and the mixture is inserted in the woman's fallopian tube.

IVF and the Spare Embryo

One of the more intriguing controversies in IVF concerns the disposition of excess embryos, those "spare" embryos that are not transferred immediately into the woman's uterus. In all but the most unusual circumstances, natural conception involves a single embryo, but IVF clinics commonly transfer multiple embryos to improve the odds that one will implant successfully. The chance that a single laboratory embryo will implant is only about 5 percent. By transferring three or four embryos at once, clinicians must balance the increased opportunity for a pregnancy against the risks of multiple births, triplets, quadruplets, and quintuplets. In the United Kingdom, for example, reproductive technologies have tripled the number of multiple births. In Australia, approximately one in every four pregnancies achieved through reproductive technologies involves twins, triplets, or quadruplets. A significant number of these infants are born prematurely. Many of them succumb during the pregnancy itself or following delivery.

Several technical solutions to the problem of multiple births may be possible. Each solution creates a new problem. The clinician can reduce the doses of fertility drugs used to stimulate the growth of eggs in the ovary, thus reducing the number of eggs available for fertilization. Unfortunately, that would also reduce the chances of producing a pregnancy. The clinician could also decide to limit the number of eggs removed from the ovary, leaving any excess behind. Those eggs, however, could continue to develop on their own and cause a potentially lethal condition called hyperstimulation.

The most practical option for the clinician is to limit the number of embryos transferred into the uterus and freeze the remainder. When the patient does not become pregnant from the "fresh" embryos, she can have the frozen embryos thawed and transferred at a later time. This procedure has two significant advantages. First, the clinician does not have to use fertility drugs to stimulate the ovaries, eliminating the risk of hyperstimulation. Second, the patient does not have to undergo multiple egg retrieval surgeries. The disadvantages of cryopreservation are numerous, but proper care and expertise can alleviate most of them. To reduce the risk that frozen embryos will be destroyed when storage facilities fail, the embryo tanks should be equipped with alarms, checked regularly, and, by necessity, have their stores of liquid nitrogen renewed. A major disadvantage to this method—for clinicians—is the lack of appropriate insurance coverage.

The use of clinic consent forms covering the disposition of excess embryos can reduce the ambiguities arising from the absence of legal guidelines covering the issue of embryo ownership. Whether clinics will actually destroy surplus embryos when a couple does not pay its storage fees, or when a prearranged storage limit has expired, or when a couple has forgotten to leave a forwarding address is unclear. Australian legislators have suggested that all unclaimed frozen embryos be put up for donation or adoption.

The easiest way to avoid the risks of a multiple pregnancy is to restrict the number of embryos transferred from the laboratory to the uterus. This often leaves the laboratory with surplus embryos which must be stored or disposed of in some manner. There is almost unanimous recognition of the special nature of these embryos but wide disagreement on how to dispose of them ethically. In Denmark, any surplus embryos must be destroyed immediately after the clinical treatment of an infertile couple. Lawmakers in the German Bundestag have forbidden the fertilization of more eggs than can be used for transfer in one in vitro fertilization cycle. In the Netherlands, scientists may, with written consent, use surplus embryos for research. In Spain, the government expects any surplus embryos to be frozen and requires clinics to have the facilities to allow them to do so. In Sweden, couples are also allowed to freeze their surplus embryos but by law they may store them only for a year. In the United States, by comparison, clinics and couples are free to make their own arrangements.

From the scientist's viewpoint, the most advantageous use of spare embryos is for research purposes. The benefits of embryo research are numerous, not only for the pure scientific knowledge to be gained but also for the improvement of currently inefficient clinical procedures. To some degree, experiments involving human embryos are everywhere controversial because they involve material that is potentially human life. "This built-in bias limiting research involving human preembryos is a necessary safeguard against premature or trivial research proposals. Such a conservative posture, however, should not preclude truly innovative research directed toward important scientific or clinical advances" (Ethics Committee 1990:63s), noted the ethics committee of the American Fertility Society. The creation of human embryos solely for the purpose of research is condemned in some countries. In a survey of fifteen national ethics bodies that had reviewed the proper circumstances for embryo research, almost half did not approve of the creation of embryos solely for research purposes (Walters 1987). In France, for example, a national ethics committee was so troubled by the idea of embryo research that it successfully imposed a moratorium on embryo experimentation. In Germany, where virtually no embryo research is performed, lawmakers made it a criminal offense to fertilize a human egg for any purpose other than to create a pregnancy in the woman who produced the egg. Italian policymakers banned embryo research for commercial purposes such as testing the effect of a new cosmetic or drug on human development. Swedish law allows couples to consent to the use of their spare embryos for research related solely to the improvement of IVF techniques. Norway prohibits all embryo research.

Other governments, most notably those of the United Kingdom, Australia, and Spain, have set up government regulatory authorities under which such experiments can proceed within a well-worked-out ethical framework that protects the interests of the couple whose gametes produced the embryo, and the embryo itself. In the United Kingdom, which has had a strong voluntary licensing system for embryo research in place since 1985, the government enacted legislation to set up a licensing authority to review all proposed embryo research. Under the law, it is a crime to perform unlicensed embryo research, but practitioners are permitted to create laboratory embryos solely for research purposes and perform experiments on them up until the fourteenth day of development. The Spanish government, under a 1988 law, permits research on nonviable embryos produced in the course of a therapeutic clinical program. Again, no research is allowed past the fourteenth day of development. The creation of embryos purely for research purposes is forbidden in Spain. In the Australian state of Victoria, any embryo research is prohibited unless approved by a standing review advisory committee in the department of health. The Victoria law was amended in 1987 to permit the creation of embryos for research on the process of fertilization prior to syngamy, which is defined in the law as "the alignment on the mitotic spindle of the chromosomes derived from the pronuclei" (Gunning 1990:11). Confusion over the precise limits of the law have led to a moratorium on virtually all embryo research in Victoria.

New IVF-Related Procedures

Several important IVF methods have been developed recently for which no guidelines have been proposed. The first set of reproductive techniques involves alternative culture methods. Embryos developing outside the body do not develop as quickly as those growing in natural conditions. To eliminate this discrepancy, some scientists have developed alternative culture conditions in which embryos are grown in the presence of fetal cells from the reproductive tract or related organs. This has been shown to promote embryonic development. The technique is widely practiced by commercial cattle embryo breeders. If the technique is not handled properly, however, the embryo can be contaminated by unwanted cellular products or even infected by viruses from the culture cells.

Other advances involve the field of micromanipulation. Robot arms can be hooked onto a microscope, allowing the embryologist to perform microscopic operations on human eggs and embryos with small glass scalpels and biopsy needles. One of the most spectacular applications of micromanipulation techniques is the development of an embryo biopsy that enables the embryologist to safely remove a single cell from an early embryo without jeopardizing the development of the remaining cells. The single cell so obtained can be genetically analyzed. If it shows no signs of an inherited defect or disease, the embryo can be transferred to a woman's uterus. Some scientists have been able to perform a similar genetic analysis on unfertilized eggs and even on single sperm cells. This preimplantation diagnosis can be used to avoid the need for later invasive prenatal tests such as amniocentesis and chorionic villi sampling (CVS), which can be performed only in the later weeks of the first trimester of a pregnancy. When the amniocentesis or CVS tests reveal an abnormality, the couple must decide then whether to undergo therapeutic abortion.

Another emerging reproductive technology utilizing micromanipulation is microsurgical fertilization, a technique in which one or more sperm is artificially introduced into the unfertilized egg. It is applicable among couples whose chances of fertilization are low, especially those who include one among the large population of infertile men. In some variations of the technique, an artificial opening is made in the membrane surrounding the egg in the hope that the channel will promote the entry of a healthy sperm cell. About twenty healthy babies have been born as a result of this procedure (Cohen et al. 1991). In other variations, a sperm cell is inserted in the space between the membrane and the egg itself. Although at least one normal birth and several pregnancies have been reported from such techniques, there are several significant concerns that make its wide clinical application unlikely anytime soon. The effect of allowing the entrance of certain spermatozoa that might under natural conditions be too unhealthy to fertilize an egg is still unclear. More than one sperm can pass through the artificial opening in the egg, and if several penetrate the egg, abnormal, "polyspermic" embryos can result. Such embryos contain an extra set of chromosomes and will therefore result in an abnormal fetus. As scientists become more proficient in the manipulation of the human egg and embryo, it is possible that they may be able to mechanically repair such abnormally fertilized eggs by simply extracting the pronucleus containing the extra chromosomes (Malter and Cohen 1989). Such a genetic repair may result in a completely normal embryo. Clinical application of these techniques is expected within the near future.

References

Australian Department of Health, Victoria, Standing Review and Advisory Committee (SRA) on Infertility. 1989. *Review of Embryo Experimentation Post Syn-*

gamy: An Information Paper. Melbourne: Victoria Department of Health (December).

Cohen, Jacques, Alexis Adler, Mina Alikani, Henry Malter, and Beth Talansky. Forthcoming. "Enhancement of Fertilization and Implantation by Micromanipulation." *The Proceedings of the First International Conference on Preimplantation Genetics.* New York: Plenum Press.

Davis v. Davis. 1989. Tenn. App. LEXIS 641.

Ethics Committee of the American Fertility Society. 1990. "Ethical Considerations of the New Reproductive Technologies." *Fertility and Sterility* (Supplement 2) 53:1s–104s.

Ford, Norman M. 1988. *When Did I Begin: Conception of the Human Individual in History and Philosophy of Science.* London: Cambridge University Press.

Gunning, Jennifer. 1990. *Human IVF, Embryo Research, Fetal Tissue for Research and Treatment and Abortion: International Information.* London: Her Majesty's Stationery Office.

Handyside, Alan. 1990. Unpublished data presented at the First International conference on Preimplantation Genetics, September 16–19, Chicago, Ill.

Hansard. 1990. *Human Fertilization and Embryology Bill: Parliamentary Debates.* London: House of Lords Official Report, 515, 35 (February 8).

Malter, Henry, and Jacques Cohen. 1989. "Embryonic Development After Microsurgical Repair of Polyspermic Human Zygotes." *Fertility and Sterility* 52: 373–380.

United Kingdom Department of Health and Social Security, Warnock Committee. 1984. *Report of the Committee of Inquiry into Human Fertilization and Embryology.* London: Department of Health and Social Security (July).

U.S. Congress, Office of Technology Assessment. 1988. *Infertility: Social and Medical Choices.* Washington, D.C.: U.S. Government Printing Office.

Walters, LeRoy. 1987. "Ethics and New Reproductive Technologies: An International Review of Committee Statements." *Hastings Center Report* 17(3):3–22.

Webster v. Reproductive Services. 1989. 57 U.S.L.W. 5023.

York v. Jones, 717 F.Supp. 421 (E.D. Va. 1989).

17

Screening Providers of Gametes and Embryos

❖

Martin M. Quigley

It has been over a hundred years since the first reported use of anonymous donor sperm to circumvent infertility due to male factors (Andrews 1985:148). Particularly in the last twenty years, the procedure of artificial insemination by donor has gained increasing recognition and application. Currently tens of thousands of children resulting from artificial insemination by donor are born in the United States each year. This procedure is now legal in the majority of states, with recognition and protection of the rights of the donor as well as the recipient couple and the resulting child. Introduction of the new reproductive technologies, including in vitro fertilization (IVF) and gamete intrafallopian transfer (GIFT), to treat otherwise untreatable infertility now has allowed the analogous use of donated oocytes, or egg cells, to alleviate infertility in couples where the woman has abnormal oocytes or nonfunctioning ovaries.

The recognition that human immunodeficiency virus (HIV) infection (acquired immunodeficiency syndrome [AIDS]) can be transmitted by donor sperm has resulted in the need for adequate selection and screening of gamete donors. The recognition that there is a period of time separating infection (and infectivity of the semen) and seropositivity (the ability to detect HIV infection by standard laboratory analysis) has led to the adoption of the use of frozen, quarantined sperm for donor insemination (AFS 1990:49).

This chapter will discuss the use of donated sperm, oocytes, and embryos in infertility treatments. Emphasis will be placed on the screening process, particularly that involving the oocyte donor, in view of the risks faced by the women donating oocytes. Because of the greater safety associated with the use of frozen sperm, as compared to fresh sperm for donor insemination, the experience of the Cleveland Clinic Foundation in switching from the use of fresh sperm to the use of frozen sperm will be examined.

Sources of Donated Gametes and Embryos

In the United States, sperm for artificial insemination has been obtained predominantly from anonymous donors. Occasionally some practitioners will utilize known donors (such as the man's brother) at a couple's request, or in situations when a compatible anonymous donor from a particular ethnic group cannot be located. Most authorities, however, frown upon the use of known donors, largely because of the theoretical risk of psychological harm to the donor, parent, and child with the involvement of a known third party in the reproductive process (Curie-Cohen, Luttrell, and Shapiro 1979:585; Joyce 1976:61). The situation with donated oocytes is somewhat different. Although some centers use only anonymous donors (Kennard et al. 1989:655), the fact that oocyte recovery entails a surgical procedure makes the recruitment of oocyte donors more difficult. Thus many centers have permitted (or encouraged) the use of known oocyte donors such as the woman's sister or friend. The potential psychological harm to the participants mentioned above is usually accepted in view of the lack of alternatives.

Other potential sources of donated oocytes include "excess" oocytes from IVF treatment cycles and oocytes incidentally removed from patients who are undergoing scheduled pelvic surgery. In the early days of IVF, a limited maximum number of oocytes were inseminated. Ideally, three or four embryos should be placed in the woman's uterus. This yields the maximum pregnancy rate with the least likelihood of a multiple pregnancy of high plurality. In order to avoid the ethical concerns of what to do with "excess" embryos, in the past most centers elected to inseminate only sufficient oocytes to result in an ideal number of embryos for uterine placement. In this scenario, there were upon occasion uninseminated oocytes that potentially could be donated. However, with the recent advent and application of embryo cryopreservation, the general practice today is to inseminate all oocytes, freezing those embryos in excess of the number desirable for uterine placement. Today, if some of the woman's oocytes were diverted to another party, her chances of becoming pregnant likely would be reduced. Thus this source of donated oocytes is less available today. While theoretically attractive, the use of oocytes harvested during otherwise indicated pelvic surgery is logistically difficult to schedule and has not become a reliable source of oocytes. Part of the problem is the rigorous screening required of potential donors (see below) and the backward approach of finding a recipient for available oocytes rather than searching for a donor for a patient who needs oocytes.

The use of donated embryos is not widespread at the present time. As discussed above, excess embryos from an in vitro fertilization cycle usually are cryopreserved for the couple's subsequent attempts at pregnancy. Although occasionally cryopreserved embryos may no longer be wanted by a couple (e.g., the Rios embryos whose "parents" were killed in a plane crash ["Australia Dispute" 1984]), the number and availability of these embryos are most likely to be so small as to not be of practical concern.

A medical procedure known as "ovum transfer" is available in a limited number of centers in the United States, however. In this process, a volunteer is inseminated with the infertile couple's man's sperm in an attempt to fertilize her oocytes naturally while in her body. Three to six days following insemination, uterine flushing procedures are performed in order to recover any fertilized embryos. Although successful pregnancies have resulted from this procedure (Bustillo et al. 1984), ethical concerns such as "retained" pregnancies and the risk of sexually transmitted diseases in the donor have restricted its use. Furthermore, the innovators of this procedure have attempted to patent the procedure and sell franchises, an approach that has not been well accepted by the medical community at large.

Risk to Participants

Sperm donors

There are no physical risks associated with sperm donation. While there have been no comprehensive studies or follow-up of sperm donors, presumably there are few, if any, psychological sequelae. Again in the absence of definitive studies, presumably sperm donors known or related to the recipient couple have a greater risk of psychological complications because of their potential subsequent contact with any resulting child.

Oocyte donors

Oocyte recovery entails a surgical procedure. Although the technique currently most utilized for oocyte recovery is ultrasound-directed needle aspiration through the vagina (Seifer et al. 1988:462), which can be done without the need for major inhalation or regional anesthesia, a woman who voluntarily submits to such a procedure still risks possible bleeding or infection. Although no direct physical risks result when a woman permits excess oocytes from an IVF cycle to be donated, she exposes herself to the risk of decreased success from her IVF cycle and exposes herself to the possibility of having her oocytes harvested a second time should she wish to continue trying to become pregnant. This is because the donated oocytes potentially could be inseminated with the man's sperm and the resulting embryos cryopreserved for an additional attempt at establishing pregnancy if the first attempt is unsuccessful, or for a subsequent pregnancy if the first attempt is successful. A woman who undergoes oocyte recovery at the time of otherwise scheduled pelvic surgery has an insignificant increase in the risk of surgical complications.

The psychological risks to any oocyte donor have not been widely studied but are probably comparable to the risks faced by sperm donors. A single follow-up study on volunteer oocyte donors has shown no short-term psychological sequelae (Schover et al. 1991:299).

Embryo donors

Although the diversion of excess embryos, either before or after cryopreservation, produces no physical risk, the possibilities of a decreased success rate and psychological risks previously noted also apply in this situation. Again, the ovum-flushing technique does expose the donor to the risk of sexually transmitted diseases (including AIDS), retained pregnancy, and, theoretically, to the risk of tubal ectopic pregnancy.

Sperm recipient

As fresh semen samples cannot be screened for infectious diseases prior to use, any recipient of donated fresh sperm is at risk of acquiring sexually transmitted diseases, including hepatitis and AIDS. With the use of frozen, quarantined sperm, this risk is minimal. There is always the chance that an abnormal child will result, but studies to date do not indicate any increase in the rate of chromosomal or other abnormalities in children resulting from artificial insemination using donor sperm (Amuzu, Laxova, and Shapiro 1990:899).

Recipients of oocytes and embryos

There is a theoretical risk of transmitting infectious disease with the use of donated oocytes or embryos. However, because of the extremely small volume of material transferred, as well as the passage of the oocyte or embryo through the several changes of culture media associated with the IVF process, the possibility of producing a sexually transmitted disease in a recipient by uterine placement of an embryo that was donated or resulted from a donated oocyte appears insignificantly small. If the oocyte or embryo is excess from an IVF cycle or left over after cryopreservation, possibly the donor will not have undergone the screening and matching process required when an individual goes through the procedure for the specific purpose of donating oocytes.

Genetic Screening for Gamete or Embryo Donors

Guidelines for screening and selection of the prospective donors have been developed by the American Association of Tissue Banks and the American Fertility Society, among others. The most recent published guidelines are from the American Fertility Society (1990). In general, the donor should not have any nontrivial malformation such as cleft lip; any non-trivial Mendelian disorder such as hemophilia; any familial disease with a known genetic component such as juvenile diabetes mellitus; should not carry an autosomal recessive gene such as the one for Tay-Sachs disease; and finally, should not have a known chromosomal rearrangement that may result in unbalanced gametes. It is not generally required that donors undergo routine chromosomal screening.

Furthermore, the donor's first-degree relatives (parents or offspring) similarly should be free of nontrivial malformations; autosomal dominant or x-linked disorders with age of onset beyond the age of the donor (such as Huntington disease); reduced penetrance (such as Marfan syndrome); or autosomal recessive disease with a high gene frequency (such as cystic fibrosis). In addition, first-degree relatives should be free from any chromosomal rearrangements other than trisomy. Finally, significant family histories of major psychoses, epileptic disorders, juvenile diabetes mellitus, and early coronary heart disease should be causes for rejection.

Who Needs Donor Sperm?

In the United States today the largest number of requests for donor sperm is from couples in which the man has previously had a vasectomy and reversal of the procedure has been unsuccessful, is not desired, or has been recommended against because of the amount of time elapsed since the vasectomy. Second most common are requests because of azoospermia (no sperm in the ejaculate) resulting either from failure of production or, more commonly, irreparable ductal obstruction. A third category of requests would be cases of male-factor infertility, including oligospermia (low sperm count), reduced motility, or other semen abnormalities that are untreatable or have been treated unsuccessfully. Finally, in a small percentage of cases donor insemination is chosen in order to avoid the risk of passing a significant genetic disease to the couple's offspring.

Sperm Donor Screening Process

At present all the sperm used for donor insemination at the Cleveland Clinic Foundation is frozen. Potential donors go through a four-stage screening process. Interested individuals are identified by advertising directed particularly to staff (interns and residents) and medical students, as well as by word of mouth. Interested individuals are given a twenty-three-page questionnaire to complete dealing with lifestyle and social, medical, sexual, and family history. An interview is then arranged with the director of the sperm bank (a Ph.D.). At the interview, the questionnaire is reviewed, ethical and legal obligations and responsibilities are discussed, and written, informed consent is obtained.

Individual who complete this stage are then asked to collect a semen sample. The minimal accepted semen analysis includes 1.7 ml volume; 40 million/ml count; 40 percent motility; 35 microns per second of velocity; and 60 percent normal morphology. If the semen meets these parameters, a semen culture for gonorrhea, morphologic examination for evidence of trichomonas vaginalis or white cells, and a cryopreservation test are performed. A successful cryopreservation test requires that the overall postthaw motility be greater than 20 percent, the postthaw recovery be at least 50 percent of the original motility, and the total postthaw number of motile sperm be a minimum of 30 million per ejaculate.

The third stage involves laboratory serologic testing for hepatitis B, syphilis, HIV, cytomegalovirus (CMV), blood type, and Rh; where indicated, a screen for Tay-Sachs disease or hemoglobinopathies is also performed. A complete medical history is then taken, and a physical examination is performed by a nurse practitioner. The physical examination includes a urethral swab for chlamydia.

Finally, semen samples are collected as frequently as possible (with a minimum of 48 hours between collections), and a semen analysis and cryopreservation check is performed on each sample. Random checks for pathogens are made during the collection process. After completion of specimen collection, the individual is retested for pathogens as described above. All semen is currently quarantined for 180 days, then the donor is recalled and retested for HIV. Only if the donor is HIV negative at the retest are the semen samples released for use.

In order to limit the likelihood of inadvertent consanguineous marriages between offspring resulting from the same sperm donor, the clinic limits each donor to a maximum of ten pregnancies. In view of the fact that some recipients require many more than the average number of inseminations to achieve a pregnancy, or wish to have additional children from the same donor, we collect enough sperm samples to perform a maximum of 175 inseminations from a single donor.

Table 17.1 summarizes the experience with our first ninety-three sperm donor candidates. Thirty-six were eliminated with the first stage in that fourteen failed to complete the questionnaire or changed their minds, nine repeatedly failed to keep appointments, three had a family history of genetically transmittable diseases, three were heavy cigarette smokers,

Table 17.1   Sperm Donor Screening Outcomes

Expressed interest, withdrew before screening	14/93	15.1%
Excluded—Lifestyle, family or personal medical history	22/79	27.8%
Excluded—Initial semen analysis	13/57	22.8%
Excluded—Poor cryosurvival	12/44	27.3%
Excluded—Detailed medical history, physical exam, laboratory screening	2/32	6.3%
Cumulative "rejection" rate	63/93	67.7%

SOURCE: Modified from Mari Schroeder-Jenkins and Susan A. Rothmann, "Causes of Donor Rejection in a Sperm Banking Program." *Fertility and Sterility* 51:903, 1989.

Table 17.2   Switch From Fresh to Frozen Semen for Insemination

1983	158 Patients	62 Patients pregnant (all fresh)
1984	159 Patients	61 Patients pregnant (all fresh)
1985	152 Patients	71 Patients pregnant (all fresh)
1986	157 Patients	69 Patients pregnant (all fresh)
1987	152 Patients	65 Patients pregnant (30 fresh, 35 frozen)
1988	153 Patients	75 Patients pregnant (5 fresh, 70 frozen)
1989	135 Patients	59 Patients pregnant (all frozen)

three used recreational drugs, two had abnormal medical histories, one had been used extensively in other donor insemination programs, and one refused to masturbate. Of the remaining candidates, twenty-five were rejected for poor pre- or postfreezing semen quality; two additional potential donors were rejected for medical history or findings during the history and physical examination. Interestingly, only 85 percent of the first 812 samples from the first 30 donors were acceptable, with about 10 percent showing inadequate initial semen analysis and 5 percent with unacceptable cryosurvival. Three potential donors (5.2 percent) had positive chlamydia cultures; two of these individuals were dropped as unreliable, and one was accepted after antibiotic treatment and subsequent negative cultures. The remainder of the laboratory tests on the donors were negative.

Switch from Fresh to Frozen Semen

Tables 17.2 and 17.3 summarize the Cleveland Clinic's experience while switching from fresh to frozen semen for the donor insemination program. Reportedly, use of frozen semen has resulted in lower overall pregnancy rates and decreased pregnancy rates per cycle, leading to an overall delay in pregnancy establishment (AFS 1990:4S). Several things are evident from the data presented in these two tables. First, it took three years to switch totally from fresh semen to frozen. This was because of the quarantine period for the frozen semen, the difficulty of attracting and screening suitable donors (as described above), and the fact that some patients wished to continue with the donor they were using currently or who had been responsible for a previous pregnancy. In spite of the change, a very consistent 38 to 49 percent of our patients became pregnant each year, regardless of whether fresh or frozen semen was utilized.

In table 17.3, the specific pregnancy rates per insemination are shown

Table 17.3   Switch From Fresh to Frozen Semen for Insemination

1986	1278 Fresh Inseminations[1] 20 Frozen Inseminations	5.0% Pregnancy/Insemination 0.0% Pregnancy/Insemination
1987	351 Fresh Inseminations[1] 460 Frozen Inseminations[2]	8.5% Pregnancy/Insemination 7.6% Pregnancy/Insemination
1988	50 Fresh Inseminations 593 Frozen Inseminations	10.0% Pregnancy/Insemination 11.8% Pregnancy/Insemination
1989	0 Fresh Inseminations 597 Frozen Inseminations (457 Cycles)	9.8% Pregnancy/Insemination 12.9% Pregnancy/Insemination Cycle

[1]Usually 3 inseminations were done per fresh cycle, corrected pregnancy rates are: 1986—11.5%/cycle (601 cycles); 1987—14.4%/cycle (155 cycles).
[2]Midyear switch from cervical to intrauterine inseminations; Cervical: 1 pregnancy/78 inseminations (1.3%)—Intrauterine: 34 pregnancies/382 inseminations (8.9%).

in more detail. Again, the pregnancy rate per insemination is remarkably consistent, but no significant differences in the rate of pregnancy were established between fresh and frozen semen. We did note, however, that frozen semen did not perform well when insemination was performed intravaginally or intracervically, only when frozen sperm was introduced directly into the uterus were pregnancy rates comparable to those seen with fresh sperm achieved (see footnotes to table 17.3).

Who Needs Donor Oocytes?

The ovaries have a dual function in establishing pregnancy. In addition to the obvious role of gamete development, the ovaries produce hormones that are necessary to uterine preparation for implantation and pregnancy maintenance until the placental shift occurs (between the eighth and twelfth weeks of pregnancy). Thus establishing pregnancy with the use of donated oocytes usually requires not only that oocytes be obtained, but also that the recipient's uterus be adequately prepared. Once pregnancy is established, exogenous hormone support must be given until placental steroidogenic function has taken over.

An estimated 1 percent of women of reproductive age do not have ovarian function. While this is a small percentage, the number of affected women numerically is very large. The largest number of these women are those who have premature ovarian failure either because of gonadal dysgenesis (being born without normal ovaries) or because they have undergone menopause prematurely, sometimes even as teenagers. In addition, some women have had successful radiation or chemotherapy for childhood malignancies which resulted in irreparable destruction of ovarian function. Other women may have had their ovaries surgically removed as treatment for pelvic infection, endometriosis, or ovarian malignancies.

The decrease in a woman's ability to become pregnant with increasing chronological age is well recognized. Much of this decrease in fertility appears to be due to the phenomenon of aging oocytes, as women's oocytes are all resident in their ovaries by the fifth month of intrauterine life. Thus a woman who is forty will have forty-and-a-half-year-old oocytes that may have been exposed to many potentially detrimental environmental agents.

Obviously, women without ovaries have no other alternative to become pregnant except the use of donor oocytes. Women over age forty who have otherwise untreatable infertility have been reported to have quite a good rate of pregnancy establishment with the use of donated oocytes (Serhal and Craft 1989). Finally, there are small groups of patients who have abnormal oocytes, as evidenced by failure of fertilization with normal sperm during in vitro fertilization, or who have genetic abnormalities that they do not wish to pass on to a child. These women also benefit from the use of donor oocytes.

Oocyte Donor Screening Process

The screening and selection process for oocyte donors is analogous in many ways to that used for sperm donors. At present, however, there is no practical way to freeze or otherwise store oocytes. Thus the oocytes cannot be collected until they are ready for use.

We were fortunate enough to obtain widespread publicity in the news media because of the innovative nature of our program ("Clinic in Ohio" 1987). We received more than 500 phone calls from interested potential donors, of whom about 100 were interested enough to make an appointment for further information. The potential donors gave a basic medical history; had physical and other characteristics (height, weight, hair color, eye color, race, national origin, religion, and education) recorded; had their blood typed and Rh determined, if unknown; and contributed a photograph to be used in the matching process. These potential donors were then placed on a waiting list until a potential recipient was ready to become pregnant. When a potential recipient was ready, the best physical match was made with our potential donors and the matching donor was recalled and offered the opportunity to go through the complete screening and oocyte donation process. Thus the potential oocyte donors were not completely screened until a matching recipient was actually ready to become pregnant.

When each donor was matched with a specific recipient, she was mailed a questionnaire similar to that used for the sperm donors. The questionnaire inquired about family health history, personal health history, and personal health habits, including sexual history. In addition, a psychological screening test was mailed to the donors. Our first thirteen donors received the Symptom Check List-90 (SCL-90) and the remainder the Minnesota Multiphasic Personality Inventory/California Personality Index (MMPI/CPI). The potential donor then went through a half-day-screening process. This included a complete medical history and physical examination by an "uninvolved" gynecologist (not a member of the IVF group), who reviewed the medical aspects of the questionnaire and ordered laboratory testing including serum CMV, syphilis, HIV, hepatitis B, and cultures for herpes, gonorrhea, chlamydia, and CMV. Informed consent was obtained by a physician team member, following which a formal, semistructured interview with a psychologist with a Ph.D. was arranged. During this interview, the psychological testing was reviewed. Finally, a representative from our bioethics department interviewed the potential donor to determine her knowledge of the procedures and risks, the validity of her informed consent, and the lack of coercion. Finally, the entire group involved in the process met together to review the screening information and make a final determination on the acceptability of the candidate. Table 17.4 lists the results of the first twenty-nine donors screened. As with the sperm donors, a significant proportion (ten of the twenty-nine) withdrew or were excluded from the program. Contrary to the experience with the sperm donors, where there were no positive CMV serologies, fifteen of the twenty-seven potential donors tested had positive CMV serology. These individuals had a convalescent serum titer performed two weeks later, along with tests of urine and cervical cultures for CMV. If there was no change in titer and the cultures were negative, they were acceptable as donors. Similar to the situation with sperm donors, one potential donor was chlamydia positive (a rate of 3.7 percent). She was treated with doxycycline, retested negative, and was accepted as a donor.

Financial Considerations

Our sperm donors are currently paid $50 for each usable specimen. Although the maximum payable for 175 samples would be more than

Table 17.4   Results of Screening Oocyte Donor Candidates

29 Screened	
12 Not used	17 Used
5 dropped out prior to start of cycle	12 underwent 1 aspiration cycle
2 excluded for medical reasons	5 underwent 2 aspiration cycles
• severe endometriosis	
• pseudotumor cerebri	
2 excluded for psychological reasons	
1 quilt in midcycle	
1 *recipient* quit	
1 *recipient* canceled for medical reasons	

$8,000, to date no single donor has received more than $3,000. A $3,000 payment would be for the collection of sixty semen samples with acceptable count and cryosurvival.

Our oocyte donors receive nothing for the screening procedure or tests involved. When actually undergoing the oocyte recovery cycle (which is analogous to the procedures involved in an IVF treatment cycle), they receive $50 a day for every day in which a blood sample is obtained or an intramuscular medication is administered; $100 a day for every day when an ultrasound examination is performed; and $350 for the day of oocyte collection. The donor cannot work on the day of oocyte collection, and some donors might not return to work until the second day following the procedure. For the average ten- to twelve-day oocyte donation process, the donors receive between $900 and $1,300.

Whether financial consideration should be given to donors of sperm or oocytes is a matter of controversy (AFS 1986). Pragmatically, it is well recognized that the only motivating factor for sperm donors is financial, and in the absence of payment, there would be little or no donor sperm available in the United States. Compared to the relatively trivial inconvenience experienced by the semen donor, oocyte donors must go through a ten- to twelve-day treatment and monitoring process in which they receive medication to induce ovarian hyperstimulation; have their ovarian response monitored by daily blood samples for estradiol and periodic ultrasound examinations; and finally undergo a surgical recovery procedure, often with associated anesthesia. Without anesthesia, there is a significant component of discomfort involved in the donation process. Although there have been no reports of significant complications to date among any of our donors, the oocyte collection procedure is invasive and carries with it a small risk of intra-abdominal bleeding or infection.

Clearly there would be few anonymous volunteer oocyte donors if financial remuneration were not available. Although the lump-sum payment of $900 to $1,300 may seem excessive, when the risks, inconveniences, and discomforts are compared to those of sperm donors (who generally receive more money, but over a longer period of time), these payments are entirely justifiable.

Since the *Roe v. Wade* decision and the improved social acceptance of one-parent families, there has been a progressive decline in the number of adoptable infants in the United States. Thus infertile couples, who previously had the ready option of adoption to begin or add to their family, are faced either with the prospect of having no children or of availing themselves of some of the newer reproductive technologies. Although pregnancy resulting from the use of donor sperm has been reported for more than a hundred years, it is only within the last twenty years that the procedure has become recognized and accepted. Using IVF technology, analogous treatments are now available for couples in which the wife needs donated oocytes.

However, the paramount issue must be the safety of all participants. Adequate screening of all donors—sperm, oocyte, and embryo—is a necessity to eliminate the risk of significant sexually transmittable diseases as well as decrease the likelihood that a child with a preventable abnormality will be born. Because of the fatal nature of HIV infection, it is not justifiable today to use anything other than frozen, quarantined semen for donor insemination.

Realistically, no such thing as a "perfect" donor exists, especially perfect donors of oocytes. Because of the trivial risks and inconveniences involved, sperm donors are generally available, although the proportion of interested donors who are conscientious and acceptable is surprisingly low. Because of the need for donors of differing physical characteristics and racial backgrounds as well as the significant inconveniences and discomforts experienced by oocyte donors, consideration should be given to continuing the encouragement of women volunteers. Without significant financial incentives, there will be few acceptable oocyte donors.

Clearly the psychological risks experienced by the participants (donors, recipients, and resulting children) needs to be studied further. With additional knowledge concerning these risks (if any), more rational decisions can be made on the wider application of these technologies.

References

American Fertility Society (AFS). 1990. "New Guidelines for the Use of Semen Donor Insemination: 1990." *Fertility and Sterility* 53 (Supplement 1):1S–13S.

American Fertility Society, Ethics Committee. 1986. "Donor Eggs in In Vitro Fertilization." *Ethical Considerations of the New Reproductive Technologies. Fertility and Sterility* 46 (Supplement 1):42S–44S.

Amuzu, B., R. Laxova, and S. S. Shapiro. 1990. "Pregnancy Outcome, Health of Children, and Family Adjustment after Donor Insemination." *Obstetrics and Gynecology* 75:899–905.

Andrews, L. B. 1984. *New Conceptions*. New York: St. Martin's.

"Australia Dispute Arises on Embryos." 1984. *New York Times* (June 11):A30.

Bustillo, M.C., J.E. Buster, S. W. Cohen, I. H. Thorneycroft, J.A. Simon, S. P. Boyers, J. R. Marshall, R. W. Seed, J. A. Louw, and R. G. Seed. 1984. "Nonsurgical Ovum Transfer as a Treatment in Infertile Women: Preliminary Experience." *Journal of the American Medical Association* 25:1171–1173.

"Clinic in Ohio Starts Egg Donor Plan." 1987. *New York Times* (July 15):10.

Curie-Cohen, M., L. Luttrell, and S. Shapiro. 1979. "Current Practice of Artificial Insemination by Donor in the United States." *New England Journal of Medicine* 300:585–590.

Joyce, D. N. 1976. "Recruitment, Selection and Matching of Donors." In M. Brudenell, A. McLaren, R. Short, and M. Symmonds, eds., *Artificial Insemination: Proceedings of the Fourth Study Group of the Royal College of Obstetricians and Gynecologists*. London: Royal College of Obstetricians and Gynecologists.

Kennard, E. A. D., R. L. Collins, J. Blankstein, L. R. Schover, G. Kanoti, J. Reis, and M. Quigley. 1989. "A Program for Matched, Anonymous Oocyte Donation." *Fertility and Sterility* 51:655–660.

Schover, L. R., J. Reis, R. L. Collins, J. Blankstein, G. Kanoti, and M. Quigley. 1991. "The Psychological Evaluation of Oocyte Donors." *Journal of Psychosomatic Obstetrics and Gynecology* 11:299–309.

Schroeder-Jenkins, M., and S. Rothmann. 1989. "Causes of Donor Rejection in a Sperm Banking Program." *Fertility and Sterility* 51:903–906.

Seifer, D. B., R. L. Collins, D. M. Paushter, C. R. George, and M. Quigley. 1988. "Follicular Aspiration: A Comparison of an Ultrasonic Endovaginal Transducer with Fixed Needle Guide and Other Retrieval Methods." *Fertility and Sterility* 49:462–467.

Serhal, P. F., and I. L. Craft. 1989. "Oocyte Donation in 61 Patients." *Lancet* I:1185.

18

National Documentation and Quality Assurance of Medically Assisted Conception: The Experience of the U.S. IVF Registry

Stuart C. Hartz, Jane B. Porter, and Alan H. DeCherney

During the early and mid-1980s, assisted reproductive technologies (ART) became increasingly accepted as viable treatments for infertility. At the same time, practitioners recognized the need to monitor the expanding use and clinical effects of these procedures.

The United States clinical community's approach to monitoring in vitro fertilization (IVF) and related practices was organized in 1985 as a collaborative effort between the Society for Assisted Reproductive Technology (SART) of the American Fertility Society (AFS) and Medical Research International (MRI). The result of this collaboration, the U.S. IVF Registry, now ending its fourth year of operations, represents a successful joint effort between a professional medical society and an independent contract research organization that receives funding support from a pharmaceutical company.

The design of the surveillance system follows a registry format capable of monitoring all U.S. clinics practicing ART. Initially the U.S. IVF Registry enrolled twenty-five clinics; currently, there are 195 member clinics out of the estimated 200 in operation in the U.S. Including 1989, the registry has documented 70,000 stimulation cycles resulting in approximately 8,200 deliveries and 10,600 babies (including frozen embryo and donor oocyte procedures).*

The registry serves as a resource for the clinical, public health, and

*See "MRI, SART, and AFS." 1990. *Fertility and Sterility* 55(1):14–23.

patient communities. The major objective of the registry is to explore the epidemiology of all ART including IVF, gamete intrafallopian transfer (GIFT), frozen embryo transfer (ET), donor oocyte transfer, and related procedures. Thus a first-order priority is to describe the use of the various procedures and the relative success of the various treatments. Another major priority is to measure the occurrence of unfavorable outcomes such as chromosomal abnormalities or congenital anomalies in the offspring resulting from ART, and any adverse experiences among the women undergoing treatment.

Design and Organization

MRI was selected as the research organization to design and implement the data collection methods; to manage, process, and analyze the data; and to publish and present the summary results to the clinical community. At the outset, the registry's integrity and also acceptance of its statistical reports depended upon a guarantee that the individual clinics would remain anonymous. Furthermore, MRI was to perform its research as an independent party, thus remaining neutral with regard to the clinical community and the current funding agent, Serono Laboratories, Inc. As a result, neither the AFS and its Society for Assisted Reproductive Technology nor Serono has access to the primary database; requests for data to address specific research questions of independent researchers are reviewed by a committee consisting of MRI, AFS, and Serono representatives.

The registry operates as a separate research project within the MRI research program. The registry utilizes MRI's capabilities in epidemiology, biostatistics, pharmacology, and computer programming. In addition, the registry's methodology is now being used in a long-term follow-up study, funded by the National Institutes of Health, of women undergoing IVF/ET.

Methodology

The initial activities of the registry were to identify the required core data set, to develop an effective data collection process, and, most important, to enroll clinics and gain their ongoing cooperation. Although these issues remain, the long-term goals center on developing a valuable database resource that can be of use to researchers and clinicians in investigating clinical and epidemiological hypotheses.

Clinic enrollment

Since the registry's goal was to enroll all of the U.S. IVF/ET clinics, MRI used clinic lists from the AFS and other sources to contact known U.S. clinics. Letters were sent to the clinic directors describing the registry and its planned operations. In addition, MRI distributed informational brochures at professional meetings.

SART clinics are required to submit their data to the registry as a condition of membership in the society. However, other registry members submit their data on a voluntary basis. The growth in U.S. membership has allowed the registry to profile the activities and results of 30, 41, 96, 135, and 163 clinics for the years 1985 to 1989 respectively.

Data collection

MRI, with clinical assistance from IVF practitioners, developed RecordKeeper©, a PC-based software program, to serve as a patient-specific data collection instrument for reporting to the registry, and as a general medical record-keeping program for clinics. The software currently records demographic information, medical/infertility history, spouse/donor information, stimulation protocols, retrieval and embryo transfer information, luteal phase support, and pregnancy and pregnancy outcome data including congenital anomalies, chromosomal abnormalities, and other adverse events.

Paper data forms also were developed, initially to collect retrospective clinic-specific summary data from clinics without computer access or that chose not to use RecordKeeper©. Presently, the paper form records the clinic's summary profile by each ART procedure: IVF with fresh oocytes, GIFT, combination IVF/GIFT, ZIFT (PROST, TPET, etc.), donor oocyte, and frozen embryo transfer (ET). The information includes the number of stimulation cycles, number of patients treated, number and type of retrieval, number and maturity of oocytes retrieved, number of embryos transferred for IVF, number of oocytes transferred for GIFT, cases of hyperstimulation, pregnancy and any outcomes, as well as congenital anomalies and chromosomal abnormalities.

In January 1987, once RecordKeeper© and the paper data forms were developed, the registry began to enroll clinics. Initially, Version 1 of RecordKeeper© and a set of paper forms were sent to forty-six clinics.

Data management

Data sent to the registry are continually screened by MRI staff. The paper forms are examined for completeness and consistency before being entered into the central database. After the data have been entered, special software is used to detect entry errors and inconsistencies.

MRI has also developed software to validate the data submitted on RecordKeeper©. These programs identify data items on patient records with missing or inconsistent information. For example, a patient record with a delivery recorded but no pregnancy indicated would be printed. These printouts are returned to the clinics for inspection and correction. When the information is corrected, the clinics send new disks back to MRI. MRI can then check the information and add it to the registry's central database.

Data are submitted to the registry several times each year. At the beginning of the year, clinics submit their results from the previous calendar year either on disk or on the paper forms. Because pregnant women have not delivered, for the most part, at this time, at least one follow-up contact is needed. Clinics that submit data via paper form indicate for each procedure the number of pregnancies that have not delivered. In the summer months, forms for collecting this incomplete information are sent to the clinics. Depending on volume, some of the data needed may be provided to MRI over the phone. The central database is updated as the information is received.

Correspondingly, for the clinics sending data via RecordKeeper©, printouts of patient records with pregnancies that have no outcome recorded are sent to the clinics. Either the information is updated and a new disk sent to the registry, or information is phoned in to MRI personnel, who then update the central database. For the treatment years 1987 and 1988, less than 2 percent of pregnancy outcomes were unknown at the completion of data collection.

A calendar year's information is complete by October of the following year. The annual *Fertility and Sterility* report, the official journal of the AFS, can then be prepared for the upcoming publication in January. For example, the 1989 data were complete by October of 1990 and appeared in the January 1991 *Fertility and Sterility*.

Confidentiality and validity

To date, the data collected by the registry have been kept completely confidential. Neither clinic names nor patient identifiers are used in reports or presentations. The registry assigns unique clinic identification codes for data submitted via paper form and disk. Clinics using RecordKeeper© are allowed to enter patient names and other identifying information. However, the copy procedure built into RecordKeeper© allows clinics to submit data to the registry with the names excluded. The results presented in publications or other presentations use pooled summary data only, so that individual clinics cannot be identified.

At the 1989 annual meeting of the AFS, SART elected to provide selected, clinic-specific results from its members to the public. The goal of releasing selected statistics is to allow patients to review the practice and success of clinics. The method for distributing this information is being developed.

Results

Four annual registry reports have been published in *Fertility and Sterility*. The first annual publication was prepared in fall 1987. Of the 88 clinics enrolled at this time, 30 and 41, respectively, were prepared to send data to the registry for publication of results of 1985 and 1986 treatments (MRI et al. 1988). A number of the clinics were relatively new and had no information to report. By the fall of 1988, 96 of the clinics reported to the registry for its second publication of 1987 treatments and related outcomes (MRI, SART, and AFS 1989) In 1989, 135 clinics reported their 1988 treatment results to the registry (MRI, SART, and AFS 1990). All of the largest clinics in the country reported their 1988 results, and it is estimated that approximately 90 percent of 1988 ART treatments were reported to the registry.

Clinics reported performing 70,267 stimulation cycles and 55,829 retrievals in the years 1985 to 1989. These stimulation cycles were performed for IVF, GIFT, ZIFT, and related procedures. Table 18.1 shows the stimulation and retrieval cycles by year and number of reporting clinics.

The total number of clinical pregnancies reported to the registry over the five years was 11,015. (The registry defines a clinical pregnancy as a rising beta hCG and gestational sac(s) within the uterine cavity documented by ultrasound.) There were 933 clinical pregnancies from 1985 to 1986, 1,976 in 1987, 3,508 in 1988, and 4,598 in 1989. The corresponding numbers of deliveries were 690 (estimated) for 1985 and 1986, 1,441 for 1987, 2,627 for 1988, and 3,472 for 1989, for a total of 8,230 deliveries. These numbers include outcomes from IVF, GIFT, ZIFT, and related procedures, and also frozen embryo and donor oocyte transfers.

Table 18.1 Annual Total Stimulation Cycles and Retrievals

Year	Clinics no.	Stimulation cycles	Retrievals No.	(%)
1985	30	3,921	2,948	(75)*
1986	41	4,867	3,832	(79)
1987	96	14,647	10,892	(74)
1988	135	22,649	17,753	(78)
1989	163	24,183	20,404	(84)
Total		70,267	55,829	(79)

*Retrievals are expressed as a percentage of stimulation cycles.

Table 18.2 Annual Clinical Pregnancy Rates for IVF and GIFT

	IVF			GIFT		
	Retrievals	Clinical pregnancies		Retrievals	Clinical pregnancies	
Year	no.	No.	(%)	No.	No.	(%)
1985	2,892	337	(11.7)*	56	3	(5.4)+
1986	3,366	485	(14.4)	466	108	(23.2)
1987	8,725	1,367	(15.7)	1,968	492	(25.0)
1988	13,647	2,243	(16.4)	3,080	846	(27.5)
1989	15,392	2,811	(18.3)	3,652	1,112	(30.5)
Total	44,022	7,243	(16.5)	9,222	2,561	(27.8)

*Clinical pregnancies are expressed as a percentage of IVF retrievals.
+Clinical pregnancies are expressed as a percentage of GIFT retrievals.

Over all years, 7,243 (16.5 percent) of 44,022 IVF retrievals and 2,561 (27.8 percent) of 9,222 GIFT retrievals resulted in clinical pregnancies (see table 18.2). For IVF, the clinical pregnancy rate increased from 11.7 percent to 18.3 percent and for GIFT, from 5.4 percent to 30.5 percent. (Note that the numbers for GIFT in 1985 were small.)

Table 18.3 presents the results of IVF deliveries associated with 1987 through 1989 treatments. The rates for clinical pregnancy and delivery increased slightly over the three years. The clinical pregnancy rate increased from 16 percent to 18 percent. Overall, 24 percent of clinical pregnancies resulted in spontaneous abortion (clinical pregnancy loss occurring prior to gestational age of twenty weeks). The ectopic pregnancy rate was 5 percent for the two-year period. (An ectopic pregnancy is defined as elevated beta hCG and gestational sac(s) implanted anywhere except in the uterine cavity.) Of the 37,764 retrievals, 4,752 (13 percent) resulted in live delivery.

Table 18.4 presents the results of GIFT deliveries associated with 1987 through 1989 treatments. The clinical pregnancy rates for the years 1987

Table 18.3   IVF Treatment Outcome (1987 to 1989)

Year	Retrievals no.	Clinical pregnancies No.	(%)	Spontaneous abortions No.	(%)	Ectopic pregnancies No.	(%)	Deliveries No.	(%)
1987	8,725	1,367	(16)*	344	(25)+	103	(7)#	991	(11)*
1988	13,647	2,243	(16)	532	(24)	116	(5)	1,657	(12)
1989	15,392	2,811	(18)	655	(23)	154	(5)	2,104	(14)
Total	37,764	6,421	(17)	1,531	(24)	373	(5)	4,752	(13)

*Pregnancies and deliveries are expressed as a percentage of retrievals.
+ Abortions are expressed as a percentage of pregnancies.
# Ectopic pregnancies are expressed as a percentage of pregnancies (clinical and ectopic).

Table 18.4   GIFT Treatment Outcome (1987 to 1989)

Year	Retrievals no.	Clinical pregnancies No.	(%)	Spontaneous abortions No.	(%)	Ectopic pregnancies No.	(%)	Deliveries No.	(%)
1987	1,968	492	(25)*	116	(24)+	30	(6)#	362	(18)+
1988	2,080	846	(27)	171	(20)	42	(5)	654	(21)
1989	3,652	1,112	(30)	247	(22)	43	(4)	848	(23)
Total	8,700	2,450	(28)	534	(22)	115	(4)	1,864	(21)

*Pregnancies and deliveries are expressed as a percentage of retrievals.
+ Abortions are expressed as a percentage of pregnancies.
# Ectopic pregnancies are expressed as a percentage of pregnancies (clinical and ectopic).

through 1989 were 25 percent, 27 percent, and 30 percent respectively. The spontaneous abortion rate varied from 24 percent to 20 percent to 22 percent over the years, whereas the ectopic pregnancy rate decreased slightly from 6 percent to 4 percent. Over the years, the delivery rates increased from 18 percent to 23 percent.

Related research and other activities

The registry attempts to disseminate its research information through a variety of means. In addition to its annual publications in *Fertility and Sterility*, MRI has presented registry data at the last three AFS annual meetings and at the previous two World Congresses on In Vitro Fertilization and Embryo Transfer, as well as several other professional meetings.

MRI cooperated with the U.S. Congress and other government officials investigating infertility issues by providing statistics and counseling on data collection methodology (Subcommittee on Regulation 1989; OTC

1988; CGO 1989). In addition, MRI was asked to testify before the U.S. Congress in 1989 at the Subcommittee on Regulation, Business Opportunities, and Energy hearing on consumer protection issues involving in vitro fertilization clinics. The chairman of this committee, Representative Ron Wyden (D-Ore.), insisted that clinic-specific data be made available to the public. He felt that the registry in its present form was not satisfactory because of center anonymity. Thus, Representative Wyden conducted an independent survey of IVF clinics in the United States in early 1989. It was heartening that the results of the Wyden survey were similar to those of the registry (Subcommittee on Regulation 1989). This finding validates the concept of an anonymous registry. MRI discussed its views on government regulation of infertility practice in an editorial co-authored by Alan H. DeCherney and Stuart C. Hartz (1988).

The registry acts as a resource for the media and for government agencies seeking statistics on ART. The registry also works cooperatively with RESOLVE, the national support group for infertile couples. In addition, MRI provides IVF researchers with registry data for presentations at professional meetings and for publications.

The methodology of the registry was reviewed by the National Institute of Child Health and Human Development (NICHD) in awarding a contract to MRI to study and follow up women who have undergone IVF and related ART treatments. The major goal of this longitudinal study is to detect and measure any possible adverse events associated with IVF and related treatments. In addition to collecting information via RecordKeeper©, questionnaires seeking more in-depth demographic data, medical histories, and current health status are completed by the women. These women are a subset of those included in the registry data. MRI believes that this study can be extended easily to closely monitor the growth and development of the offspring resulting from ART.

Because of MRI's success with the registry and the NICHD study, MRI was asked by the Society of Reproductive Surgeons of the AFS to act as a coordinating center for its large, multicenter, randomized clinical trial of alternative treatments for endometriosis.

The U.S. IVF Registry has been of immeasurable clinical help. It has allowed physicians and other interested parties to monitor the number of ART cycles performed, as well as success rates, with emphasis on clinical pregnancy, spontaneous abortion, ectopic pregnancy, multiple gestation, and delivery. The new reproductive technologies represent a unique aspect of medical care in the United States. This is because they have come under strict scrutiny, both at the regulatory level and in terms of the evaluation of results. The establishment of the U.S. IVF Registry has been extremely beneficial in both of these areas. In fact, as an offshoot of the registry, embryo laboratories in the United States soon will be monitored by an association of pathologists in order to assess quality assurance. This will include the monitoring of results as well.

In addition to collaborating on the establishment of the registry, the AFS has set up revised minimal standards for the performance of IVF, GIFT, and related procedures (AFS 1990). These standards will ensure clinic uniformity in the performance of the new reproductive technologies. Clinics that adhere to these minimal standards are eligible for membership in SART.

The moves by Representative Wyden and SART toward reporting clinic-specific results have some inherent problems. These include pressure to manipulate statistics when economic considerations are important, and they also bias the selection of patients. Some clinics might select only those patients with a high chance of success, for example, young women with tubal disease. These same clinics might reject older women or couples in which the male is oligospermic. Thus a registry that provided clinic-specific results might provide deceptive advertising for some clinics. Failure to achieve uniform reporting would be troublesome.

The fact that the registry's results appear to be consistent from year to year is encouraging. This validates the registry's data collection and reporting methods. Although the number of cycles reported in the United States has quadrupled, success rates have remained relatively stable, increasing only slightly.

Unfortunately, the registry's limited resources prevent MRI from performing on-site audits of the submitted data. At the 1989 annual meeting of the AFS, members of SART initiated plans to evaluate alternative methods for conducting such data reviews.

In the future the registry can be utilized not only to assess success rates and, in a remote fashion, quality assurance, but to monitor new techniques such as cryopreservation and genetic engineering. In addition, it offers a productive venue for multicenter studies, since only a few centers in the United States generate enough cycles to make meaningful statements when treatment protocols are changed or new ideas advanced.

Although an unusual concept in the practice of medicine, the registry has been very successful in describing the practice of ART. With longevity, the IVF Registry will become more valuable, as data quality continues to improve and trends can be detected. Its future success and usefulness will depend on an active and effective research program. This will help to maintain quality and also justify its cost.

References

American Fertility Society (AFS). 1990. "Revised Minimum Standards for In Vitro Fertilization, Gamete Intrafallopian Transfer, and Related Procedures." *Fertility and Sterility* 53:225.

DeCherney, Alan H., and Stuart C. Hartz. 1989. "Assisted Reproduction: Registration Vis-à-Vis Regulation." *Fertility and Sterility* 51:568–570.

Medical Research International (MRI), Society for Assisted Reproductive Technology (SART), and American Fertility Society (AFS). 1988. "In Vitro Fertilization/Embryo Transfer in the United States: 1985 and 1986 Results from the National IVF-ET Registry." *Fertility and Sterility* 49:212–215.

Medical Research International (MRI), Society for Assisted Reproductive Technology (SART), and American Fertility Society (AFS). 1989. "In Vitro Fertilization/Embryo Transfer in the United States: 1987 Results from the National IVF-ET Registry." *Fertility and Sterility* 51:13–19.

Medical Research International (MRI), Society for Assisted Reproductive Technology (SART), and American Fertility Society (AFS). 1990. "In Vitro Fertilization/Embryo Transfer in the United States: 1988 Results from the IVF-ET Registry." *Fertility and Sterility* 53:13–20.

Medical Research International (MRI), Society for Assisted Reproductive Technology (SART), and American Fertility Society (AFS). 1991. "In Vitro Fertilization/Embryo Transfer in the United States: 1989 Results from the IVF-ET Registry." *Fertility and Sterility* 55:14–23.

Subcommittee on Regulation, Business Opportunities, and Energy of the Committee on Small Business, House of Representatives. 1989. *Consumer Protection Issues Involving In Vitro Fertilization Clinics.* Serial Number 101-05 (March). Washington, D.C.: U.S. Government Printing Office.

U.S. Congress, Committee on Government Operations (CGO). 1989. *Infertility in America: Why Is the Federal Government Ignoring a Major Health Problem?* House Report 101-389. Washington, D.C.: U.S. Government Printing Office.

U.S. Congress, Office of Technology Assessment (OTC). 1988. *Infertility: Medical and Social Choices.* OTA-BA-358. Washington, D.C.: U.S. Government Printing Office.

19

Parity for the Donation of Bone Marrow: Ethical and Policy Considerations

*Warren Kearney and Arthur L. Caplan**

Parity for Donation of Tissue and Organs

A California couple recently made public the fact that they had conceived a child in the hope that she would serve as a bone marrow donor for their seventeen-year-old daughter, who has chronic myelogenous leukemia (CML). No suitable, HLA-matched marrow donor exists within the family.** Prior to the conception, no matched donor had been found in the course of numerous searches of existing computerized registries of unrelated persons who had indicated their willingness to serve as marrow donors. The parents, both of whom are in their forties, decided to reverse the husband's vasectomy in order to try to conceive. The result-

*The authors wish to gratefully acknowledge the helpful suggestions and comments of the following people: Bonnie LeRoy, University of Minnesota; Haavi Morreim, University of Tennessee; Joel Frader, University of Pittsburgh; Karen Gervais, Beth Virnig, Steven Miles, University of Minnesota Center for Biomedical Ethics; and in particular, Pamela Ely, University of Minnesota Department of Hematology, and Dorothy Vawter, Center for Biomedical Ethics.

**HLA is the designation for those genetic markers on human cells that play the most important roles in determining whether tissues are recognized as "self" or "foreign," thus determining whether tissues will be rejected in a foreign host. In bone marrow transplants, there is a distinct advantage in having as close a match in HLA markers between donor and recipient as possible, and this match by far and away is most likely to be found within biological relatives.

ing child, a girl, was born last year. As reported in the media, the baby was born and was a full HLA match. The Transplant was carried out without any known complications.

The case generated a tremendous amount of publicity and commentary because of its novelty. While the conception of a child in the hope of securing a bone marrow donor is a rare event, the California case is not the first such attempt. At least forty families in the United States have conceived a child in the hope of locating a marrow donor. The publicity attendant with the California case may encourage other families searching for donors to try to procreate for the purpose of finding a donor of bone marrow. Progress in successfully performing allogeneic marrow transplants may lead other families to pursue this option.

Terminology

Situations in which women become pregnant and give birth in the hope of obtaining tissue (or organs) from their child for transplantation to others can be described as parity for donation. Parity is the medical term used to refer to a woman who has given birth to a living child. This usage indicates the important point that the practice not only involves the intentional conception of a child, but the subsequent birth of the child and its planned participation as a live donor of marrow.

Parity for donation can be seen as one of a more general set of possible reproductive strategies for obtaining organs or tissues that may be termed conception for donation. Conception for donation could involve the elective termination of an intended pregnancy to obtain tissues or fluids from fetal remains (Vawter et al. 1990). Conception for donation may also involve the procurement of fluids or tissue while a fetus is still in utero, with either a subsequent decision to electively abort or to bring the fetus to term. The creation of an embryo for the purpose of donating it to another couple or person who want a child but cannot conceive an embryo (Elias and Annas 1987), or to make an embryo available for the purposes of research or tissue procurement (Robertson 1990), constitute other instances of conception for donation.

The term donation implies that the person providing marrow is making a voluntary choice. To some, it suggests a choice that newborns or very young children cannot make. James Childress has argued that the term donation is not appropriate for referring to situations in which the person who provides organs or tissues is not capable of voluntary, informed consent (1989). He suggests using the term source whenever consent is not possible or practical (1989).

Newborns and young children are not considered competent to give consent for donation of tissues or organs. Parents usually have been accorded a proxy decision making status when consent is sought for procuring organs or tissues from a newborn or young child for transplant, even to someone within the same family. Donation in this context refers to the decision of parents to permit procurement and transplant. Parental surrogacy is grounded in the presupposition that parents can best determine and act upon the best interest of their child.

In this discussion, the term donation has been retained for two reasons. The term is widely used to describe surrogate decision making by parents in situations of organ or tissue procurement involving their own children and is invested with great psychological force. For these authors, the term correctly reflects the underlying beneficent intent of parents and clinicians in a complex situation. Within the context of parity for donation, important questions may arise about the ability of parents to make surrogate or proxy decisions for their child, but retaining the customary usage avoids begging the question by avoiding negative suppositions about the motives parents may have in conceiving a child with the intent to create a tissue or organ donor.

In addition, this usage also avoids the ethical presumption of dismissing a widely used ethical practice, parental surrogacy, as being irrelevant to conceiving children for donation of tissue. Parity for donation has arisen in the context of accepted practices of procurement by parental surrogacy of transplant organs from incompetent children. While the applicability of parental surrogacy, proxy consent for live donation, and their underlying presumptions may require defending in the context of parity for donation, it is most productive to consider the difficulties raised within the accepted framework rather than reject the accepted framework at the outset.

Embryo donation, which has occurred in certain surrogacy arrangements in the United States and other nations (Bartels et al. 1990), and parity for donation are the only reported instances of conception for donation. Public response to the California case has been largely a search among ethical and clinical practices for established rules and approaches, such as principles of reproductive privacy or prohibitions against using people as means to an end, that would classify or judge the practice. We believe that parity for donation (as well as conception for donation in general) presents complex ethical and public policy questions. Because of certain unique features, parity for donation provides an unusually clear opportunity to examine several ethical problems, both for clinical medicine and general society. Among them are the moral status of fetuses, the moral status of young children, the adequacy of current proxy consent, and the status of both women's and parental control and domain over reproductive capacity.

Rationale for Parity for Donation of Bone Marrow

The rationale for undertaking parity for marrow donation is to provide the stem cells of a fully HLA-matched donor for transplant to a biological relative. This follows from the substantial increase in morbidity and mortality in marrow transplants performed with marrow that is less than fully HLA matched or which originates from unrelated donors (Anasetti et al. 1989; Hansen et al. 1987; Beatty et al. 1985). For leukemia and lymphoma, the rate of graft failure when using partially HLA-matched marrow rises to six times that of fully matched marrow transplants (Anasetti et al. 1989:199). For chronic myelogenous leukemia, the survival rate using fully matched, unrelated marrow appears to be two-thirds that of fully matched, related marrow, and for mismatched, unrelated marrow transplants the rate falls to 40 percent of the rate of fully matched, related marrow transplant (McGlave et al. 1990). The morbidity due to graft versus host disease rises sharply with increasing degrees of HLA mismatching, from approximately 35 percent for related, fully matched marrow transplants to 85 percent for a related, haplomatched marrow transplant (Kaminski 1989:443).

Currently, the majority of patients with illnesses potentially treatable by bone marrow transplants cannot find suitable HLA-matched donors within their own families (Beatty et al. 1988). Many marrow transplant centers will, if the nature of the disease permits, offer the option of an unrelated transplant to persons needing a bone marrow transplant. In order to find an unrelated, HLA-matched donor, it is necessary to search the existing public and private registries in the United States and other nations to see whether a matching donor exists.

The current prospects for finding a donor are poor. One center reports that even when an unrelated matched donor is found for a patient, on average nine potential donors are searched for each identified match. The number of prospective donors who have been fully tissue typed in existing registries in the United States, such as in the registry sponsored by the National Marrow Donor Program (NMDP) and other private registries, is too small to permit a high probability of locating an unrelated, HLA-matched donor, even for relatively common tissue types. As of June 1, 1990, 148,082 people were registered as potential donors with the NMDP, which operates the largest registry. Of these, 32,186 (23.8 percent) have been fully tissue typed (Coppo 1990).

The failure to find a fully matched donor in the existing registries means that patients and their families can either arrange to pay for the completion of tissue typing for prospective donors who are known to be partially compatible, or attempt to find and recruit new donors and pay for their tissue typing. Either strategy rapidly becomes prohibitively expensive, since donor recruitment campaigns are expensive and tissue typing costs can be as high as two hundred dollars for each person who agrees to be typed. This search process often involves great personal expense or is conducted with funds raised privately through various types of campaigns.

Within the constraints of a given registry size, the odds for finding a matched, unrelated donor vary widely for people of different ethnic backgrounds and HLA type. For people with a common HLA pheno-type, the chances of finding a matched donor in a registry the current size of the NMDP are more than 50 percent (Beatty et al. 1988). Depend-ing on HLA phenotype, the odds of finding an unrelated donor in the existing registries vary between one in one hundred and one in 1 million (Coppo 1990). Because of the nonrandom distribution of HLA alleles, the odds for members of racial and ethnic minorities in the United States finding a compatible donor in the nation's existing registries, which currently are based on largely Caucasian populations, are disproportion-ately low (Beatty et al. 1988). For these people with uncommon HLA phenotypes, large increases in the size of the volunteer donor pool may not greatly improve their odds of finding a match (Beatty et al. 1988:718).

For the families of many patients, particularly those without substan-tial financial resources or those of diverse, non-Caucasian ethnic back-ground, the relatively high odds (described below) of producing an HLA-matched donor by parity for donation may appear to be a reason-able alternative to the odds and expense associated with finding an unrelated donor. When combined with the improved odds of a desirable outcome of the transplant procedure made possible by a related, fully HLA-matched donor, parity for donation may look even more desirable.

Practical Limits on Marrow Donation from Newborns

The success of parity for donation depends on giving birth to a healthy child who is HLA-matched with the potential recipient in time to provide a transplant. For a number of diseases there is sufficient time between the diagnosis of an illness and the time needed to conceive a child, complete pregnancy, and allow the child to grow to a sufficient size to permit the withdrawal of sufficient amounts of marrow. The youngest donor of marrow known to the authors (not in a case of parity for donation) is a child six weeks old. Many bone marrow transplant programs report to us that their earliest attempts to obtain marrow from young infants occur at three or four months postterm. Thus parity for donation usually may be possible only when the person needing the transplant has the prospect of at least a year's survival time in stable condition from the time of conception of the donor. Many acute conditions, such as severe aplasia or acute myelogenous leukemia, may not permit such a wait.

The success of bone marrow transplantation is, in part, a function of the number of cells transplanted per kilogram of the recipient's body weight. The need for a sufficient number of cells raises questions about the age and size potential infant donors must reach in order to safely remove a large enough volume of marrow to achieve engraftment. The determination of how much marrow is enough also depends upon the extent to which there is a disparity in the size of the donor and the recipient (as in the California case where the would-be recipient is a seventeen-year-old woman).

The availability of cord blood, obtained at birth from the umbilical cord or placenta, may enhance the prospects for successful marrow or stem cell procurement from a very young infant. Stem cells may be obtained from cord blood with no known risk to the newborn (Nathan 1989). The number of totipotent stem cells contained in umbilical cord blood is unknown and thus so is the likelihood of a permanently engrafted marrow transplant using cells from this source (Linch and Brent 1989). Cord blood is known to be relatively rich in committed stem cell precursors and may contain sufficient totipotent stem cells to permit permanent engraftment for a recipient of comparable size. Transplant of cord blood to one patient, a five-year-old boy, has recently been reported, with evidence of trilineage engraftment (Gluckman et al. 1989). For larger recipients, where permanent engraftment is less likely, a transplant of stem cells from cord blood might provide a temporary "bridge" graft that could allow the donor to grow to a size where a sufficient quantity of marrow could be procured to allow permanent engraftment.

A number of questions remain about utility of this procedure (Linch and Brent 1989). The transplantation of cord blood may pose risks to. recipients. The possible intermingling of neonatal cells with maternal cells in cord blood may cause graft versus host disease (GVHD) (Linch and Brent 1989). In addition, bridge grafts using cord blood may require the recipient to undergo the full, ablative pretransplant regimen of radiation. Should the graft fail, the recipient would then be left in a life-threatening, immunocompromised state, raising the possible need for

procurement of marrow from the infant donor much earlier than anticipated if the patient is to survive.

Creating a Suitable Donor

The genetics of HLA inheritance are such that odds associated with
parity for donation of successfully producing an HLA-matched donor for
a sibling are one in four (25 percent). If the potential recipient's illness is
a sex-linked disorder, these odds are modified by the three in four
chance of producing an undiseased child: the odds for producing a
suitable donor then fall to three in sixteen (.25 × .75, or approximately
19 percent). The odds of producing a match can be increased through an
incestuous conception between a parent and a child.

On average, parity for donation will result in more haplomatched and
unmatched children than matched potential donors. In the unlikely event
that the parties involved feel it is necessary and acceptable to transplant
haplomatched marrow, perhaps because of the desire to use a related
rather than an unrelated, mismatched donor or for reasons of urgency,
then the odds for producing a suitable donor for a sibling rise to three in
four.

In this way, the odds for producing a healthy, suitable donor *and*
curing or ameliorating the patient's condition may be approximated.
Cure rates after bone marrow transplantation differ for various illnesses,
but for malignant diseases the best rates occur in certain forms of leukemia; for CML they are approximately 60 percent (Jandl 1987:671–725).
Under optimistic genetic and therapeutic assumptions, parents begin the
effort of parity for donation with a 15 percent chance of successfully
curing a recipient of CML (.25 × .60). It should be clear that this may
not be the calculation that any individual parent initially looks to for
guidance. Parents undertaking parity for donation may take the success
of the conception effort as a given or as irrelevant, either out of hope or
out of the willingness to accept a new child regardless of the outcome of
the matching. They may then compare odds for a favorable outcome for
donation from a related, fully HLA-matched donor with the odds of
finding an unrelated, matched donor and the odds of a poorer outcome:
such a comparison will more clearly favor parity for donation.

Technological advances in tissue typing may provide the means for
raising these odds. If accurate tissue typing in utero became widely
available, parents might choose to terminate pregnancies in which the
fetus did not have the desired HLA type. Techniques have evolved
allowing the HLA typing of fetuses in utero. These techniques have been

developed in efforts to improve prenatal diagnosis of congenital disorders, to provide genetic evidence of paternity, and to refine HLA matching of unrelated bone marrow donors. Expression of HLA antigens can be induced and enhanced on cultured chorionic villus and amniotic cells (Callaway et al. 1986; Maurer et al. 1987; Pollack et al. 1989). Other techniques use polymerase chain reaction (PCR) amplification of specific DNA sequences and subsequent identification of HLA alleles by allele-specific oligonucleotide (ASO) probes or restriction fragment length polymorphisms (RFLP) (Uryu et al. 1990; Riisom et al. 1988; Howell et al. 1990; Maeda et al. 1989). The accuracy of these HLA typing methods seems to compare favorably with standard typing techniques (Maeda et al. 1989).

These techniques could be applied to chorionic villi samples obtained as early as nine weeks in the gestational period (Callaway et al. 1986), allowing identification of the HLA status of a conceived donor in the late first trimester. At some point in the future, it may become possible to utilize such diagnostic techniques in conjunction with in vitro fertilization, cell culture, and embryo biopsy to identify and selectively implant suitably HLA-matched embryos.

For now, the techniques for in utero HLA typing are still investigational, and their reliability is likely to be dependent on the experience of individual research laboratories. While the prospect of electively aborting pregnancies based on the determination of fetal HLA phenotype may soon exist, not even a single case of parity for donation in which an elective abortion was performed after in utero HLA tissue typing has been identified.

There are also risks associated with parity for donation for some couples and conceived infants. For some inherited diseases, there is a risk of having another child with the same disease for which a marrow donor is sought. While the vast majority of hematopoietic malignancies show no measurable heritable trend, several of the heritable metabolic disorders do. One case in which parity for donation for a sibling with severe combined immunodeficiency disorder (SCID) resulted in a second child with the same condition has been described to the authors.

Extent of the Practice of Parity for Donation: Results of a Telephone Survey

No registry keeps track of the practice of conception for donation. In order to better understand the extent and nature of the practice of conceiving children as live marrow donors, the authors conducted a telephone survey of transplant physicians and transplant coordinators at fifteen of the twenty-seven approved bone marrow transplant centers, including the ten largest. The results indicated more than forty cases of attempted parity for donation of marrow occurred between 1984 and 1989, including eight cases in which the child went on to serve as a donor. No results were available on the outcomes of the transplants, but no complications to the donors were known. These figures probably represent an underestimate, as many respondents pointed out that parents would not always be likely to inform transplant teams that a new baby had been conceived with donation in mind.

The survey yielded some interesting anecdotal descriptions of behaviors and outcomes in attempts at parity for donation, as well information about policies and attitudes toward parity for donation among transplant institutions. One center reported an instance of parity for donation in which a woman became pregnant by means of artificial insemination using sperm obtained from her ex-husband. Another center reported a case in which a family had had three children in the hope of finding a donor for another child within the family. None of the children conceived for this purpose were compatible donors. Two centers reported cases in which an adult recipient had located an unrelated donor but decided to delay transplantation until a pregnancy had ended and tissue typing could be performed on the newborn. In one case the prospective recipient was the father of the child. In neither case was the child a compatible donor.

No center contacted had formal policies regarding parity for donation, nor did they keep formal statistics on the practice. Most of the respondents indicated that they were uncomfortable raising the option of parity for donation with families seeking donors. Personnel at each of the seven centers where parity for donation was reported indicated that it was the families who raised the option or decided on their own to procreate for this purpose. Personnel at six other programs noted that families are likely to realize the option of parity for donation exists without prompting from health care personnel.

No center in the poll routinely offers or performs in utero tissue typing in situations where parity for donation is known to have occurred. Three centers reported cases in which in utero tissue typing was done in order to expedite the donation of marrow for potential family recipients who were in failing health.

Respondents at seven of the transplant centers, including six of the seven where parity for donation is reported to have occurred, indicated that they would have no ethical objection to utilizing a child procreated in this manner as a donor. Respondents at five of the transplant centers indicated that they would have ethical objections to using such a child as a donor. Transplant coordinators expressed more reservations about the practice than did transplant physicians. Personnel at two centers indicated that they would follow the policies of their centers should parity for donation become known, although neither center had a policy with respect to parity for donation. One transplant coordinator stated that before any child resulting from parity for donation would be accepted as a donor, the approval of the institution's ethics committee would have to be obtained, but for exactly what purpose was not clear.

The policy of transplant centers varied when no suitable bone marrow donor could be found within the family and when searches of existing registries failed to locate a possible matched, unrelated donor. All centers reported that they would continue efforts to search existing registries. A variety of other options were available, including offering the option of donation using haplomatched, related donors or unrelated, mismatched donors, referring families to centers where transplants involving mismatched donors are attempted, and assisting families in the preparation of genealogical trees to help locate more distant relatives who might be approached about their willingness to be tissue typed. No center reported having a policy which would suggest or urge parity for donation as a therapeutic alternative.

Many of the respondents indicated that their greatest concern about parity for donation is the safety of the donor. They noted the risks inherent in removing large amounts of marrow from an infant for transplantation to an adolescent or adult recipient, the dangers associated with anesthesia and replacement blood transfusions, and the risks associated with the need to perform repeat or multiple harvests in situations in which insufficient amounts of marrow are obtained or initial grafts fail. A few transplant physicians noted that they were troubled by efforts to procure marrow that had resulted in inadequate amounts of marrow being obtained, especially in light of the risks involved for both donor and recipient. About half of the transplant physicians noted that there was insufficient knowledge about how much marrow would be sufficient when small children were used as donors for adolescents or adults. Several respondents offered the observation that they were troubled by the fact that an infant cannot consent to the donation of marrow. Two transplant coordinators associated with transplant centers where parity for donation has occurred observed that it was important that families clearly understand the poor odds they face and that their decision not be the result of the extraordinary emotions and pressures involved when a relative is dying for want of a donor.

Ethical Considerations in Parity for Donation

Ethical criticism has centered on objections to the use of babies as sources of spare organs and tissues ("spare parts" [Doris 1990:23]). Parity for donation (and by extension conception for donation) has been cited as a violation of a basic moral principle that human beings ought not be treated only as means to serve the ends of others. Some critics of the couple in California argue that the motive of saving a child is not a sound moral reason to try to conceive another child ("children are not medicine" [Spector 1990:D1]).

Defenders of the behavior of the couple in California and of the practice of parity for donation have emphasized the right to privacy of reproductive choice on the part of parents, and the right to have a child to save another child, free from moral criticism (Dershowitz 1990). Some have suggested that it is wrong to even raise ethical questions about the motives parents bring to the conception of children (Dershowitz 1990; Wecht 1990).

Parity for donation raises a number of important and complicated issues that are not captured by invoking specific principles or rights. The claim that a child has been created solely from the motive of exploiting its potential as a donor does not reflect any empirically based information about the motives of parents who have engaged in parity for donation, nor do such claims capture the underlying psychological complexities that certainly surround conception and birth in these circumstances.

The complexity of the ethical issues raised extends beyond those concerning the donor child. Parity for donation raises at least six areas of potential ethical concern. These include the potential risks of harms or wrongs to the prospective donor; the standards and procedures for obtaining valid proxy consent for donation; risks of wrongs and harms to the donor's mother; risks of wrongs and harms to the family and questions of familial duty; the appropriateness of "value neutrality" on the part of health care providers; and the morality of elective abortion for unsuitable donors.

Wrongs and harms to children

Objections to parity for donation represent a challenge to the privacy of parents to make reproductive decisions for themselves and their intended children, as well as to their role in making medical decisions for their children's best interests. Challenges of this sort have arisen in areas such as surrogate motherhood (Krimmel 1989) and prenatal sex selection (Wertz and Fletcher 1989).

Unlike prenatal sex selection and surrogate motherhood, parity for donation employs no new technology beyond existing transplant techniques. No new kinds of social practices are defined, such as the contracting for surrogate motherhood. No obviously new social relations are defined, such as the relationship between the surrogate mother and the family who contracts for the child, or the possible reduction of a child to a commodity some claim this contract entails (Krimmel 1989). In parity for donation, ethical problems arise from the novel order of events. The deliberate decision to try to conceive an HLA-matched child who will serve as a bone marrow donor reverses the usual order of events, where an existing child is discovered to be HLA-matched after the need for a donor arises. Since the production of the match is an accident in either case, the ethical difference arises from the intent behind the deliberate attempt at producing this accident and whatever results from this intent.

In the ethical analysis of parity for donation, an important distinction can be made by separating potential wrongs from harms resulting from the act. Harms involve the risk of injury, disability or death to another. Wrongs connote a different type of injury, one which derives from violation of certain principles. Wrongs consist, for example, in violations of a person's dignity, privacy, liberty or self-respect, as well as the results of that violation.

A wrong may also result from violating a societal principle, rather than a principle related to a particular individual, and the resulting wrong may be independent of any particular effect on the individuals involved in any particular case. Because of this violation, the act could be claimed to be inherently unacceptable, regardless of claims that in a particular case all the individuals involved came out well or happy. Thus prenatal sex selection is said to violate a societal principle of sex neutrality and to be unacceptable regardless of whether or not particular resulting families are happy (Krimmel 1989). Similarly, surrogate motherhood has been labeled fundamentally wrong because it objectifies children as commodities (Wertz and Fletcher 1989), or employs a woman's reproductive capacity as a commercial resource.

Potential wrongs to donor child

Parity for donation has been criticized as being fundamentally wrong, regardless of the outcome of a particular case, due to the fear that children who are created as a result are inherently wronged because they are conceived with an explicit purpose to serve. Those who voice concern about wronging potential donors seem to have in mind Kant's instructions in *Foundations of the Metaphysics of Morals*:

> Every rational being exists as an end in himself and not merely as a means to be arbitrarily used by this or that will. . . . The practical imperative, therefore, is the following: Act so that you treat humanity, whether in your own person or in that of another, always as an end and never as a means only. (1959:46–47)

It is not clear, however, that there is any simple and direct path between Kant's widely cited metaphysical axiom and understanding what it means practically to improperly "use" another human being (Beck 1959; Davis 1984). It does seem clear that using others is a part of most daily human interactions. The Kantian proscription is against using people *solely* as a means to an end. Using another human being does not appear automatically unacceptable if certain conditions for respecting the intrinsic rights and values of the person are met; this is one of the principles underlying informed consent in donation for transplant.

In this sense, parity for donation does not appear to inherently violate any fundamental social values. Nothing inherent in the intent to produce a compatible child donor rules out valuing, raising, and loving the child for itself. Objectifying a child by treating him or her only as a source of marrow, a kind of tissue farm, would be a tragic wrong. However, it is unclear how such extreme behavior would look in practice. Objecting to parity for donation as wronging a child donor because it necessarily means the child is valued only as a means to someone else's end makes an unjustified a priori judgment about the motives and intentions of parents. Parents who undertake parity for donation do so in the hope of finding a marrow donor. This does not mean that their only motive in having a child is marrow donation or that their only way of viewing and treating their child is as a source of marrow for another. In lieu of any evidence to the contrary, there is no reason to presume that parents will treat a child who results from parity for donation *solely* as a means to helping another.

However, the intent in parity for donation to conceive a child with a specific purpose in mind serves as a warning that wrongs and harms may occur to the potential donor as a result of the circumstances surrounding the attempt. In the immediacy of the desire to save the life of a family member, there may be an undue emphasis on the conceived child's purpose in saving another life. This could arise from the parents themselves, their families, or others in their community; and it could be inadvertently promoted by similar feelings expressed by health care providers.

The prospective donor child might be wronged in several ways. Regardless of success or failure of the matching or of the transplant procedure, a child might be born into a family that cannot afford or did not plan for another child before the need for a donor arose. The attempt at parity for donation might fail, either because the child is not a suitable donor or the procedure fails despite a suitable match. Parents may be faced with having to cope with a new child at a time when they have lost another child or close family member. The confusion or guilt which may follow in the wake of failure could be transferred to the donor child with untoward effects, either in early bonding or later, as the child grows up under the shadow of having failed in an important task. Even if the transplant procedure is a success, it would be important that the child not come to feel as though his or her worth had depended upon this curative mission. These are risks to the sense of self-image and self-worth of the children involved.

Potential harms to donor child

For adult bone marrow donors, the risk to their health in donating marrow essentially is that associated with general anesthesia and blood transfusion. As long as the potential donor's health is good, the risk of harm associated with donation is extremely small. Timing of the procedure to procure marrow can be coordinated with the needs of the patient without increased risk to the donor. This may not always be the case with the young infant donor.

Relatively few infants less than two years of age have served as bone marrow donors. Experience with the procedure in this group is thus smaller, and risks, while probably not quantifiable, may be higher than for adults. Various illnesses have varying natural histories, and the optimal time of transplant may occur when the donor is quite young. The risk of harms may be heightened by disparities in size between the potential donor and the recipient. Acquiring sufficient numbers of cells for successful engraftment of a significantly larger recipient may entail increased risks due to the need to remove a greater volume of marrow from a small donor, including a larger number of replacement transfusions and the need to undertake repeated harvest procedures. Should a bridging graft with cord blood be attempted, early failure of the graft would certainly increase the feeling of urgency to procure marrow from a young donor much earlier than anticipated.

The risks for a donor child are further increased if the donor is born with or acquires medical problems that in themselves increase the risk of adverse outcomes from marrow procurement. In families in which a parent is a carrier of a heritable disease, parity for donation carries an inherent risk of harm to the extent of the odds of producing a child with disease. With increasing age of the mother, there is an independent risk of producing a child with a congenital malformation.

Parents and transplant professionals may not be able to adequately represent the best interests of the child in weighing the risks of harms associated with being a donor. A singular concentration on providing a successful donation and transplant may place the potential donor at risk if parents do not adequately weigh the risk of harm to one of their children against the benefits that might be obtained for another family member, or are not appropriately aided in this by the transplant team.

Proxy consent

Any living organ or tissue donor undergoes a medical risk not related to a therapy for his or herself. In parity for donation, there are two kinds of such nontherapeutic medical risks. One is the basic risk of the procurement procedure under what would be optimal circumstances for the donor; the other is any measurably increased risk due to particular circumstances, such as large disparity in size between donor or recipient, coincident illness in the donor, or a need to do the procedure earlier than would be optimal.

Questions about both the process and justification for informed consent using incompetent children as transplant donors are not restricted to parity for donation. Questions have been raised in court cases regarding donation of nonrenewable organs such as kidneys by incompetent children or by those who are mentally retarded (*Strunk v. Strunk* 1969; *Little v. Little* 1979), and in general discussion over the principles (Ramsey 1975; Kass 1979; McCormick 1974).

Some argue that since no meaningful informed consent can be obtained for young children, it is impossible for a proxy to try to guess or infer what a child would consent to in terms of facing risks of harms or wrongs. If consent is held to be the only basis for nontherapeutic medical interventions involving infants and young children, it is argued that no child should be involved in any procedure involving more than minimal, trivial risk (Ramsey 1975; Kass 1979). Others argue that while it may not be possible to make a substituted judgment for an incompetent child, it can still be in the child's best interest to participate in some medical interventions such as tissue or organ donation (*Strunk v. Strunk* 1969; McCormick 1974).

In practice, parents are allowed to give proxy consent for the donation of organs and tissues from infants and children on the presumption that they have the best interests of their child at heart, even when the recipient is their own child. However, when so close to the realization of their intended rescue and having overcome the odds against producing a suitable donor, the dilemma of mediating between what may be conflicting interests among members of the same family challenges this presumption. It seems unreasonable to assume that parents will always be capable of making appropriately considered proxy decisions for potential donors. A similar argument can be constructed for the physicians and transplant team members who seek a donor for their patient.

Parity for donation may require considering a new standard and procedure for assuring informed proxy consents. If consent is grounded in making a judgment about what is in the best interest of a child, then decisions to allow a child to be a marrow donor may require oversight and approval by a third party who is specifically charged with protecting the interests of the child. This might be a physician or health care professional not involved in the care of the prospective recipient, or a designated committee. The third-party mandate would be to provide an unequivocal advocacy for the interests of the child. In cases in which more than minimal risk to prospective child marrow donors is believed to be involved, review and approval by a court of law may be appropriate.

A change in the proxy consent process for marrow donation does not end the ethical issues in the realm of consent. Unless there are sound arguments that can justify allowing a child to assume either the basic risk of the procurement, or any particular increased risk above this basic risk, for the sake of saving a relative's life, the process by which proxy consent is reached may be insufficient justification for the consent.

One standard often applied is that the child donor's best interests can be served by undergoing such risk. In some cases, such as a court allowing a mentally retarded young man to donate a kidney to his brother, the justification is peculiar to the circumstances, in this case the measurable contribution of the older brother to the donor's quality of life (*Strunk v. Strunk* 1969). In general, such arguments turn on the relationship of the child to the family or the moral community at large. The act of donation may confer a privileged moral status on a child donor that justifies being submitted to increased risks. The child donor eventually derives a moral benefit from entry into the moral community at an early age, a benefit which accrues and becomes consciously appreciated as the donor matures (McCormick 1974).

Nancy Jecker argues that there may be different ethical principles governing relations and duties within a family than those which obtain for the impersonal relationships among strangers (1990). In parity for donation, these duties might justify the assumption or imposition (in the case of proxy decisions) of increased risk. However, strictly speaking, it might well be argued that the newborn child is still essentially a stranger to the family and the community, and that these obligations may only arise over time. Loving feelings by the family toward the new child may not automatically be a source of obligations for the child to the family. The presumed benefits of entering the family under such salutory emotional circumstances rest on speculation, and not all familial relationships end up being beneficial (Morreim 1990; English 1985). Alternatively, the fact that the child is cared for by the family may be argued to create a quid pro quo obligation.

In medical ethics, the principle of nonmaleficence (do no harm) is often felt to take priority over the principle of beneficence (do good). If it could be shown that the risks of wrongs or harms associated with parity for donation were minimal or trivial, then a duty of beneficence might govern donation, even for an incompetent child.

Insufficient attention has been devoted to the analysis of family duties and the duty of beneficence to arrive at a firm consensus regarding the morality of consent to donation of marrow on the part of a minor child. However, the growing interest in using living donors, some of whom are not able to give voluntary, informed consent to donation, as sources of organs and tissues makes it imperative that more attention be given to the ethics of imposing risks on the incompetent for the purposes of organ or tissue donation.

Wrongs and harms to women

Parity for donation carries risks for wronging or harming not only the donor child, but also the women who might potentially bear a lifesaving donor. Parity for donation represents a new possibility for saving a life by a deliberate reproductive act. Under certain circumstances, the option of becoming pregnant and bearing a child might be seen not as a choice but as an obligation. This could occur explicitly as a matter of public moral debate, or implicitly and privately through the pressures of guilt and persuasion which might arise in individual families or within the religious or cultural milieu in which the woman lives. In this way a woman becomes a means to a relative's ends, out of proportion to her value as a person.

The result of transforming parity from a choice to a duty would be a compromise in the autonomy of a woman over her reproductive abilities. This interpretation may convert what is arguably a supererogatory moral act—deliberately becoming pregnant, with the attendant risks (especially for older women) and the subsequent assumption of parental responsibility for another child—into an ordinary moral duty.

If parity for donation were to be seen as a duty on the part of women, the relationship of health care providers to the family of the patient might be compromised. The very suggestion that parity for donation is a therapeutic possibility would represent the beginning of a process of coercion. Since the extent to which the state has an interest in controlling women's reproductive capacities is not settled in the United States, the possibility exists of legal action to try to compel pregnancy in circumstances where parity for donation was the only option for saving a life.

A woman who might attempt parity for donation also faces the possibility of unusually strong feelings of guilt or depression over the failure of the effort. She may develop similar feelings over her refusal to undergo the attempt, or over her physical or financial inability to undergo the risks of parity for donation.

Obligations of families

Many of the same concerns about the ethical pressures on individual women to attempt parity for donation may be extended to the family unit. Families may be unwilling to undertake procreation for donation for any one of a variety of personal reasons, including the inability to afford the rearing of one or more new children produced in the attempt. The suggestion that parity for donation might be a therapeutic option may cause families who choose not to attempt it to feel guilt that they did not exhibit sufficient concern or love for a needy family member. Such families may also become the object of tacit professional or community opprobrium for failing to pursue all possible courses of action to "save" their family member. Arguments that families "should" undergo the attempt may be extending the definition of family obligations.

The moral difficulties for transplant providers and counselors

Most of the health care professionals contacted in our telephone poll reported disquiet at the idea of raising the option of parity for donation with families. Many insist that parents can figure this option out for themselves without information from the transplant team. Whether that is so or not is a matter for further inquiry. However, it is reasonable to wonder why transplant teams should not include this option as a routine component of counseling families about the strategies they can pursue to locate HLA-matched donors. Is it really nondirective, or value-neutral to omit this option? Would transplant teams remain neutral about a family member who raised the option of an incestuous conception in order to maximize the chances of locating a suitable donor? Nor is it obvious what legal or moral basis exists for refusing to perform a transplant from a child known or suspected to be a product of deliberate conception.

The question of whether counseling can or should be nondirective is complicated by the potential for very different perspectives on the odds for success. What may seem like low initial odds for success to an outsider may seem like high odds to a family that believes the choice is between these odds and certain death for a child. For some parents, the existence of any possibility for success may amount to no choice at all. Whether it is possible for a counselor to achieve a neutral position in such situations without interjecting personal feelings or seeming resistant to the family is not clear.

Transplant teams also must consider the stance they adopt toward discussing and counseling families about parity for donation. Families who do decide to pursue this strategy may feel that they have a special claim upon the resources of the transplant team should a suitably matched donor be created. Many potential recipients do not benefit from marrow donation because they lack the money to pay for the transplant or the search for a matched donor. Families who engage in parity for donation with the tacit or explicit support of a transplant team may expect the team to minimize any financial barriers to performing the transplant that exist, should a potential donor be created.

Elective abortion and parity for donation

The continued development of techniques for in utero HLA matching may permit the early termination of pregnancies when a mismatched potential donor has been conceived. Advocating or allowing this practice may involve advancing claims for the autonomy of women to new limits. It might also be argued as a clear instance of complete objectification and use of the fetus, in violation of the Kantian principle previously discussed. Many of the ethical reasons often given in defense of the morality of elective abortion—the priority of the mother's interests in controlling her body, the fact that conception was not undertaken in a planned, voluntary manner, or that parents were unprepared and unable to bear the cost of raising a child—might need reconsideration or might not apply when parity for donation is involved. Though selective abortion on the basis of HLA compatibility may not be seen as "trivializing" abortion in the way prenatal sex selection is argued to, this degree of objectification of the fetus may represent a problem, even for advocates of abortion.

However, attempts to directly limit the ability to electively abort unsuitable donors would require a burdensome degree of regulatory or legal oversight into the motives for reproduction and the motives for abortion. Specific, practical attempts to prohibit abortion when a fetus is created who cannot be a marrow donor may constitute unwarranted interference in areas of personal choice still held as private and protected by legal precedent. Indirect attempts to regulate abortion in such circumstances, by specific wording in informed consent documents or through counseling, may also been seen as unduly intrusive.

If regulating abortion for selection of unsuitable donors is desirable, a practical regulatory approach may be to forbid prenatal testing for HLA typing in situations of parity for donation. Such a policy has its own regulatory and oversight difficulties. The techniques currently are under development for a wide variety of accepted prenatal testing purposes. The practical difficulties in preventing selection of fetal donors by HLA typing might be similar to those encountered by genetic counselors when programs forbid parents to use prenatal information for sex selection.

Suggested Guidelines

Parity for donation of bone marrow remains a rare event, but it has important ethical and public policy implications for the children and families involved, for our understanding of personal and familial duties, and for designing mechanisms to protect the interests of incompetent children. The ethics of parity for donation are further complicated by the fact that it will be exceedingly difficult, and perhaps undesirable, to control or regulate the reproductive practices of parents who desire to aid a dying family member. Attempts to make policy regulating parity for donation should consider at what point in the process policy will be practical and acceptable.

All centers performing bone marrow transplants should develop a specific approach and set of policies concerning parity for donation. This may involve nothing more than stating an unwillingness to perform transplants from donors known to result from parity for donation. The willingness or unwillingness of the center to perform such transplants should be clear to the families of all patients for whom it might be relevant, to avoid misunderstandings after an attempt has been made by the parents. However, centers considering restrictive policies should be aware that they are entering murky waters by setting limits on what are acceptable motives for reproduction and are not necessarily avoiding ethical difficulties by the attempt. Restrictive policies may discriminate against families and patients in which parents are in some sense "found out," or are honest about their reproductive motives.

The full breadth of counseling needs for parents, donors, and patients should be anticipated. These include genetic, psychological, and pastoral counseling. Technical aspects of parity for donation including the genetic odds, as well as center-specific information on transplant outcomes, must be readily available in accessible language to counselors and families. The goals of counseling should include at least the following: parents should understand fully the probabilities of success; the risks of adverse outcomes, including those of pregnancy for the mother; the danger of wrongs to the child, the mother, and the family; and the probabilities and costs associated with unrelated marrow transplants. The counseling process should be acutely sensitive to the optimistic weight endorsement by health professionals can give to even the most remote chances of saving a life.

For the time being, attempts at parity for donation should be viewed as an unusual and supererogatory behavior not to be equated with providing a potential recipient with a "fair chance." Those who counsel families should make it clear that some of the hardest ethical choices associated with parity for donation begin once a child is born. The possibilities for guilt and confusion in the event of failure in the effort, or in the decision not to attempt parity for donation, should be anticipated.

Because of the powerful and important role of physicians and other members of the immediate health care team in the lives of patients eligible for bone marrow transplants, it is difficult to specify suggestions for their role in the process of informing families about the possibility of parity for donation. On the one hand, suggesting that these personnel neither instigate or suggest the option, and that discussions and counseling be carried on by others, such as transplant coordinators and various counselors might seem wise. However, the fine line between objectivity and an unacceptable degree of aloofness from patients and families may be practically untenable and present an ethical dilemma for some. This role should be a part of discussions among members of every center performing bone marrow transplants.

Whether in utero HLA typing of potential donors should be available in these situations should be openly discussed. At the very least, the status of the various techniques in development, from research tools to standardized techniques and including the reliability, specificity, and operator dependency, should be clarified in the literature prior to offering it to parents. Centers and laboratories with demonstrated expertise should be certified and this expertise made known to families.

Every marrow transplant center which accepts children resulting from parity for donation should consider adopting a public mechanism for assigning proxy decision makers for prospective child donors. At a minimum, this may require assigning potential donors their own physician who is independent from the team caring for the potential recipient and knowledgeable as to the risks of donation. An independent oversight committee, such as an ethics committee, should routinely play a role in monitoring the welfare and interests of prospective donors, perhaps with final authority to disapprove either the donation or the transplant.

Most parents who seize upon the strategy of parity for donation will do so with very mixed motives and mixed feelings. They have discovered that they, and not the medical profession, control a potentially lifesaving therapeutic tool: their reproductive capacity. This demands care and thoughtfulness on the part of health care providers in assuring that parental decisions are well informed and that appropriate safeguards and support mechanisms are in place for all family members.

References

Anasetti, C., D. Amos, P. G. Beatty et al. 1989. "Effect of HLA Compatibility on Engraftment of Bone Marrow Transplants in Patients with Leukemia or Lymphoma." *New England Journal of Medicine* 320(4):197–204.

Bartels, D. M., R. Priester, D. E. Vawter, and A. L. Caplan. *Beyond Baby M.* Clifton, N.J.: Humana.

Beatty, P. G., R. A. Clift, E. M. Mickelson et al. 1985. "Marrow Transplantation from Related Donors Other than HLA-Identical Siblings." *New England Journal of Medicine* 313 (13):765–771.

Beatty, P. G., S. Dahlberg, E. M. Mickelson et al. 1988. "Probability of Finding HLA-Matched Unrelated Marrow Donors." *Transplantation* 45(4):714–718.

Callaway, C., C. Falcon, G. Grant et al. 1986. "HLA Typing Used with Cultured

Amniotic and Chorionic Villus Cells for Early Prenatal Diagnosis or Parentage Testing without One Parent's Availability." *Human Immunology* 16:200–204.

Childress, J. 1989. "Ethical Criteria for Procuring and Distributing Organs for Transplantation." *Journal of Health Politics, Policy and Law* 14(1):91–101.

Coppo, P. 1990. National Marrow Donor Program. Personal communication.

Davis, N. 1984. "Using Persons and Common Sense." *Ethics* 94:387–406.

Dershowitz, A. 1990. "Don't Rush to Judge These Parents." *Boston Herald* (February 26):23.

Doris, M. 1990. "Infants for Spare Parts? No." *Boston Herald* (February 26):23.

Elias, S., and G. Annas. 1987. *Reproductive Genetics and the Law*. Chicago: Year Book Medical Publishers.

English, J. 1985. "What Do Grown Children Owe Their Parents?" In C. H. Sommers, ed., *Vice and Virtue in Everyday Life*, pp. 460–467. San Diego: Harcourt Brace Jovanovich.

Gluckman, E., H. E. Broxmeyer, A. D. Auerbach et al. 1989. "Hematopoietic Reconstitution in a Patient with Fanconi's Anemia by Means of Umbilical-Cord Blood from an HLA-Identical Sibling." *New England Journal of Medicine* 321(17):1174–1178.

Hansen, J. A., P. G. Beatty, C. Anasetti et al. 1987. "Treatment of Leukemia by Marrow Transplantation from Donors Other than HLA Genotypically Identical Siblings." *Progress in Bone Marrow Transplantation*. New York: Alan R. Liss, pp. 667–675.

Howell, W. M., P. R. Evans, D. A. Sage, C. M. Lambert, P. J. Wilson, and J. L. Smith. 1990. "The Use of Polymerase Chain Reaction (PCR) Gene Amplification and Synthetic Oligonucleotide Probes for HLA-DP Typing Bone Marrow Transplantation." *Bone Marrow Transplantation* 5(1):66–67.

Jandl, J. 1987. *Blood: Textbook of Hematology*. Boston: Little, Brown.

Jecker, N. S. 1990. "Conceiving a Child to Save a Child: Reproductive and Filial Ethics." *Journal of Clinical Ethics* 1(2):99–103.

Kaminski, E. R. 1989. "How Important is Histocompatibility in Bone Marrow Transplantation?" *Bone Marrow Transplantation* 4:439–444.

Kant, Immanuel. 1959. *Foundations of the Metaphysics of Morals*. Translated with an introduction by L. W. Beck. New York: Macmillan.

Kass, L. R. 1979. "Making Babies Revisited." *The Public Interest* 54:32–60.

Krimmel, H. T. 1989. "Surrogate Mother Arrangements from the Perspective of the Child." In J. Arras and N. Rhoden, eds., *Ethical Issues in Modern Medicine*, 3d ed., pp. 376–383. Mountain View, Calif.: Mayfield Publishing.

Linch, D. C., and L. Brent. 1989. "Can Cord Blood Be Used?" *Nature* 340:676.

Little v. Little. 1979. 576 S.W. 2d 493 (Texas Cir. Ct. App. 1979).

McCormick, R. A. 1974. "Proxy Consent in the Experimentation Situation." *Perspectives in Biology and Medicine*. 18:2–20.

McGlave, P. B., P. Beatty, R. Ash, and J. M. Hows. 1990. "Therapy for Chronic Myelogenous Leukemia with Unrelated Donor Bone Marrow Transplantation: Results with 102 Cases." *Blood* 75(8):1728–1732.

Maeda, M., H. Inoko, A. Ando, N. Uryu, and K. Tsuji. 1989. "HLA-D Typing of

Heterozygotes Using Restriction Fragment Length Polymorphism in the HLA-DQ Gene Region on the Basis of Standard Band Patterns Derived from HLA Homozygotes." *Human Immunology* 25:195–205.

Maurer, D. H., C. Callaway, S. Sorkin, and M. S. Pollack. 1987. "Gamma Interferon Induces Detectable Serological and Functional Expression of DR and DP but Not DQ Antigens on Cultured Amniotic Fluid Cells." *Tissue Antigens* 31:174–182.

Morreim, E. H. 1990. Personal communication.

Nathan, D. G. 1989. "The Beneficence of Neonatal Hematopoiesis." *New England Journal of Medicine* 321(17):1190–1191.

Pollack, M. S., C. Callaway, S. Sorkin, A. Zaafran, and D. Maurer. 1989. "Differential Induction of Class II HLA Molecules on Cultured Amniotic Fluid and Chorionic Villus Cells by Gamma Interferon." *Transplantation Proceedings* 21(1):635–636.

Ramsey, P. 1976. "The Enforcement of Morals: Nontherapeutic Research on Children." *Hastings Center Report* 6(4):21–30.

Riisom, K., I. J. Sorensen, B. Moller, T. A. Kruse, B. Graugaard, and L. U. Lamm. 1988. "HLA-DR Typing Using Restriction Fragment Length Polymorphism (RFLP) with One Enzyme and Two Probes." *Tissue Antigens* 31: 141–150.

Robertson, J. A. 1990. "Prior Agreements for Disposition of Frozen Embryos." *Ohio State Law Journal* 51(2):407–424.

Spector, M. 1990. "Birth Raises Tough Ethical Questions." *Washington Post* (May 1).

Strunk v. Strunk. 1969. 445 S.W. 2d 145 (Ky., 1969).

Uryu, N., M. Maeda, M. Ota, K. Tsuji, and H. Inoko. 1990. "A Simple and Rapid Method for HLA-DRB and -DQB Typing by Digestion of PCR-Amplified DNA with Allele Specific Restriction Endonucleases." *Tissue Antigens* 35:20–31.

Vawter, D., W. Kearney, K. G. Gervais, A. L. Caplan, D. Garry, and C. Tauer. 1990. *The Use of Human Fetal Tissue: Scientific, Ethical and Political Concerns.* Minneapolis: University of Minnesota Center for Biomedical Ethics.

Wecht, C. 1990. Letter to the editor. *American Medical News* (May 30).

Wertz, D. C., and J. C. Fletcher. 1989. "Fatal Knowledge? Prenatal Diagnosis and Sex Selection." *Hastings Center Report* 19(3):21–27.

20

Pitting the Fetus Against Its Mother

Martha A. Field

The newest technique in the assault against women's independence is pitting the fetus against the mother. A potential conflict between fetus and carrier is fairly obvious when the question is abortion and the scope of the pregnant woman's right to choose to terminate fetal life. But the approach of viewing fetus and mother as adversaries has recently become prevalent also in discussions about the mother's conduct and medical treatment during pregnancy. There is a new tendency to view the mother as the fetus's opponent and to allow decisions concerning her conduct to be made by the state, the medical profession, or even her employer rather than by her.

The approach is a clever one, if the goal is to undermine women's independence. The asserted aim—to protect the health of newborns and children—is so appealing and indeed universally espoused that it is almost embarrassing to take "the women's rights position." A frequently heard disclaimer is "Even though I'm a feminist, I can't support allowing women to produce cocaine-dependent babies." The implication is that promoting decision making by women must entail a view that women have a "right" to harm their offspring. In fact, no one believes that women or anyone else should produce brain damage or other serious health problems in babies to be born, and all would be attracted by legislation that seemed effectively to prevent that from happening. The issue is not about a "right to choose" such a horrible outcome but rather about who will bear the responsibility to protect against it. It is also about whether pregnant women, like other persons, can make decisions concerning their own medical treatment or whether someone else will do that for them.

All the evidence to date shows that decision making by anyone other than the pregnant woman not only carries risks of being highly intrusive, especially to poor women, but also is utterly ineffective in producing healthier offspring. In fact, such regulation, unaccompanied by other obvious and more effective efforts to improve the health of offspring, is far more antiwoman in aim and effect than it is pro-newborn.

Is such regulation even legally permissible? Until very recently there was little relevant judicial precedent. The rulings that are emerging support the right of the woman to decide on her own treatment whether she is pregnant or not. This essay endorses that approach.

A leading judicial opinion is *In re A.C.*, decided in April 1990 by the Court of Appeals of the District of Columbia sitting *en banc*. The story was a particularly dramatic and horrible one and so it captured much public attention.

In June 1987 the District of Columbia courts imposed a cesarean upon a dying woman, contrary to her wishes as well as the wishes of her husband, parents, and doctors, and even knowing that the operation would hasten the woman's death. Angela Carder, the woman involved, had been diagnosed as having bone cancer at age thirteen. She underwent extensive treatments and operations over the years, which included having her leg amputated. At age twenty-seven she had married and become pregnant, and her cancer had been in remission for three years. Twenty-five weeks into her pregnancy, Ms. Carder went for a routine checkup, and the doctors told her she had a large tumor in her lung and might have only days to live. Because she was pregnant, Carder's own wishes as to how she might want to die or live her remaining days were not respected.

Carder was admitted to George Washington Hospital with a prognosis of "terminal." Five days later her condition worsened, and the hospital decided to try to save the unborn child. The hospital took this position through its lawyers and over the objections of Ms. Carder, her family, and her own doctors. And it did so even though the fetus was only twenty-six weeks developed and might not be able to survive after delivery.

The hospital's doctors told the judge that there was a 50 to 60 percent chance of survival for the baby and less than a 20 percent chance that it would be born with a handicap. They also informed the court that the operation would hasten Carder's death. The hearing obtaining an order from the superior court, together with an appeal (which was decided in telephone consultation by three judges on the court of appeals), took a total of six hours, during which time Carder was being prepared for surgery.

When the court of appeals refused to stay the order for surgery, the operation was performed. The baby, a girl, died two hours later, and Angela Carder died two days after that. Surgery was listed on her death certificate as a contributing factor.

It is important not to lose sight of the human dimension of these stories. Carder's mother tells of being called from her daughter's bedside when the hospital said the family was needed for a short meeting: "They did not tell us it was a court hearing. It took all day. Poor Angie, first she's told she's dying and the next thing everybody abandons her and leaves her alone in her room. . . . Then even before the hearing was over they started prepping her for surgery. She was already in so much pain. We told the judge she didn't want the surgery, that we didn't want her to suffer anymore, that we didn't think the baby would live. But they didn't listen. After the surgery and after they told her the baby was dead, I think Angie just gave up" ("Drama in the Womb," *Los Angeles Times*, December 25, 1987).

Five months after the operation and deaths, a panel of the District of Columbia Court of Appeals wrote an opinion seeking to justify the court's decision (*In re A.C.*, 533 A.2d 611, 1987). While the panel expressed condolences to Ms. Carder's family, it accepted the hospital's position that it had not been necessary to respect her right to decide on her own treatment: "The Caesarean section would not significantly affect A. C.'s condition because she had, at best, two days left of sedated life; the complications arising from the surgery would not significantly alter that prognosis. The child, on the other hand, had a chance of surviving delivery" (533 A.2d at 617). The approach is startling not only for the cavalier attitude with which it treats the wishes of the dying, but also for the precedent it could set for removing organs before death from unwilling donors.

Indeed, Carder's own doctors (who together with the obstetricians had opposed the hospital administration's decision to force surgery on her) had not given up on prolonging her life, and afterward Carder's father commented, "For 14 years our daughter was considered terminally ill and what right did the court have to decide that her life was over?" (*Los Angeles Times*, December 25, 1987).

This opinion by the court of appeals panel was later vacated and heard by the court of appeals *en banc*. It was not until two and a half years later that the court issued its opinion, but that now stands as the fullest and

leading explication of the law on this subject. In May 1990, the *en banc* court held that the earlier decision had been erroneous and that "in virtually all cases the question of what is to be done [concerning a woman pregnant with a viable fetus] is to be decided by the patient—the pregnant woman—on behalf of herself and the fetus" (*In re A.C.*, 573 A.2d at 1237). The court emphasized that the right is not lost because a woman is ill, or even dying. The court also said that if a woman is not competent to form her own judgment, then a substituted judgment procedure may be used, but there too the issue is what the patient herself would want, not others' predilections.

The *en banc* court went to some lengths not to criticize the earlier tribunals, pointing out the difficulties of making quick decisions in an atmosphere of emergency. Nonetheless, it held that the prior decisions were erroneous. The courts had mistakenly not recognized that if Carder *was* competent, she had the authority to decide on her treatment. They also did not make findings concerning *whether* she was competent (or whether instead she was too sedated and semiconscious to be able to understand what was happening and to make her own decisions). And they did not use the substituted judgment procedure that would have been required if Carder was not in fact competent to decide.

The *A.C.* case was highly unusual in several respects: the operation was performed when all agreed it would shorten the mother's life; the mother was dying; and the mother was white and middle class. There had been many decisions forcing cesareans before *A.C.*, most of them involving women without funds (Kolder, Gallagher, and Parsons 1987).

Despite the many prior judicial orders forcing cesarean sections, the *en banc* court could find only one appellate court decision that was reported. That was a well-known 1981 case, *Jefferson v. Griffin Spalding County Hospital Authority*, decided by the Supreme Court of Georgia. Mrs. Jessie Mae Jefferson had refused to submit to a cesarean, which the doctors said she needed, because of her religious conviction that surgery was wrongful. The hospital where Mrs. Jefferson had been seen went to court to obtain permission to force surgery upon her, explaining that "defendant has a placenta previa; that the afterbirth is between the baby and the birth canal; that it is virtually impossible that this condition will correct itself prior to delivery; and that it is a 99 percent certainty that the child cannot survive natural childbirth (vaginal delivery). The chances of defendant surviving vaginal delivery are not better than 50 percent" (*Jefferson*, 274 S.E.2d at 459).

The differences from *A.C.* are obvious. First, the Jefferson child was

fully viable, the defendant being in her thirty-ninth week of pregnancy. Moreover, it was entirely clear that Mrs. Jefferson both was competent and had declared her choice. In A.C., by contrast, the *en banc* court of appeals found it was unclear whether Carder was able to decide and whether she in fact had expressed a choice; it faulted the trial court for not making findings concerning these subjects. Finally, unlike A.C., the *Jefferson* patient herself was predicted to be at risk without the operation; it was supposedly to benefit her as well as her child, and was not seen as being detrimental to her.

In *Jefferson* the Georgia Supreme Court allowed the hospital to force the operation in order to save the life of mother and child. It used the legal mechanism of granting the state's Department of Human Resources temporary custody of the fetus, saying it was not receiving proper parental care. It ordered Mrs. Jefferson to submit to an ultrasound, a cesarean section, any necessary blood transfusions, and related procedures considered necessary by the attending physician to sustain the life of the child (274 S.E.2d at 459).

Before the operation could be performed, however, Mrs. Jefferson gave birth naturally. Despite the dire predictions that had been made, mother and child both emerged healthy, more battered by litigation than by childbirth. The *Jefferson* case is by no means unique in this respect; courts usually grant hospital requests for emergency cesareans, but when they have denied them, in many instances the natural delivery has been successful.*

Jefferson is unusual in that the cesarean was predicted to be beneficial to the mother as well as the fetus. A more typical forced-cesarean decision is *In re Madyun*, decided by the District of Columbia Superior Court

---

*Another case in which the doctors predicted dire results without a cesarean—results that did not materialize—involved a thirty-five-year-old indigent woman in New York City who had had ten children already. The hospital said a cesarean was necessary because the umbilical cord was wrapped around the neck of the baby and it would strangle during the birth. But civil court judge Margaret Taylor refused to order surgery, saying that pregnant women, like other people, have a right to decide whether to undergo surgery and cannot be forced to do so for the benefit of another person, even their own child. After the order was denied, the mother delivered a healthy child (*see* Lewin 1987).

In still another case in which an order was obtained, doctors were surprised that the baby when finally delivered by cesarean was much healthier than the fetal monitoring had led them to expect. The doctors concluded "that a more asphyxiated infant with poor neonatal outcome did not result after so long a duration of apparent fetal distress simply underscores the limitations of continuous fetal heart monitoring as a means of predicting neonatal outcome" (Bowes and Selgestad 1981:211). Kolder, Gallagher, and Parsons (1987:1192–1196) report six cases in which forced cesareans w sought where the prediction of harm to the fetus was inaccurate.

in 1986 and affirmed by the Court of Appeals in an unreported order.* Ayesha Madyun, age nineteen, had been in labor for two days when she arrived at the hospital to give birth to her son. Eighteen hours later, when the birth was still not progressing, doctors decided they needed an emergency cesarean to save the unborn infant. Madyun, distrustful of surgery, refused to consent, but the doctors won a court order to force the surgery upon her, and the operation was successfully performed.

The ground for forcing the surgery in *Madyun* and in many other forced-cesarean cases was that despite her competence and her clearly declared wishes, the state had a right to order the surgery in order to protect the viable fetus, the child to be born. The adult was expressly denied the right "to gamble [with] the life or death of an unborn infant." "To ignore the undisputed opinion of a skilled and trained physician to indulge the desires of the parents the court cannot do. Indeed, even if the religious beliefs of the parents were the primary or sole reason for refusing a caesarean, the state had a compelling interest in ensuring this infant could be born" (573 A.2d at 1263). The court found there were risks to the mother from the cesarean procedure but that they were "minimal" (.25 percent) in comparison to "significant" risks to the fetus from delaying the procedure.

Unlike Carder's case, which fortunately is unique, the Madyun story is fairly typical. The cesarean rate in the United States has reached what some physicians have called alarming proportions.** Doctors who believe a cesarean should be performed can usually obtain the consent of the woman on whom they would operate, but in those rare cases in which women persist in their objections, the doctor may go to court to obtain an order for surgery. In most cases that have been brought, doctors have prevailed rather easily. One interesting 1987 study reported twenty-one instances since 1981 of doctors going to court to get a cesarean over the mother's refusal, all but three of which the doctors won; in 88 percent of the cases the order to operate was received within six hours, and in almost 20 percent it was received in less than an hour (Kolder, Gallagher, and Parsons 1987:1192–1193).

A central issue expressly left open by the *en banc A.C.* opinion is whether that court would adhere to the earlier, and more typical, *Mad-*

*D.C. Super. Ct., July 26, 1986. The case was first officially reported when it was placed in the appendix to the *en banc A.C.* decision (*In re Madyun,* as reported in *In re A.C.,* 573 A.2d at 1259).

**In the past sixteen years the percentage of cesareans in this country has quadrupled so that today almost one birth out of four is a cesarean. The rate of cesarean section delivery in this country increased from 4.5 per one hundred deliveries in 1965 to 22.7 per one hundred deliveries in 1985 (Taffer, Placek, and Liss 1987:955).

yun decision or would reject it. The court of appeals' refusal to say whether *Madyun* was rightly decided (573 A.2d at 1252*n*23) does not square easily with the court's insistence elsewhere in its opinion that "in 'virtually all cases' " the wishes of the patient must be controlling:

> We do not quite foreclose the possibility that a conflicting state interest may be so compelling that the patient's wishes must yield, but we anticipate that such cases will be extremely rare and truly exceptional. . . . We need not decide whether, or in what circumstances, the state's interests can ever prevail over the interests of a pregnant patient. We emphasize, nevertheless, that it would be an extraordinary case indeed in which a court might ever be justified in overriding the patient's wishes and authorizing a major surgical procedure such as a caesarean section. Throughout this opinion we have stressed that the patient's wishes, once they are ascertained, must be followed in "virtually all cases," unless there are "truly extraordinary or compelling reasons to override them." Indeed, some may doubt that there could ever be a situation extraordinary or compelling enough to justify a massive intrusion into a person's body, such as a caesarean section, against that person's will. Whether such a situation may someday present itself is a question that we need not strive to answer here. (573 A.2d at 1253)

The separate opinion of Judge Belson points out the contradiction between the court's limiting intervention to the "truly extraordinary" case and its professing not to decide whether to disturb *Madyun*. For himself, Belson would "ordinarily" respect a patient's wishes but would allow the state to override a pregnant patient's wishes more readily than the majority would and would give more weight to the interests of unborn life (573 A.2d at 1253–1257).

Before evaluating the pros and cons of forcing cesareans on nonconsenting women, let us consider two other types of cases prevalent today that similarly involve controls on decision making by pregnant women but which are not typically situated in the hospital delivery room. First there are the cases involving controlling the conduct of the pregnant woman throughout her pregnancy, cases most frequently involving the use of drugs (legal or illegal) by pregnant women but also involving more broadly the disobeying of doctor's orders, which can cover a wide range of subjects as diverse as diet, bed rest, sexual practices, and prenatal visits.

Public attention was first called to this type of state regulation by the prosecution of Pamela Rae Stewart, a twenty-seven-year-old mother of two who lived in California and was herself a battered woman. Stewart had been warned by her doctor that hers was a problem pregnancy and was instructed to seek medical attention at the first sign of bleeding. She also was told to refrain from sex with her husband. But when her bleeding started, she disregarded the medical advice, stayed home with her husband, had sexual intercourse, took amphetamines, and waited twelve hours before going to the hospital. Her son was born with extreme brain damage and died six weeks later.

The prosecutor brought criminal charges against Ms. Stewart, claiming that her conduct violated a California statute prohibiting a parent "without lawful excuse" from willfully omitting "to furnish necessary clothing, food, shelter or medical attendance, or other remedial care for his or her child" (California Penal Code, Sec. 270, West 1970 and Supp. 1988). Ms. Stewart's prosecution was thrown out on the basis that even though the statute expressly provided that a "child conceived but not yet born is to be deemed an existing person insofar as this section is concerned," it was not intended to apply to a mother's refusal to obey doctors' orders.* But the *Stewart* case was well publicized, and that attempt to punish a mother for having disobeyed doctors' orders during pregnancy stirred the imaginations of many to uses that could be made of their own state's criminal laws or abuse-and-neglect laws, or to laws the state legislatures could design that would expressly prohibit "fetal abuse" by the pregnant woman. Since then, prosecutions and child removals for drug use during pregnancy, and even detentions of pregnant women thought "likely to abuse" their fetus, have been reported with increasing frequency.

The relatively recent discovery that excessive drinking of alcohol by pregnant women can cause severe mental and physical problems for their offspring, and the growing problem of babies born with crack, heroin, or cocaine addiction have led to increased concern that pregnant women respect the interests of fetuses they plan to deliver. Moreover, the "war on drugs" has led to testing of even apparently healthy newborns, and the large numbers discovered to have traces of illegal sub-

---

*The court's interpretation of the statute was a permissible one, but it certainly was not the only possible one. The language concerning fetuses in the statute had been added in 1925, when the statute applied only to fathers, and it was intended to impose liability upon the father who refused to provide support to the pregnant woman. Later the statute was amended so that it applied to mothers as well as fathers. According to the court's ruling, the effect of the amendment was to make women as well as men financially responsible for the expenses of pregnancy, but not to impose upon women an obligation to obey doctors' orders. *See,* generally, "Maternal Rights and Fetal Wrongs: The Case Against Criminalization of 'Fetal Abuse,'" *Harvard Law Review* 101:994–1112n1, 1988.

stances in their blood or urine have caused concern. The upshot is a growing attitude that women must be regulated while pregnant and punished for any conduct they have engaged in that is inimical to their fetus.

Pregnant women should not ingest substances (legal or illegal) that are harmful to the fetus, and certainly they have no moral "right to choose" to do so. But even those eager to regulate have had trouble devising a satisfactory remedy. A wide range of methods is being tried. In the Pamela Rae Stewart case and in many others, the approach was not coercion before birth (as in the forced-cesarean cases) but instead punishment after the fact (after the birth and death of her son). A prosecution under the state's general child abuse provisions was not a possibility because the California Court of Appeals in an earlier case had held that fetuses were not within the intended scope of the California child abuse law.* Other states, however, interpret their existing statutes to include protection for the unborn,** and state legislatures may craft new laws explicitly regulating "fetal abuse." Already Florida has convicted a woman who ingested cocaine during pregnancy of delivering drugs to a minor (*State v. Johnson*), and Massachusetts filed similar charges against a woman when cocaine was found in the urine of her healthy newborn son (*Commonwealth v. Pellegrini*).*** In other states women have been charged with crimes of child abuse, child neglect, or fetal endangerment for similar conduct, and with manslaughter in a case in which the newborn died.

A different approach is removal of the child from the mother rather than punishment of the mother as such. In states where the fetus is not considered to be a child within the meaning of the child abuse-and-neglect laws, the theory for the removal is that drug use during pregnancy is probative of continuing unfitness on the part of the parent.****

*In *Reyes v. Superior Court*, 75 Cal. App. 3d 214, 141 Cal. Rptr. 912 (1977), the California Court of Appeals held that because the statute does not expressly mention fetuses, the provisions of the general child-abuse law, sec. 273a, do not apply to fetal abuse.

**A Colorado case applying Colorado's abuse-and-neglect laws to the unborn is reported in Bowes and Selgestad (1981:209–214). See also *In re Vanessa F.*, 76 Misc. 2d 617, 351 N.Y.S.2d 337 (1974); *In re Baby X*, 97 Mich. App. 111, 293 N.W.2d 736 (1980); *In re Smith*, 128 Misc. 2d 976, 492 N.Y.S.2d 331 (Fam. Ct. 1985); *In re Ruiz*, 27 Ohio Misc. 2d 31, 500 N.E.2d 935 (1986)—all cases considering certain conduct during pregnancy as neglect, resulting in the removal of the child after birth.

***The prosecution was later thrown, with the Superior Court judge saying that the statute covering distribution to minors does not apply to ingestion during pregnancy. She also said that if the statute did apply, it would be an unconstitutional intrusion into the relationship between fetus and mother. *See* Coskley (1990).

****See, e.g., *In re Baby X*, 97 Mich. App. 111, 293 N.W.2d 736, 739 (1980).

In many of these cases children are removed from their mother at birth, but because they are not immediately free for adoption they are sent into foster care.

Given the sad realities of the foster care system, some children will be significantly worse off than they would be if they stayed with their mothers. This is especially so because the *degree* of drug use is frequently not a factor in the initial removal. In one shocking case, a mother who was not a drug user lost custody of her newborn for nine months because she followed a nurse's advice and took marijuana during the delivery to relieve the pain of her contractions. When THC was found in the newborn's urine, the mother lost custody and was unable to regain it for nine months, during which time she had to attend a rehabilitation program that she did not need (see *In the Matter of Ryan*).

Both the punishment and the child-removal approaches involve after-the-fact remedies—not coercion before birth (as in the forced-cesarean cases). In other contexts as well, courts have occasionally tried to control the childbearer during pregnancy—an approach that intrudes considerably upon the pregnant woman but which at least often has the virtue of preventing the particular harm that is feared. Sometimes this is accomplished by preventive detention in the form of holding in prison a pregnant drug user whose offense would otherwise be viewed as minor (like a first offense for passing a bad check) thereby preventing her from pursuing her habit during pregnancy. Occasionally, the detention for pregnancy is more direct—for example, in Wisconsin a young woman was ordered detained during pregnancy because she "tended to be on the run" and "lacked motivation" ("Girl Detained to Protect Fetus," *Wisconsin State Journal*, August 16, 1985). In one Massachusetts case a judge ordered a woman locked up because he could not find a treatment program that would take pregnant addicts (*Commonwealth v. Pellegrini*). Detentions also have been ordered in Colorado and Illinois for pregnant women with diabetes.* Civil libertarians view such detentions with dismay. The medical community is divided in its reaction, but detention does have widespread support. One study reports that 46 percent of heads of fellowship programs in maternal-fetal medicine thought that women who refused medical advice and thereby endangered the life of the fetus should be detained (Kolder, Gallagher, and Parsons 1987:1196).

As well as controlling and punishing errant mothers-to-be, laws may regulate the means of discovering which pregnant women use forbidden substances. Minnesota, for example, has passed a law requiring doctors

---

*See Kolder, Gallagher, and Parsons (1987:1193), reporting court-ordered hospital detentions in Illinois and Colorado of women with diabetes who were thirty-one to thirty-three weeks pregnant.

to report substance abuse by pregnant women (just as they are required in Minnesota and other states to report suspected child abuse). The administrative and judicial system is then supposed to force treatment upon the woman (Minn. Stat. Sec. 626.5561, enacted June 1989). Most states lack such regulation, so reporting is at the physician's discretion. As an alternative detection measure, many hospitals test some newborns at birth. Theoretically, testing of all newborns might be required, but in practice whether to test is usually left to medical discretion. Illinois does not require testing, but in a 1988 statute it required notification if the test is performed and the newborn's blood or urine is positive (Ill. Ann. Stat. ch. 23, para. 2053, Smith Hurd, 1988). Many jurisdictions are considering how broadly to mandate measures of detection and require cooperation from the medical profession. Surveillance and reporting by neighbors is an additional possible means of control.

To date, most enacted and proposed regulation has centered on illegal drugs and, to a lesser extent, alcohol, but as the above examples show, it need not be so limited. The concern also covers other substances and habits discovered to be harmful to developing life and could easily include, for example, cigarette smoking, ingestion of caffeine, use of hot tubs, inordinate weight gain, and failure to get adequate bed rest, to name but a few of the manifold possibilities. Some have suggested state surveillance of pregnant women who stay outside the prenatal care system during the third trimester of pregnancy.* Indeed there is no logical stopping place once the state assumes the role of making medical-lifestyle decisions for the woman. Why not, as evidence of its healthiness accumulates, let doctors *require* breastfeeding instead of simply encouraging women to try it? Why should not government *require* home care for children if that is considered preferable to day care?

A final type of regulation, passed upon by the United States Supreme Court during its 1990 term, concerned barring women from certain workplaces because of a supposed concern for fetuses they may be carrying— or even concern for fetuses they might in theory produce. In the case presenting this issue, *UAW v. Johnson Controls*, the United States Court of Appeals for the Seventh Circuit, sitting *en banc*, upheld by a 7–4 vote an automotive battery plant's "fetal protection policy" barring women from jobs that would expose them to lead unless the women could prove it was not possible for them to bear children. The policy was applied even to women in their forties and fifties with no plans for childbearing but unable to come up with the requisite proof of incapability (McNamara 1989a:1). Women who had struggled to get equal opportunity

*Twenty-six percent of the maternal-fetal specialists surveyed in one interesting study approved of state surveillance (Kolder, Gallagher, and Parsons 1987:1194).

for high-paying jobs found themselves barred by this approach, even though all the evidence of hazard to reproduction that the company could come up with showed lead to be equally hazardous to the reproductive systems of the men.* As Judge Frank Easterbrook pointed out in his dissent, through a supposed concern for "fetal rights" the company managed to institute just the sort of sex discrimination in employment that women thought they had successfully conquered with the demise of laws restricting female labor and with congressional legislation providing for nondiscrimination in employment (886 F.2d at 145–152, Easterbrook, J., dissenting).** Another obvious problem with the policy was the incentive it created for women to get sterilized in order to keep their jobs.***

The type of regulation involved in *UAW v. Johnson Controls* went beyond the other types of regulation mentioned in this essay because it was applied to women not currently pregnant, and even to women who had no intention of becoming pregnant, and most probably no ability to do so. (The company's presumption of fertility extended to all women under age seventy!) Medical regulations also could be broadly applied in this way. If the movement to control the woman in order to protect the fetus became entrenched, we logically should expect compulsory medical regimes—vitamin therapies, testing for certain genetic conditions, and bans on cigarette smoking or obesity as well as bans on exposure to certain conditions in the workplace—extending to all women of childbearing years or younger, and designed to perfect their future reproductive capacity and to protect their future offspring.

In fact, however, the Seventh Circuit's approach did not carry the day. In March, 1991, the Supreme Court of the United States in a rare unanimous pronouncement reversed the court of appeals and held the company's policy impermissible sex discrimination and discrimination against pregnancy, both in violation of Title VII of the Civil Rights Act of

* *See also* Brody (1981:C1); *Wright v. Olin Corp.*, 697 F.2d 1172 (4 Cir. 1982); Levy and Wegman (1983:308).

** Easterbrook believed that Title VII—relating to discrimination in employment—gives parents the power to make occupational decisions affecting their families; it does not give that power to courts or to employers (886 F.2d at 136).

*** As of 1979, an estimated 100,000 jobs were already closed to women, ostensibly to protect future offspring (Williams 1981:647).

For other instances in which companies have been permitted to deny equal employment to women on the ground that their work sites are particularly hazardous to fetuses, see *Wright v. Olin Corp.*, 697 F.2d 1172 (4 Cir. 1982), and *Oil, Chemical and Atomic Workers International Union v. American Cyanamid*, 741 F.2d 444 (D.C. Cir. 1984). See also *Hayes v. Shelby Memorial Hospital*, 726 F.2d 1543 (11 Cir. 1984). For critical discussion, see Cherner-Mareval (1985:939); Sor (1986:141); Stellman (1977:160); Scott in Chavkin (1984:180); Stellman and Henifin (1982:117); and Becker (1986:1219).

1964. Particularly relevant to our inquiry was Justice Blackmun's observation that the worker is the relevant decision maker here:

Johnson Controls' professed moral and ethical concerns about the welfare of the next generation do not suffice to establish [an excuse for their policy]. Decisions about the welfare of future children must be left to the parents who conceive, bear, support, and raise them rather than to the employers who hire those parents. Congress has mandated this choice through Title VII, as amended by the Pregnancy Discrimination Act. (111 S.Ct. at 1207)

Although the law in this area is still unformed, *Johnson Controls* thus joins with the *en banc A.C.* decision in suggesting that the right to decide belongs to the pregnant patient, not to the doctor, the courts, or the employer.* It is appropriate that the wishes of the pregnant woman should be controlling. Many of the proposed controls and limits upon her behavior may be highly desirable, but they should be put into effect by persuading her of their merits, not by attempting to force them upon her.

The coercive regulation of women's conduct and medical treatment denies the competence of women as decision makers. To force the pregnant woman to have an operation without her consent is an unprecedented intrusion into the right to choose which is otherwise invariably granted to competent adults. The Supreme Court has affirmed that the right to decide on one's own medical treatment, and to refuse unwanted treatment, is protected by the due process clause of the United States Constitution (*Cruzan v. Missouri Department of Health*).** In pregnancy, of course, the fate of the fetus is affected as well as the fate of the carrying mother, but it is clear in our law (rightly or wrongly)*** that an individual has no obligation to undergo any medical risk, including a minimal one, even in order to confer substantial benefit upon another.**** It would be

---

*The Massachusetts Superior Court has reached the same result. *See* n. 7 above.

**All Justices supported this position except for Justice Scalia, who did not believe that the issue had constitutional dimensions (110 S.Ct. at 2859, Scalia, J., concurring).

*** *See*, generally, "Coerced Donation of Body Tissues: Can We Live with *McFall v. Shimp?*" *Ohio State Law Journal* 40:409–440, 1979 (suggesting that in some circumstances compelled donations should be required).

****See *McFall v. Shimp*, 10 Pa. D. & C. 3d 90 (Allegheny Ct. Comm. Pleas 1978). The case involved cousins, but the court made clear that it was not the closeness or the distance of the relationship that was important but rather that no person would be forced to be a donor for another. The plaintiff suffered from a rare bone marrow disease and would not survive without a compatible donor, and it was stipulated that his cousin the defendant was the only person who was a suitable donor. The court based its decision upon "[t]he common law [which] has consistently held

surprising to elevate the interests of the unborn fetus even above the interests of a fully formed child who may, for example, be dependent for continuation of his life upon a bone marrow donation from a parent who is the only person who is a suitable donor; forcing cesareans would give the fetus a greater claim to parental sacrifice than the fully formed child.

It is hard to resist the conclusion that the various coercive regulations at issue depend for their support on the fact that they fall exclusively upon women. Only women, of course, become pregnant, so in that sense there is a ready explanation for this limitation on the controls; there is no way to prove or disprove the frequent claim that "if men became pregnant, abortion would be a sacrament." But one does not have to engage in this degree of fantasy to notice that when the same principle that supposedly requires regulating pregnant women would impinge upon men, the principle has not been followed. The familiar example is that of a father who has a kidney his son desperately needs to survive and who is not required to give that kidney to his son even when any risk to himself is deemed insubstantial; the requirement is not imposed even though most fathers in that situation would readily choose to act as donor.

But even in other contexts the asymmetry between what is asked of pregnant mothers-to-be and the fathers of offspring is striking. Pamela Rae Stewart is prosecuted for endangering her fetus by not following doctor's orders, but her husband is not prosecuted for beating her while pregnant—to the detriment of both fetus and mother. Known drug use during pregnancy, even on an occasional or one-time basis, is probative that the mother will abuse or neglect the child that is born and on that basis warrants removal from the mother in some jurisdictions, but the father's drug habit receives much less attention and does not result in removal of the child at birth—even though statistically fathers are much more likely to abuse their children than mothers are. Suggestions that regulations might make men actually help pregnant women get necessary bed rest—by assuming more responsibility for their other children, for example, or cutting down on their work hours—would be met with derision. And the exposure to lead, which renders males more vulnerable to reproductive risks than women (because spermatogenesis is continuous and dividing cells are most vulnerable), resulted in women being

---

to a rule which provides that one human being is under no legal compulsion to give aid or to take action to save that human being or to rescue. . . . For our law to *compel* the Defendant to submit to an intrusion of his body would change every concept and principle upon which our society is founded" (10 Pa. D. & C. 3d at 91; emphasis in original). The risks to the bone marrow donor were small. *See* Steinbrook (1980:11–14) and Meisel and Roth (1978:5–6).

removed from high-paying jobs that then were reserved for men. If the risk of lead poisoning were taken seriously and men's reproductive risks to their future offspring were taken into account, the solution of increasing the safety of the workplace would doubtless be adopted. But when a way is found to place the cost of "safety" solely upon women, improving the safety of the workplace seems too expensive.

Not only do the regulations, somewhat irrationally, fall exclusively upon women, but also they fall disproportionately upon the poor and minority populations. There are strong indications of a class dimension to the issue of whether to coerce the pregnant woman. The rare cases in which doctors go to court to force their views upon their patients are those in which the patient is poor or has an ethnic or cultural background very different from the doctor's own; most forced cesareans have been performed on poor women who are members of racial minorities, many of whom did not speak English (Kolder, Gallagher, and Parsons 1987:1195). Forcing intervention is indeed a sign of the doctor's disrespect for the patient and the doctor's failure to understand her attitudes.

The same racial disparities exist when one looks at state intervention on the basis of maternal drug use during pregnancy. A study of one Florida county found that a larger number of white women than black women use drugs (and even a slightly higher percentage) but black women are reported for drug use in the context of childbirth ten times more frequently than white women are (Chasnoff, Landress, and Barrett 1990:1204). Much of the explanation (similar to the explanation for the underreporting of middle-class child abuse) is that white, middle-class women are not suspected or tested by their doctors.

Both these discriminatory aspects of coercive regulation and its potential intrusiveness should give lawmakers pause, but the most compelling reason for avoiding coercive governmental regulation of pregnancy is that it simply will not work to accomplish its professed goal of producing healthier infants. Instead, it will be counterproductive. Women ordered to report for cesarean delivery may go into hiding rather than comply and thus will not receive other medical help for themselves and their fetus. Even before a coercive order is issued against them, women who want to control their own medical treatment may avoid prenatal care altogether, or at least medical assistance in the birth itself. Similarly, women who fear that doctors will spot their addictions to drugs or alcohol will avoid prenatal care altogether, or if they do see a doctor will not disclose their habits for fear that they will be arrested or that their newborn will be taken from them. As a result, they and their fetuses will not have access to what help is available.

In some ways the most difficult issue concerning forcing medical treatment, such as cesareans, is the one still left open by the *en banc* court in *A.C.*—that is, whether intervention should never be forced over the patient's wishes or whether coercion is still possible in extraordinary cases. If the latter, there are of course many difficult issues concerning how to delineate the extraordinary situations—issues that would be resolved over time on a case-by-case basis. They might, for example, limit intervention to cases where the fetus is fully developed and only an operation away from birth; or to cases where intervention was necessary to benefit the mother as well as the child; or at least to cases where the forced medical intervention posed no risk to the mother (or perhaps alternatively no "significant" risk). Undoubtedly much ink would be spilled and much argument spent on which of these, or other, formulations was the appropriate one. But the preferable approach may well be the other one the *A.C.* court described: that the wishes of the patient are invariably the controlling factor; that if her doctor or others in the medical establishment disagree with those wishes then the appropriate course is to try to persuade the patient to change her mind—but not to force unwanted intervention. This approach would treat the pregnant woman like other patients, despite the fact that she carries a fetus.

One reason for adopting a per se rule against forced intervention is that, as *A.C.* itself illustrates, an authority to intervene designed for use only in the clearest cases will not always be so limited in application. It is extremely difficult to delineate any logical stopping place for regulation of the mother-to-be once the responsibility for decision making is shifted to the state or to the medical profession. It is also noteworthy that rules regulating the mother typically elevate the interests of the fetus above all other considerations (the mother's religious beliefs or her concerns for her other children, for example), although that is not the way even the best of parents make decisions concerning the treatment and welfare of their already-born children.

While forced intervention will on occasion serve to protect the health of a particular newborn, it will do more harm than good by scaring others away from the health care system. In addition, it is a misuse of judicial processes to buttress a doctor's judgment with a court order obtained in circumstances in which there is no opportunity for deliberation, for careful fact-finding and analysis. The forced-cesarean cases, for example, are often "heard" while the fetus is, according to testimony, rapidly declining; the hearings may even be held in the hospital room. Any right to appeal that is honored in such a situation is at best perfunctory.

It is also important to bear in mind that doctors do make mistakes, albeit inadvertently. This has repeatedly been shown in their predictions of the need for cesareans, as discussed above, but doctors have also advised mistaken therapies. In the 1960s, for example, many prescribed DES (diethylstilbestrol) to prevent miscarriages; the drug turned out to be carcinogenic to unborn daughters. Similarly, they prescribed thalidomide as a sleeping medication, and it turned out to cause severe birth defects. More recently, the phenobarbital routinely administered to children with seizures has proven detrimental to their developing IQ (Farwell et al. 1990:364).

Courts lack the ability to know which of the doctors' judgments are dependable—a problem that is exacerbated in emergency hearings (where both sides of a controversy may not be presented) but that also exists even in more relaxed settings. Although doctors themselves often cannot know what will occur without the intervention, "When obtaining an order becomes an objective in itself, an incentive to overemphasize the consequences of nonintervention may exist" (Kolder, Gallagher, and Parsons 1987:1195).

Many physicians, moreover, do not want the authority to coerce their patients; they are content to rely upon their ability to persuade a pregnant woman as they would their other patients, and when faced with a veto of their advice they would not go to court to override that veto. The American College of Obstetricians and Gynecologists anticipated the en banc A.C. opinion when it adopted a policy that doctors are "almost never" justified in going to court to compel treatment for a pregnant woman (American College of Obstetricians and Gynecologists Policy Statement, issued August 1987; reported in Lewin 1987). The statement reflects the reluctance of many physicians to enter into an adversarial relationship with their patients. They recognize that it would be self-defeating for the state to exert control and that even those coercive measures that appear most effective would almost certainly do more harm than good (even from the sole perspective of preventing prenatal harm) by frightening pregnant women away from the health care system.

The same approach of relying on the mother-to-be herself as decision maker should apply when the issue is the conduct of the mother during pregnancy. Drug use by pregnant women is a terrible tragedy, but it would be self-defeating to enlist the medical profession in an effort to punish the mother for misconduct during pregnancy or to remove her child because of conduct during pregnancy. The most significant contribution to date of the campaign against use of drugs in pregnancy is not the arrests or child removals but the publicity, which has educated the public that use of drugs and alcohol (and some other substances) can be harmful to a developing fetus. Pregnant women and others are much more aware of those facts today than they were a decade ago. Women who have decided to have a child of course have an important interest in having the child born as healthy as possible. This is a subject on which the interests of the state, the mother-to-be, and the fetus are in harmony. In this setting, at least the first lines of attack should be education and persuasion.

If the means were available to mothers-to-be to care well for the developing fetus, the vast majority would choose that course. Unfortunately, the movement to punish the mother—by imprisonment or child removal—is not part of any general campaign to produce healthier babies. Infants' health has never been a national priority in the United States. In 1985 our infant mortality rate ranked nineteenth in the world, behind all major industrialized nations and even behind countries with far fewer resources, such as Singapore or Spain. Moreover, when only the black infant mortality rate is considered, the United States ranked twenty-eighth (Geronimus 1986:1416; Children's Defense Fund 1988). If the movement to punish women reflected an all-out-effort to leave no stone unturned in an effort to produce healthier offspring, one might feel more sympathy toward it. Instead it seems to be the only pebble that has even been touched.

Before attempting coercive controls, government should at least attempt to give women the means to provide for their developing fetuses. Widespread voluntary compliance with recommended practice might well be accomplished by educating women about prenatal care and the needs of their fetuses—more compliance than any compulsory model could achieve. Certainly, providing free prenatal care to those who cannot afford to pay would make a vast difference. Women who have contact with doctors can be told of the fetus's needs and will often be persuaded of the importance of a healthy regimen. The leading factor associated with neonatal mortality is low birthweight, which studies show is significantly reduced by prenatal care, especially for high-risk women (Division of Health Promotion and Disease Prevention 1985:8; *see also* American Academy of Pediatrics Task Force on Infant Mortality 1986:1155; Dott and Fort 1975:854; National Health Program 1985:259). But state and federal funding for prenatal care is hopelessly inadequate, and for many in this country prenatal care is simply not available today (Greater New York March of Dimes; Leu 1986:561–563). Prenatal care seems to our legislators too expensive to provide, even though the expenses we incur without it, including elaborate rescue operations for babies born prematurely, are even greater. Daniel Callahan, director of the Hastings Center, has described this as "craziness" but explains it by an American preference for high technology and the results it accomplishes rather than for the comparatively undramatic gains that could be made by generally available prenatal care (Thompson 1990:81–82).

Education and persuasion are not, of course, effective tools in all situations. If the pregnant mother acts as she does out of religious conviction, it may not be possible to get her to change her mind. Education and persuasion are similarly ineffective in cases of addiction (and the criminal law is ineffective here as well). A serious effort to cut down on harm to fetuses that will be born would have to include the provision of good substance-abuse programs, free of charge, to all pregnant women who wanted them, or even to women desiring to become pregnant (or open to all people, for that matter).

Such programs are not available today, even though it is recognized that the number of pregnancies complicated by maternal substance abuse has risen sharply. While punitive efforts have been made and publicized, no effort has been made to reach out to high-risk communities to offer treatment, and even pregnant addicts who seek help cannot find centers that will take them, or else they are told they must wait six or eight months for their treatment to begin (Brody 1988, quoting Dr. Janet Chandler). Many programs actually discriminate against pregnant women, whose treatment may be complicated by the need to take account of the effects of withdrawal on the fetus; one reason is the programs' fear of liability (Chavkin 1990:483–487).* The result is that even those addicted mothers-to-be who desperately want to break their habit in order to protect their fetus are denied the means to do so.

Few funds are available to help alcohol or drug abusing pregnant women, even though that could do much more to prevent fetal harm than could any criminal law (Schachter 1986). Such programs would, of course, be expensive. A principal utility of the compulsory model seems to be creating the impression of acting to prevent fetal harm while actually refusing to dedicate the resources that would be needed to make a significant improvement.

The coercive measures that some propose in the war against "fetal abuse" may seem inexpensive by comparison, but they are ineffective at best, counterproductive at worse. That the coercive measures being promoted are so inadequate raises suspicions that as well as protecting fetuses, control of women is part of the point here. The coercive effort may represent a backlash against women and the rights to decision

---

*See also McNamara (1989b:1, 11) and Lewin (1990), both reporting on the above New York City survey by Dr. Wendy Chavkin of Columbia University School of Public Health, which found that of the existing seventy-eight treatment centers, 54 percent did not accept pregnant women and 87 percent would not treat pregnant women on Medicaid addicted to crack cocaine.

making they have recently won in the area of reproduction, as much as any bona fide attempt to deal with problems of fetal abuse.

Of course I do not suggest that there are any quick or perfect solutions, nor do I minimize the considerable problem of finding any remedies that work, especially when addiction is involved. Even rehabilitation that is apparently successful does not prevent later recidivism. One nurse from a neonatal intensive unit has suggested the expedient of offering "these mothers a week's supply of free drugs if they would let us take out their uterus" (Hundley 1989). If we are not so draconian as to sterilize, however, there is no real alternative to funding meaningful treatment. Even if we punish the woman or remove the child, many women will keep using drugs and having babies. Moreover, it should be of some relevance that treatment not only benefits the addict's offspring, it benefits the addict herself.* In focusing on the tragedy of drug-addicted newborns, some people talk as if the women who produced them want to take drugs and want to harm their babies, that all they need is to decide to get off drugs for the benefit of their offspring. When that scenario in fact exists—when options have been offered and not pursued—child removal may perhaps be appropriate. But in a setting where no treatment exists that is available to her, it is perverse to punish the woman rather than to help her and to help produce a healthy child. Society will not even save money by using a punitive rather than a treatment approach; it is even more expensive *not* to provide care for pregnant addicts than it is to provide it (U.S. Congress, Senate, July 31, 1989, statement of Dr. Ira Chasnoff, President NAPARE).

Until rules are adopted, the coercive approach will doubtless sometimes be followed by administrators and judges faced with distressing events and hopeful of helping a child-to-be. The punitive approach also has political appeal and may sometimes be pursued by prosecutors or legislators in order to benefit their own careers. If we are to develop a sensible and sensitive approach in this country, it will fall primarily to health care professionals and legislators to put that approach into effect. Courts may place some outer bounds on what lawmakers can do (finding some degree of individual decision making protected by women's liberty and privacy interests), but it is not at all clear that the appropriate resolutions of these issues are constitutionally dictated. Moreover, the current stance of the United States Supreme Court that states should be given wide leeway for choice and experimentation in areas of developing

---

*For discussions of the almost incredible disinterest in the plight of drug-addicted women and the problems that produced their dependency, *see*, e.g., Chavkin (1990:485) and Pollit (1990:418); "the worst thing about fetal rights is that it portrays a woman as having only contingent value."

social policy suggests that the primary solution will not be found in federal constitutional law (see *Webster v. Reproductive Health Services* and *Cruzan v. Missouri Department of Health*).

As a matter of policy and even of constitutional law, a mother-to-be should be permitted to decide whether to accept medical treatment, and her own decision should be controlling.

Of course there is risk in leaving the behavior of pregnant women unregulated. Some women will harm some fetuses in ways they clearly should not—through alcohol and drug abuse, for example (of course, some will do so even if government does regulate). And many women will be negligent about some things that they ought to do for the sake of their fetus—taking their vitamins, drinking their milk and orange juice, keeping their weight down (or up, if they go to a doctor of the opposite persuasion), and so on. Generally, however, women who intend to give birth will try not to harm their child, especially if they are taught how to avoid harm. Coercive state regulation promises to do more harm than it could effectively redress, and there are better ways to use the state's resources than in a pregnancy-regulatory program.

Pregnancy is a personal event. It should not be made into a legal event as well—an occasion for governmental intervention. There is no need for the law to regulate pregnancy and no net benefit from its doing so. Mother and fetus ideally and normally are in a supportive relationship, not a competitive one, but attempts to regulate the mother to protect the fetus or to punish the mother for misconduct toward the fetus tend to make them legal adversaries. Such attempts also put the mother-to-be and her doctor in a potentially adversarial relationship and would tend to frighten away from the health care system many of the women most in need of prenatal care.

Instead of adopting legal rules and constraints to govern the mother-to-be, the law should leave her to decide in accordance with the rules that govern the decision making of all other competent adults. If the real goal is not control of women but protection of the child-to-be and the creation of a newborn population as healthy as possible, then the appropriate means are education and persuasion, free prenatal care, and good substance-abuse rehabilitation programs, available free of charge to pregnant women. These remedies appear more expensive in the short run than the coercive approaches and therefore are more difficult to put in place—but unlike the coercive measures, they will truly help to produce healthy infants.

References

American Academy of Pediatrics Task Force on Infant Mortality. 1986. "Statement on Infant Mortality." *Pediatrics* 78:1155–1160.

Becker, Mary. 1986. "From *Muller v. Oregon* to Fetal Vulnerability Policies." *University of Chicago Law Review* 53:1219–1273.

Bowes, Watson A., Jr., and Brad Selgestad. 1981. "Fetal Versus Maternal Rights: Medical and Legal Perspectives." *Obstetrics and Gynecology* 59:209–214.

Brody, Jane. 1981. "Sperm Found Especially Vulnerable to the Environment." *New York Times* (March 10):C1.

Brody, Jane, 1988. "Widepsread Abuse of Drugs by Pregnant Women Is Found." *New York Times* (August 30):I1.

California Penal Code, Sec. 270 (West 1970 and Supp. 1988).

Chasnoff, Ira J., Harvey J. Landress, and Mark E. Barrett. 1990. "The Prevalence of Illicit Drug Use During Pregnancy and Discrepancies in Mandatory Reporting in Pinellas County, Florida." *New England Journal of Medicine* 322:1201–1206.

Chavkin, Wendy. 1990. "Drug Addiction and Pregnancy: Policy Crossroads." *American Journal of Public Health* 80:483–487.

Cherner-Mareval, Wendy. 1985. "Occupational Safety and Health." *Temple Law Quarterly* 58:939–975.

Children's Defense Fund. 1988. *The Health of America's Children: Maternal and Child Health Data Book.* Washington, D.C.: Children's Defense Fund.

"Coerced Donation of Body Tissues: Can We Live with *McFall v. Shimp?*" *Ohio State Law Journal* (1979), 40:409–440.

Commonwealth v. Pellegrini, D.C. Mass., Brockton Div., August 25, 1989.

Coskley, Tom. 1990. "Judge Rejects Charge that Woman Gave Drug to Her Unborn Child." *Boston Globe* (October 17):1.

Cruzan v. Missouri Department of Health, 110 S.Ct. 2841 (1990).

Division of Health Promotion and Disease Prevention. 1985. *Preventing Low Birthweight.*

Dott, A., and A. Fort. 1975. "The Effect of Availability and Utilization of Prenatal Care and Hospital Services on Infant Mortality Rates." *American Journal of Obstetrics and Gynecology* 123:854–860.

"Drama in the Womb: A Matter of Life and Death Winds Up in Court." 1987. *Los Angeles Times* (December 25):5A-5.

Farwell, J., et al. 1990. "Phenobarbital for Febrile Seizures—Effects on Intelligence and on Seizure Recurrence." *New England Journal of Medicine* 322:364–369.

Geronimus, A. T. 1986. "The Effects of Race, Residence, and Prenatal Care on the Relationship of Maternal Age to Neonatal Mortality." *Journal of American Public Health Association* 76:1416–1421.

"Girl Detained to Protect Fetus." *Wisconsin State Journal* (August 16, 1985): sec. 3–2.

Greater New York March of Dimes. "The Campaign for Healthier Babies: Fighting the Problem of Low Birth Weight in New York City."

Hayes v. Shelby Memorial Hospital, 726 F.2d 1543 (11 Cir. 1984).

Hundley, T. 1989. "Infants: A Growing Casualty of the Drug Epidemic." *Chicago Tribune* (October 16): sec. 1, p. 1.

Ill. Ann. Stat. ch. 23, para. 2053 (Smith Hurd 1988).

In re A.C., 533 A.2d 611 (District of Columbia, Court of Appeals, 1987), vacated and remanded 573 A.2d 1235 (1990; *en banc*).

In re Baby X, 97 Mich. App. 111, 293 N.W.2d 736 (1980).

In re Madyun (District of Columbia Superior Court, July 26, 1986), as reported in appendix to *In re A.C.* (573 A.2d at 1259).

In re Ruiz, 27 Ohio Misc.2d 31, 500 N.E.2d 945 (1986).

In re Smith, 128 Misc.2d 976, 492 N.Y.S.2d 331 (Fam. Ct. 1985).

In re Vanessa F., 76 Misc.2d 617, 351 N.Y.S.2d 337 (1974).

In the Matter of Ryan, New York Supreme Court, Family Court, 2d Dept. (MO #889).

Jefferson v. Griffin Spalding County Hospital Authority, 247 Ga. 86, 274 S.E.2d 457 (1981).

Kolder, Veronica, Janet Gallagher, and Michael Parsons. 1987. "Court-Ordered Obstetrical Interventions." *New England Journal of Medicine* 316:1192–1196.

Leu, Lori. 1986. "Legislative Research Bureau Report: A Proposal to Strengthen State Measures for the Reduction of Infant Mortality." *Harvard Journal of Legislation* 23:559–578.

Levy, Barry, and David Wegman. 1983. *Occupational Health: Recognition and Prevention of Work-Related Diseases*. Boston: Little, Brown.

Lewin, Tamar. 1987. "Courts Acting to Force Care of the Unborn." *New York Times* (November 23):A-1.

Lewin, Tamar. 1990. "Drug Use During Pregnancy: New Issue Before the Courts." *New York Times* (February 5):1–1, 12.

McFall v. Shimp, 10 Pa. D. & C. 3d 90 (Allegheny Ct. Comm. Pleas, 1978).

McNamara, Eileen. 1989a. "Factory and Fertility." *Boston Globe* (October 17):1.

McNamara, Eileen. 1989b. "Fetal Endangerment Cases on the Rise." *Boston Globe* (October 3):1, 11.

"Maternal Rights and Fetal Wrongs: The Case Against Criminalization of 'Fetal Abuse.' " *Harvard Law Review* (1988), 101:994–1112.

Meisel, Alan, and Loren Roth. 1978. "Must a Man Be His Cousin's Keeper?" *Hastings Center Report* 10:5–6.

National Health Program. 1985. "The Cost Effectiveness of Prenatal Care." *Clearing House Review* 19:259–264.

Oil, Chemical and Atomic Workers International Union v. American Cyanamid, 741 F.2d 444 (D.C. Cir. 1984).

Pollitt, Katha. 1990. " 'Fetal Rights': A New Assault on Feminism." *Nation* (March 26):409–418.

Reyes v. Superior Court, 75 Cal. App. 3d 214, Cal. Rptr. 912 (1977).

Schachter, Jim. 1986. "Help is Hard to Find for Addict Mothers: Drug Use 'Epidemic' Overwhelms Service." *Los Angeles Times* (December 12):II-1.

Scott, J. 1984. "Keeping Women in Their Place." In Wendy Chavkin, ed., *Double Exposure*. New York: Monthly Review Press.

Sor, Yvonne. 1986. "Fertility or Unemployment." *Journal of Law and Health* 1: 141–228.

State v. Johnson, 89–890 CFA, Fla. Cir. Ct. Seminole Co. (1989).

Steinbrook, Robert. 1980. "Unrelated Volunteers as Bone Marrow Donors." *Hastings Center Report* 10:11–14.

Stellman, Jeanne, and M. Henifin. 1982. "No Fertile Women Need Apply." In Ruth Hubbard, M. Henefin, and B. Fried, eds., *Biological Women: The Convenient Myth.* Cambridge, Mass.: Schenkman.

Taffer, Selma, Paul Placek, and Teri Liss. 1987. "Trends in the United States Caesarian Section Rate and Reasons for the 1980–1985 Rise." *American Journal of Public Health* 77:955–959.

Thompson, D. 1990. "Should Every Baby Be Saved?" *Time* (June 11):81–82.

UAW v. Johnson Controls, 886 F.2d 871 (7 Cir. 1989), rev'd 111 S.Ct. 1196 (1991).

U.S. Congress, Senate. 1989. *Hearings Before the Committee on Government Affairs. Missing Links: Coordinating Federal Drug Policy for Women.* 101st Cong., 1st sess.

Webster v. Reproductive Health Services, 57 U.S.L.W. 5023 (1989).

Williams, Wendy. 1981. "Firing the Women to Protect the Fetus." *Georgetown Law Review* 69:641–704.

Wright v. Olin Corp., 697 F.2d 1172 (4 Cir. 1982).

About the Contributors

Henry Aaron, Ph.D., is director of economic studies at the Brookings Institution and a professor of economics at the University of Maryland, College Park. He is co-author of *Painful Prescription: Rationing Hospital Care.*

W. French Anderson, is chief of the molecular hematology branch of the National Heart, Lung, and Blood Institute, National Institutes of Health, and editor-in-chief of the journal *Human Gene Therapy.*

Robert H. Blank, Ph.D., is a professor of political science at Northern Illinois University and the University of Canterbury, Christchurch, New Zealand. He has published fourteen books including *Rationing Medicine, Life, Death and Public Policy,* and *Regulating Reproduction.* He is currently a member of the advisory committee on neuroscience research for the U.S. Congress Office of Technology Assessment.

Andrea L. Bonnicksen, Ph.D., is professor of political science at Northern Illinois University. Dr. Bonnicksen was a Rockefeller Foundation Fellow at the Institute for the Medical Humanities, University of Texas Medical Branch. She is the author of two books, *Civil Rights and Liberties: Principles of Interpretation* and *In Vitro Fertilization: Building Policy from Laboratories to Legislatures.*

Daniel Callahan is the co-founder and director of the Hastings Center. He has a Ph.D. in philosophy from Harvard and a B.A. from Yale, and also holds honorary degrees from the University of Colorado and the University of Medicine and Dentistry of New Jersey. He is a member of the advisory board on scientific integrity of the U.S. Department of Health and Human Services. He is the author, most recently, of *What Kind of Life: The Limits of Medical Progress*.

Arthur L. Caplan, Ph.D., is director of the Center for Biomedical Ethics at the University of Minnesota where he is also professor of philosophy and a professor of surgery. He was formerly associate director of the Hastings Center.

Jacques Cohen, Ph.D., is Scientific Director of the Center for Reproductive Medicine and Infertility, New York Hospital, Cornell University Medical Center.

Alan H. DeCherney, M.D., is John Ely Professor in the Department of Obstetrics and Gynecology at the Yale University School of Medicine and director of the Division of Reproductive Endocrinology at Yale. He is the editor-in-chief of *Assisted Reproduction Reviews* and is on the editorial boards of numerous journals.

Martha A. Field, J.D., is professor of law at Harvard University Law School. She recently published *Surrogate Motherhood* (Harvard, 1990) and is working on a book about the reproductive rights of persons with handicaps.

Stuart C. Hartz, Sc.D., is president of Medical Research International, Inc., associate professor of community health at Tufts School of Medicine, and adjunct associate professor of public health at Boston University School of Medicine.

Robert Lee Hotz is an editor and science writer for the *Atlanta Journal-Constitution*. He is author of *Designs on Life: Exploring the New Frontiers of Human Fertility* (Pocket, 1991).

Warren Kearney, M.D., is an associate at the University of Minnesota's Center for Biomedical Ethics. He completed his residency in internal medicine at the Montreal General Hospital, where he served on the ethics consult committee. He is currently in the M.P.H. program at the University of Minnesota.

David J. Kears is agency director of the Alameda County Health Care Services Agency. In that capacity, he directs six departments (mental health, public health, alcohol and drugs, environmental health, and two 300–bed county hospitals) and 3,000 employees that comprise the agency. Mr. Kears reports directly to the Board of Supervisors and is responsible for coordination, development, and implementation of county and state health care policies. He holds a master of social work degree from the University of California, Berkeley.

John Kitzhaber, president of the Oregon State Senate, received his M.D. degree from the University of Oregon Medical School in 1973. He was appointed an associate professor at the Oregon Health Sciences University in Portland in 1988. The senator is currently a practicing emergency physician in Roseburg. He recently finished serving as project direct for a research grant through the Oregon Health Sciences University concerning the integration of health outcomes research into health care delivery systems.

Daniel E. Koshland, Jr., Ph.D., is the editor of *Science* and a professor of molecular and cell biology at the University of California, Berkeley. He has received numerous awards, the most recent of which was the National Medal of Science.

Nancy Lamontagne, Ph.D., is the director of the Cystic Fibrosis Research Program and program director for Metabolism, Metabolic Research Program of the Division of Diabetes, Endocrinology and Metabolic Diseases, NIDDK, National Institutes of Health.

Rodger G. Lum, Ph.D., is assistant agency director of the Alameda County Health Care Services Agency. He received his Ph.D. in clinical psychology from the University of California, Berkeley in 1979. From 1979 to 1988, he was executive director of Asian Community Mental Health Services in Oakland, California. He has published articles and chapters on Asian-American mental health.

J. Michael McGinnis, M.D., has served since 1977 as Deputy Assistant Secretary for Health and director of the Office of Disease Prevention and Health Promotion in the U.S. Department of Health and Human Services. He also holds the rank of Assistant Surgeon General in the Commissioned Corps of the U.S. Public Health Service. Dr. McGinnis is responsible for policy formulation and program coordination for national initiatives in disease prevention and health promotion. His most recent contribution is *Healthy People 2000* issued in 1990 by Secretary Louis W. Sullivan. He is a Fellow of the American College of Epidemiology and the American College of Preventive Medicine, and has held faculty appointments as adjunct professor of public policy at Duke University and instructor in medicine at George Washington University.

Paul Menzel, Ph.D., is professor of philosophy at Pacific Lutheran University, Tacoma, Washington. He is author of *Medical Costs, Moral Choices: A Philosophy of Health Care Economics for America* (Yale, 1983), *Strong Medicine: The Ethical Rationing of Health Care* (Oxford, 1990), and articles on the philosophical dimensions of health policy.

John C. Moskop is professor of medical humanities at the East Carolina University School of Medicine in Greenville, North Carolina, where he has taught since 1979. His publications include the edited volumes *Ethics and Mental Retardation*, *Ethics and Critical Care Medicine*, and *Children and Health Care: Moral and Social Issues*, as well as articles on ethical issues in death and dying, organ transplantation, AIDS, and the allocation of health care.

Dorothy Nelkin, Ph.D., is a University Professor at New York University, teaching in the Department of Sociology and the School of Law. Her research focuses on the social and political implications of controversial areas of science, technology, and medicine.

Jane B. Porter, M.S., is an epidemiologist at Medical Research International, Inc., and project manager of the U.S. IVF Registry. She has extensive experience in the drug epidemiology/research field.

Martin M. Quigley, M.D., is chief of the Division of Reproductive Endocrinology and Infertility, Department of Obstetrics and Gynecology, Mt. Sinai Medical Center, Cleveland, Ohio. He is the past president of the Society for Assisted Reproductive Technology of the American Fertility Society.

William B. Schwartz, M.D., is Vannavar Bush University Professor and professor of medicine at Tufts University, and senior physician at the New England Medical Center. He is co-author of *Painful Prescription: Rationing Hospital Care*.

Janice A. Sharp, Ph.D., J.D., is an associate with Christie, Parker and Hale, where she specializes in biotechnology patent law. Before joining this firm, she spent ten years in academic and industrial research in molecular biology.

Michael A. Stoto is with the Institute of Medicine of Deputy Director of the Division of Health Promotion and Disease Prevention the National Academy of Sciences. He recently directed the Institute's effort in support of the Public Health Service's Healthy People 2000 project. His current projects address a number of issues in health statistics, public health, and AIDS. Stoto received a Ph.D. in statistics and demography from Harvard University, and was formerly an associate professor of public policy at Harvard's John F. Kennedy School of Government.

Robert A. Weinberg, Ph.D., is a member, Whitehead Institute for Biomedical Research in Cambridge, Massachusetts, and is a professor of biology at the Massachusetts Institute of Technology.